Children of Substance-Abusing Parents

Dynamics and Treatment

T0255016

Shulamith Lala Ashenberg Straussner, PhD, CAS, is a professor at New York University (NYU) Silver School of Social Work. She is also the Director of their Post-Master's Certificate Program in the Clinical Approaches to Addictions.

Among her 16 books are: *Clinical Work with Substance-Abusing Clients* (2nd Ed., Guilford Press, 2004—selected by Psychotherapy Book Club); *Understanding Mass Violence: A Social Work Perspective* (coedited with Norma Phillips; Allyn & Bacon, 2003); *Urban Social Work: Policies and Practice in the Cities* (coauthored with N. Phillips; Allyn & Bacon, 2002); *International Aspects of Social Work Practice in the Addictions* (coedited with Larry Harrison; Haworth Press, 2003); *The Handbook on Women and Addictions* (coedited with S. Brown; Jossey-Bass, 2002); *Ethnocultural Factors in Addictions Treatment* (Guilford, 2001); and *Gender and Addictions: Men and Women in Treatment* (coedited with E. Zelvin; Jason Aronson Press, 1997). She is the founding editor of the *Journal of Social Work Practice in the Addictions* (Taylor & Francis).

Dr. Straussner has been a Fulbright Senior Scholar at the Academy of Labour & Social Relations in Kiev, Ukraine, a visiting professor at Warsaw University in Poland, and the recipient of the Lady Davis Fellowship to Hebrew University in Jerusalem. Previously, she was a Fulbright Senior Scholar to Israel (2003) and a Visiting Professor at Omsk State University, Siberia (2000). In June 2008 she received the Lifetime Achievement Award from the NYC Chapter of the National Association of Social Workers (NASW) for her contributions to the field of addictions.

Dr. Straussner served on the National Center on Substance Abuse Treatment panel on workforce issues, and was the Northeast Regional Director for federally funded multimillion dollar national Project Mainstream, an interdisciplinary project to improve health professional education on substance abuse. During 2005–2006, she chaired the National Association for Children of Alcoholics (NACoA) Social Work Initiative on developing core competencies for working with families and children affected by addiction. She is a past chair of the NASW Section on ATOD and vice president of the NYC Chapter of the NASW. Dr. Straussner has a private therapeutic and supervisory practice in New York City and lectures and consults throughout the United States and abroad.

Christine Huff Fewell, PhD, LCSW, CASAC, is an adjunct associate professor at Silver School of Social Work at NYU, where she teaches in the areas of clinical practice and substance abuse and in the Post-Master's Certificate Program in the Clinical Approaches to Addictions. She is codirector of the Specialized Substance Abuse and Co-Occurring Disorders Focused Learning Opportunity and Seminar.

Dr. Fewell is Associate Editor of the *Journal of Social Work Practice in the Addictions* and a peer reviewer for the *Clinical Social Work Journal*. Recent publications include "Using a Mentalization-Based Framework to Assist Hard-to-Reach Clients in Individual Treatment" (in S. Bennett and J. K. Nelson [Eds.], *Adult Attachment in Clinical Social Work: Practice, Research, and Policy*. New York: Springer, 2010), *Impact of Substance Abuse on Children and Families: Research and Practice Implications* (coedited with S. Lala Ashenberg Straussner, Haworth Press, 2006), *12-Step Groups as a Treatment Modality* with Betsy Spiegel (in S. L. A. Straussner [Ed.], *Clinical Work with Substance-Abusing Clients*, 2nd Ed., Guilford Press, 2004), and *The Mental Health Needs of Children of Alcohol and Substance Abusers* (in *Update*, Newsletter of the New York State Chapter, NASW, September 2005). In June 2008, she received the Lifetime Achievement Award from the NYC NASW for her contributions to the field of addictions. Dr. Fewell has served on the New York State Board for Social Work and currently consults with students and faculty about licensing issues in New York State and conducts review courses related to the licensing exam.

Dr. Fewell is a graduate and member of the Institute of Psychoanalytic Training and Research (IPTAR), and a Fellow of the International Psychoanalytic Association. She maintains a private practice providing psychotherapy and supervision in New York City and Hastings-on-Hudson.

Children of Substance-Abusing Parents

Dynamics and Treatment

Shulamith Lala Ashenberg Straussner, PhD, CAS
Christine Huff Fewell, PhD, LCSW, CASAC

Editors

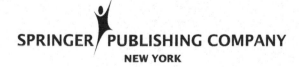

SPRINGER PUBLISHING COMPANY
NEW YORK

Springer Publishing Company, LLC
11 West 42nd Street
New York, NY 10036
www.springerpub.com

Acquisitions Editor: Jennifer Perillo
Senior Editor: Rose Mary Piscitelli
Composition: S4Carlisle Publishing Services

ISBN: 978-0-8261-6507-7
E-book ISBN: 978-0-8261-6508-4

11 12 13/ 5 4 3 2 1

The author and the publisher of this Work have made every effort to use sources believed to be reliable to provide information that is accurate and compatible with the standards generally accepted at the time of publication. The author and publisher shall not be liable for any special, consequential, or exemplary damages resulting, in whole or in part, from the readers' use of, or reliance on, the information contained in this book. The publisher has no responsibility for the persistence or accuracy of URLs for external or third-party Internet Web sites referred to in this publication and does not guarantee that any content on such Web sites is, or will remain, accurate or appropriate.

CIP data is available from the Library of Congress

Special discounts on bulk quantities of our books are available to corporations, professional associations, pharmaceutical companies, health care organizations, and other qualifying groups.

If you are interested in a custom book, including chapters from more than one of our titles, we can provide that service as well.

For details, please contact:
Special Sales Department, Springer Publishing Company, LLC
11 West 42nd Street, 15th Floor, New York, NY 10036-8002
Phone: 877-687-7476 or 212-431-4370; Fax: 212-941-7842
Email: sales@springerpub.com

Printed in the United States of America by Hamilton Printing

Dedication

To those who as children suffered from
substance abuse in their families
and to those who have dedicated themselves
to healing them.

Contents

Contributors   *ix*
Foreword by Sis Wenger, NACA   *xi*
Preface   *xiii*
Acknowledgments   *xv*

PART I: CONCEPTUAL OVERVIEW OF THEORY AND PRACTICE

1. Children of Substance-Abusing Parents: An Overview   *1*
   Shulamith Lala Ashenberg Straussner

2. An Attachment and Mentalizing Perspective on Children of
   Substance-Abusing Parents   *29*
   Christine Huff Fewell

3. Dynamics of Substance-Abusing Families and Implications for
   Treatment   *49*
   Wendy K. K. Lam and Timothy J. O'Farrell

**PART II: ISSUES ACROSS THE LIFE SPAN OF CHILDREN
    OF SUBSTANCE-ABUSING PARENTS**

4. Prenatal Impact of Alcohol and Drugs on Young Children:
   Implications for Interventions With Children and Parents   *77*
   Elizabeth C. Pomeroy and Danielle E. Parrish

5. Treatment Issues and Interventions With Young Children and
   Their Substance-Abusing Parents   *101*
   Jeannette L. Johnson, Jan Gryczynski, and Jerry Moe

6. Treatment Issues and Interventions With Adolescents From
   Substance-Abusing Families   *127*
   Judy Fenster

7. Treatment Issues and Psychodrama Interventions With Adults
   Who Grew Up With Substance-Abusing Parents   *153*
   Tian Dayton

PART III: PROGRAMS FOR INTERVENTION ACROSS THE LIFE SPAN AND SETTINGS

8. Prevention and Intervention Programs for Pregnant Women Who Abuse Substances   *171*

   Iris E. Smith

9. Programs for Young Children With Substance-Abusing Parents   *193*

   Alissa Mallow

10. Programs for Adolescent Children of Substance-Abusing Parents in School and Residential Settings   *207*

    Ellen R. Morehouse

11. Interventions With College Students With Substance-Abusing Parents   *223*

    David F. Venarde and Gregory J. Payton

12. Programs for Children of Parents Incarcerated for Substance-Related Problems   *243*

    Audrey L. Begun and Susan J. Rose

PART IV: CONCLUSION

13. Stories From the Inside: Life as the Child of a Substance-Abusing Parent   *269*

    Anonymous, Christopher H. Acker, Claudia Narváez-Meza, and Peter X

    Index   281

Contributors

Christopher H. Acker, MSW, LSW
Clinician, Bridgewater, New Jersey

Audrey L. Begun, MSW, PhD
Associate Professor, College of
Social Work, The Ohio State
University, Columbus, Ohio

Tian Dayton, PhD, TEP
Director, New York Psychodrama
Training Institute, Editor in Chief
of *The Journal of Psychodrama,
Sociometry and Group Psychotherapy*,
New York, New York

Judy Fenster, PhD, LCSW
Associate Professor, School of
Social Work, Adelphi University,
Garden City, New York

Jan Gryczynski, MA
Research Associate, Friends
Research Institute, Inc.,
Baltimore, Maryland

Jeannette L. Johnson, PhD
Research Professor, School of
Social Work, State University
of New York at Buffalo,
Buffalo, New York

Wendy K. K. Lam, PhD
Project Leader, Child Health,
Duke Translational Medicine
Institute, Duke University,
Durham, North Carolina

Alissa Mallow, DSW, LCSW
Vice President, Quality Improve-
ment, Promesa, Inc.,
Bronx, New York

Jerry Moe, MA
National Director of Children's
Programs, Betty Ford Center,
Rancho Mirage, California

Ellen R. Morehouse, LCSW
Executive Director, Student
Assistance Services Corporation,
Tarrytown, New York

Claudia Narváez-Meza, MSW, MFA
Trauma Recovery Clinician,
The New York Society for the
Prevention of Cruelty to Children,
New York, New York

Timothy J. O'Farrell, PhD, ABPP
Professor of Psychology, Chief,
Families and Addiction Program,
Harvard Medical School,
Department of Psychiatry at the
VA Boston Healthcare System,
Brockton, Massachusetts

Danielle E. Parrish, PhD, MSW
Assistant Professor, Graduate
College of Social Work,
University of Houston,
Houston, Texas

Gregory J. Payton, PhD
Lecturer, Teachers College,
Columbia University,
New York, New York

Elizabeth C. Pomeroy, PhD, LCSW
Professor and Codirector, Institute
for Grief, Loss and Family Survival,
School of Social Work,
University of Texas at Austin,
Austin, Texas

Susan J. Rose, PhD
Associate Professor of Social Work
and Scientist with the Center for
Addiction and Behavioral Health
Research, Helen Bader School
of Social Welfare, University of
Wisconsin-Milwaukee,
Milwaukee, Wisconsin

Iris E. Smith, PhD, MPH
Associate Professor, Behavioral
Sciences & Health Education,
Rollins School of Public Health,
Emory University,
Atlanta, Georgia

David F. Venarde, PsyD
Deputy Director, Counseling and
Wellness Services, Student Health
Center, New York University,
New York, New York

Foreword

Nearly 19 million children (one in four) in the United States live with a parent who abuses or is dependent on alcohol. Additional millions of children and adults have been and continue to be impacted by other parental substance abuse.

These children often grow up in homes characterized by unpredictable and even chaotic behavior. While many are highly resilient, others are often at higher risk for emotional, physical, and mental health problems, such as depression, anxiety, eating disorders, and suicide attempts. They may suffer from low self-esteem and have difficulty in school. They are also much more likely than other children to become addicted to alcohol or other drugs themselves. These issues do not end in childhood. Adult children of alcohol- or other substance-using parents often continue to demonstrate adverse emotional, behavioral, and mental health consequences. They are also at high risk to develop a substance use disorder or marry someone who has one, thereby passing on the problems into the next generation.

Social workers and other health and mental health professionals have a long history of working with young and adult children of alcohol- and other drug-abusing parents, and in the last three decades have helped to develop a significant body of research-based knowledge and clinical wisdom. This knowledge has led to the development of core competencies for mental health professionals that can guide them in providing increasingly effective interventions and support programs for impacted young and adult children and their families.

Children of Substance-Abusing Parents: Dynamics and Treatment is a necessary reference for all mental health professionals and students who need to understand and treat this population. It offers an invaluable look at treatment options and programmatic interventions across the life span and fills an important gap in the current literature. The contributors include a wide range of experts who provide up-to-date, evidence-based clinical and programmatic strategies for working with children of alcohol- and other substance-abusing parents of any age and in almost any practice setting.

This highly recommended book is a valuable resource for all practitioners and students concerned about this very large, but often hidden, group of individuals and families.

Sis Wenger
President/CEO
National Association for Children of Alcoholics

Preface

It is estimated that 27 million children in the United States live with a parent who abuses or is dependent on alcohol or other substances. Additional millions of young and adult children have been and continue to be impacted by parental substance abuse. Thus, is it a rare social worker or other health and mental health professional or educator who does not encounter such an individual in their everyday practice and even in their own private life. This book is intended as a clinical reference for all those encountering young and adult children of substance-abusing parents regardless of the setting.

Each of the chapters is written by an expert familiar with both the most recent research studies as well as the application of theory and research to clinical practice. Throughout the book, clinical examples guide the reader in how to best intervene with the particular group of children of substance-abusing parents the authors are addressing.

In addition to providing important evidence-based information and guidance to working professionals, this book can be used by both undergraduate and graduate students in a variety of fields, ranging from social work to psychology, nursing, medicine, and education. This edited book is divided into four parts:

Part I provides an overview of the existing state of knowledge regarding children of substance-abusing parents and examines the developmental effects of alcohol and other drugs on children and implications for practice. Chapter 1 by Straussner provides a general introduction and overview of the issues in this field and is followed by Fewell's chapter focusing on the latest theoretical conceptualization affecting parent-child interaction, that of mentalization and how it can be applied to clinical practice. The final chapter in this section, by Lam and O'Farrell, identifies the dynamics typically found in substance-abusing families and their implications for family treatment.

The four chapters in Part II explore treatment issues across the life span of children of substance-abusing parents beginning with the prenatal impact and spanning the life cycle. The emphasis is on those individuals who need treatment in a clinical setting. Chapter 4 by Pomeroy and

Parrish provides the latest research data on the prenatal impact of substances on newborns and the implications for effective interventions. It is followed by a chapter focusing on treatment issues and intervention with young children and their substance-abusing parents written by Johnson, Gryczynski, and Moe. Chapter 6 by Fenster identifies the treatment issues and interventions with adolescents from substance-abusing families, while the next chapter written by the expert on psychodrama, Tian Dayton, identifies treatment issues and psychodrama interventions with adults who grew up with substance-abusing parents.

Part III of this book focuses on programmatic interventions for children of substance-abusing parents across the life span. The first chapter in this section, Chapter 8 by Smith, focuses on prevention and early intervention programs for substance-abusing pregnant women, and is followed by Mallow's chapter on exemplary programs designed for young children with substance-abusing parents. Morehouse's Chapter 10 describes a variety of school-based and residential programs aimed at adolescent children of substance-abusing parents, youngsters who are often at great risk to become the next generation of substance-abusing parents. Chapter 11 by Venarde and Payton discusses the large, often overlooked, population of college students with substance-abusing parents. These authors provide examples of effective interventions specifically designed for this age group. Begun and Rose conclude this section with an important chapter focusing on the growing number of children with substance-abusing incarcerated parents.

The final section of this book includes four brief, real-life personal accounts of individuals who grew up in substance-abusing families. Their vivid and poignant descriptions of their early traumatic lives reflect both the pain experienced by children of all ages who grew up with a substance-abusing parent as well as the resilience that is found in many such children and which allows them to go on and succeed in life and become caring professionals.

Given the limited literature on this important topic, we strongly believe that this book makes a critical contribution to those working with or concerned about the millions of young and adult children whose parents abuse or have abused alcohol and other substances.

Acknowledgments

Writing and especially editing a book is always a communal endeavor. We would like to thank all the authors who made this book possible and who were willing to keep revising the chapters to make it into a coherent book. We also would like to thank Jennifer Perillo, Senior Acquisitions Editor at Springer Publishing Company, who first approached us about a book on this topic and has been a constant source of support, and Sis Wenger, CEO/President of the National Association for Children of Alcoholics, for all her work on behalf of children of alcohol- and other drug-abusing parents.

Shulamith Lala Ashenberg Straussner
Christine Huff Fewell

1

Children of Substance-Abusing Parents: An Overview

Shulamith Lala Ashenberg Straussner

Addiction does not begin and end with the abuser; it sends shock waves through an entire family unit. The reach of substance abuse also extends to schools, communities, health and welfare agencies, the justice systems, and to society at large. We all shoulder the costs. Children of substance abusers suffer the most—from direct effects on their physical and mental health to influences on their own use of tobacco, alcohol, or drugs.

(CASA, 2005, P. 1.)

INTRODUCTION

According to the latest U.S. government data, approximately 22.3 million persons 12 years or older, or 9% of the U.S. population, met the diagnostic criteria for alcohol or other substance dependence (AOD) or abuse (Substance Abuse and Mental Health Services Administration [SAMHSA], 2008). Of these, 15.5 million were dependent upon or abused alcohol, 3.7 million were dependent upon or abused illicit drugs, and 3.2 million were dependent upon or abused both alcohol and illicit drugs. However, as indicated in the quote above, addiction, or the abuse and dependence on alcohol and other drugs, "does not begin and end with the abuser." Millions of family members are impacted by substance abusers, including an estimated 27 million children who live with a parent who

1

abuses or is dependent upon alcohol or illicit drugs (National Center on Addiction and Substance Abuse at Columbia University [CASA], 2005). More critical is the fact that substance abuse by parents is more likely to involve the most developmentally vulnerable of all children, those who are the youngest: According to SAMHSA (2008), almost 14% of children living with a substance-abusing parent were aged 5 or younger, compared with 9.9% of youths who were aged 12–17.

Children of alcohol and other drug-abusing parents, who will be referred to as children of substance-abusing parents or COSAPs, run a risk of multitude of short- and long-term problems and are likely to become the next generation of individuals who are alcohol and/or drug dependent, thus perpetuating this cycle into the future (Hussong et al., 2008). However, since COSAPs exhibit not only problematic behaviors, but also strengths or resilience, careful individual assessment of each family and each child is required. Help needs to be age and culturally appropriate and systemic, and must take into account the needs of the individual child and his or her family members.

The purpose of this chapter is to provide an overview of the dynamics of families with substance-abusing parents, the impact on their children, and the most effective treatment approaches for children of various ages, ranging from those impacted by prenatal maternal substance use to older children, adolescents, and adults. Such children are found in every socioeconomic and ethnic and racial group in the United States (SAMHSA, 2008; Straussner, 2001) and in every setting ranging from preschools to community agencies, to colleges and universities, to hospitals and mental health facilities, and in the private offices of mental health clinicians.

UNDERSTANDING SUBSTANCE USE DISORDERS

Every day millions of Americans use alcohol and other drugs; however, not everyone experiences a problem due to such use. It is therefore helpful to conceptualize the use of such substances as ranging on a continuum from nonproblematic social use to substance misuse or abuse to dependence or addiction (Straussner, 2004).

Although there is no generally accepted distinction that differentiates between the "use" and "abuse" of a substance, the fourth edition of the American Psychiatric Association's (APA, 2000) *Diagnostic and Statistical Manual of Mental Disorders (DSM-IV-TR)* classifies all mood-altering substances under the category of substance-related disorders, which is further differentiated into two substance use disorders: *substance abuse* and *substance dependence.* The *DSM* defines "abuse"[1] as the continued use of a substance despite experiencing social, occupational, psychological, or physical problems; recurrent use in situations in which use is physically hazardous, such as driving while intoxicated; and a minimal duration of disturbance of at least 1 month. "Substance dependence," which is synonymous with the term "addiction," may vary in severity from mild to severe, and refers to compulsive and continued use despite adverse consequences. Depending on the particular substance, it typically implies the existence of an initial increase of tolerance to the drugs, that is, that more and more of the substance is required to achieve the same effect. Once dependence or addiction develops, the individual cannot wait too long between doses without experiencing craving and symptoms of physical withdrawal (Doweiko, 2009).

IMPACT OF SUBSTANCE ABUSE ON THE FAMILY SYSTEM

The concept of family as a system has long been accepted in substance-abuse literature and clinical practice (Nichols, 2011). The basic definition of a family system dynamic is that a change in the functioning of one family member is automatically followed by a compensatory change in other family members. Consequently, in a family in which one of the members becomes a substance abuser, profound and significant implications for the rest of the family can be anticipated as familial roles are shifted and generational boundaries are crossed. For example, as a substance-abusing parent becomes unable to fulfill his or her role, other family members, including the children, may begin to fill the existing vacuum and assume the missing parental roles and responsibilities, often at the expense of their own development (Straussner, 1994).

Given the generally different roles assumed by fathers and mothers, it is important to closely examine the differential impact on the family when the father or mother, or both, have a substance abuse problem (Edwards, Eiden, & Leonard, 2004).

Paternal substance abuse, particularly alcohol, is often correlated with domestic violence, child emotional and physical abuse, incest, and poverty (Donohue, Romero, & Hill, 2006; Gruber & Taylor, 2006). Although alcohol abuse by husbands/fathers has existed throughout the ages, the impact today is more profound since traditional extended family members

---

[1]It appears that the next edition of the *DSM* (*DSM-5*), which will be published in 2013, will no longer use the terms alcohol or drug "abuse" or "dependence." The diagnostic term is likely to be Substance Use Disorder with qualifiers of "moderate" or "severe" depending on the number of criteria met.

who used to provide emotional and physical support with childcare are likely to live far away, and the mother is more likely to be experiencing the stresses of the labor force or be herself more dysfunctional due to her own use of alcohol or other substances (Grucza, Bucholz, Rice, & Bierut, 2008).

Many women, whether they have a substance abuse problem themselves or not, tend to remain in relationships with substance-dependent men. On the other hand, men, in general, tend to leave women who have a substance abuse problem, leaving the women with limited financial and emotional resources that make it difficult to care for themselves, much less their children (Straussner & Brown, 2002). Moreover, many substance-abusing women come from homes where they were physically and/or sexually abused and where parenting was poor or nonexistent. As a result, their own parenting behavior may be markedly deficient, and they may have difficulty in developing a healthy attachment to their infants and young children (see Fewell, Chapter 2, this volume; Pederson et al., 2008). Many such women are reported to child welfare services and often lose custody of their children. Finally, women are likely to have other family members who are alcohol and drug users; consequently, even if they do seek and obtain help, their recovery is made difficult by the fact that they tend to return to environments that are not supportive of their continued abstinence (Greenfield et al., 2007).

With the growing number of women with substance abuse problems, it is more common to find families in which both parents have alcohol and other drug problems. In such situations, the child is essentially parentless and likely learns to take care of himself or herself. Unfortunately, depending on the child's age, he or she may become a "parentified child" (Fitzgerald et al., 2008), who becomes a caretaker of his or her own parents and siblings even at the cost of his or her own development. For example, the 15-year-old eldest daughter in a family with an alcoholic father and a pill-addicted mother may take over the responsibilities of making sure that her younger sister gets to school on time and is picked up safely after school, even if it means that she cannot attend the afterschool choir practice that she loves so much, while her 14-year-old brother gets an afterschool job at a neighborhood grocery store in order to bring in money and leftover food for the family.

Although the above descriptions focus on traditional families, similar dynamics may occur in families where the parents are gay or lesbian. Unfortunately, though there is a large body of literature on gay and lesbian substance abusers (see Senreich & Vairo, 2004), the literature on gay/lesbian families with substance-abusing parents and their children is sparse.

Given the differential impact of the various substances on individuals, it is important to examine those differences in more detail.

IMPACT OF DIFFERENT SUBSTANCES ON THE FAMILY

The most commonly abused substances impacting on family life are alcohol and other sedative-hypnotics (sleeping pills and tranquilizers); opiates, in particular heroin, and more recently, prescription pain medications such as Oxycodone; stimulants such as cocaine (including crack) and methamphetamine; and cannabis (marijuana and hashish). Due to their different legal and social status, addictive potential, and differential effects on the brain, the impact on the family will vary depending on which substance is being abused (Straussner, 1994). Although there has been an increasing trend toward multiple substance use, most individuals tend to have a definite preference for a given substance.

Since alcohol and other sedative-hypnotics are usually obtained legally, the lifestyles and ethnic backgrounds of families who abuse them vary widely, reflecting the population at large. Although it is possible for adolescents and young adults to have severe alcohol problems, in general dependence on alcohol develops slowly and usually tends to interfere with a person's functioning after adult independence has been achieved. Thus alcohol abusing individuals are very likely to marry and have children before the insidious impact of their addiction on family life is fully recognized.

Although the effects of alcohol abuse by a spouse or parent vary considerably from family to family, common patterns of familial interaction and behavior have been described in the literature (see Gruber & Taylor, 2006). Families of individuals with alcohol-use disorders are often characterized by communication problems, conflict, chaos and unpredictability, inconsistent messages to children, breakdown in rituals and traditional family rules and boundaries, and emotional, physical, and sexual abuse (see Lam & O'Farrell, Chapter 3, this volume). Moreover, it is not uncommon for family members to engage in behaviors that maintain and perpetuate the substance use by protecting the individual from any negative consequences. For example, the wife of a man suffering from a hangover after a night of drinking may call his employer to say that he is sick with the flu and will not be able to come to work that day. This dynamic has been termed "enabling" (Zelvin, 2004). Another important and somewhat more controversial concept is that of "co-dependency." It is defined as "an exaggerated dependence upon a loved object or, by extension, external sources of fulfillment . . . Co-dependent individuals are 'people pleasers' who . . . tend to rescue others at the expense of their own needs" (Zelvin, 2004, pp. 269–270). While codependent individuals can be found in any dysfunctional family, they are more typically found in a substance-abusing one. All these issues will have to be addressed in the treatment process when working with substance-abusing families (O'Farrell & Fals-Stewart, 2006; Steinglass, 2009).

Unlike alcohol, nonprescription opiate use is illegal and many opiate abusers grow up in dysfunctional and often physically abusive families with alcohol and/or opiate abusing parents and even grandparents. Due to the highly addictive nature of opiates, individuals become affected by them at an earlier age than alcohol, frequently before completing their education and functioning as self-supporting adults. Consequently, they are more often connected to their dysfunctional family of origin and less likely to form and/or maintain a stable family of procreation of their own (Straussner, 1994).

In general, opiate abusers are more likely to be members of minority or disenfranchised, low-income groups and/or characterized as having an antisocial personality with poor superego development (Kaufman, 1994). Since the time and effort necessary to obtain drugs and to pay for the addiction are considerable, the lifestyle associated with opiate addiction is highly unstructured and generally characterized by poverty and illegal activities that tend to have a severe negative impact on family life. A series of live-in partners, prostitution, and incarcerations are fairly common.

The impact of AIDS resulting from intravenous heroin use or sexual relations with a HIV-infected individual has had a profound effect on family life of opiate users in the United States (Lester et al., 2009). Of the estimated 1 million people in the United States living with HIV/AIDS, about one-third were infected directly or indirectly due to injected drug use. Intravenous drug abusers (IVDA) or sexual contact with IVDAs accounts for the vast majority of HIV/AIDS cases in women, particularly black women, and their children (National Institute on Drug Abuse, 2006).

In addition to HIV/AIDS, the use of dirty, shared, and reused needles results in various systemic infections. Illnesses such as hepatitis C, anemia, tuberculosis, heart disease, diabetes, and pneumonia are also common among heroin abusers, whereas cocaine use affects the cardiovascular system, resulting in blockages in blood circulation, abnormal heart rhythms, and strokes. Prostitution, a frequent means of support for drug-dependent women, leads to a high incidence of sexually transmitted diseases (Friedman & Wilson, 2004).

The impact of cocaine use on the family system is less known with much of the research limited to studies of perinatal and child-related issues. It is likely that familial impact of cocaine varies depending upon the route of administration, socioeconomic class, and gender of user (Straussner, 1994). Since the cost of loose, snortable cocaine is high, users tend to be trend-setting and high-income individuals. Cocaine's expense and high potential for addiction may lead to stealing from the family and workplace, business bankruptcies, and legal repercussions. Moreover, the common psychological side effects of increased paranoia and suicidal ideation wreck havoc on family life (Ockert, Baier, & Coons, 2004).

The use of a low-cost, but even more addictive, smokeable form of cocaine known as crack tends to be more common among low-income families, paralleling the familial dynamics seen with heroin abusers. The use of crack in the United States has had a particularly destructive and tragic impact on African American families and communities, due in part to the high rate of use among black women (SAMHSA, 2008; Straussner, 1994), thereby diminishing their availability to maintain familial and community life.

Little is known about the impact of marijuana on family life. Since the addictability and the cost of marijuana is not as high as for some of the other substances, the impact on the family appears to be more subtle. Clinically, marijuana-abusing individuals appear to be less socially interactive and more inner-focused making them less physically and emotionally available to the family.

THE IMPACT OF SUBSTANCE-ABUSING PARENTS ON CHILDREN

COSAPs can range from those exhibiting severe emotional and behavioral problems to resilient children who do well in life. In a well-known longitudinal study, Werner and Johnson (2004) followed children of alcoholics for over a 30-year period beginning at age 2. These researchers found that it was the availability of support systems within the extended family or in the community that significantly affected the development of the children into adulthood. Strong extended family support and the maintenance of family routines were the important mediating factors on the potential for positive outcomes for the child (Gruber & Taylor, 2006; Lam, Fals-Stewart, & Kelley, 2008).

Nonetheless, though some COSAPs are relatively well adjusted, many become dysfunctional with high risk of developing their own substance abuse and/or establishing their own substance-abusing family systems in adulthood (Anda et al., 2006; CASA, 2005; Peleg-Oren & Taichman, 2006). It is important to keep in mind that the impact of parental substance abuse varies depending, as pointed out previously, upon whether the abuser is the father, the mother, or both parents; the quality of parent–child attachment; the coping abilities of the nonaddicted parent; the age when parental substance abuse is most problematic; the physical and psychological status of parents and other family members; the availability of extended family and other support systems; the existence of sexual and physical abuse; the economic and health care resources of the family; and inborn ego strength or resiliency (Straussner, 1994).

Recent neurological and psychological studies reveal that children who grow up in violent and otherwise traumatizing households suffer not just from the psychological impact, such as emotional dysregulation and difficulties in social relationships (Eiden, Colder, Edwards, & Leonard, 2009; Fewell, Chapter 2, this volume) but may also have permanent neurological changes affecting them for the rest of their lives (Dayton, Chapter 7, this volume; van der Kolk, 2003).

ISSUES ACROSS THE LIFE SPAN OF CHILDREN OF SUBSTANCE-ABUSING PARENTS

A critical factor in determining the impact of parental substance abuse and the most helpful intervention is the age of the child. The following sections explore the impact of parental substance abuse on children at different ages and discuss the best interventions for a given age.

Impact of Prenatal Substance Use

While there are some indications that *paternal* substance use is detrimental to the fetus and newborn child, such impact has yet to be fully explored (Klonoff-Cohen & Lam-Kruglick, 2001). On the other hand, there is a growing knowledge about the consequences of maternal substance abuse during pregnancy. The impact of fetal exposure to substances is determined by many factors, including the gestation age of the fetus at exposure, the dosage and frequency of substance intake, other substances consumed simultaneously, mother's nutrition, and environmental factors (Nadel & Straussner, 2006). Substances used by the mother are transmitted to the fetus during pregnancy and may result in the birth of an addicted baby or, depending on the substance used and the timing, in permanent physiological and neurological damage (Azmitia, 2001). It is important to note that though substance use during pregnancy can be very destructive, for many women pregnancy and motherhood can function as a motivating factor in seeking treatment, although fear of losing custody of their children or lack of childcare resources are frequent treatment obstacles (Greenfield et al., 2007).

Alcohol consumed by pregnant women is the most frequently used destructive substance for the developing fetus. Although much of the early research focused on a singular disorder titled fetal alcohol syndrome (FAS), more recent research has revealed a continuum of developmental outcomes known as fetal alcohol spectrum disorder

(FASD), which is believed to affect approximately 1% of all children born in the United States (Centers for Disease Control and Prevention [CDC], 2009). This continuum, which includes FAS and the milder fetal alcohol effects (FAE), can range from subtle neurobehavioral effects to hyperactivity to central nervous system and information processing problems to facial deformities to profound mental retardation. In fact, FASD is now recognized as one of the leading causes of mental retardation and birth defects (CDC, 2009).

The use of illicit drugs, particularly heroin, is also associated with maternal complications and adverse outcomes for infants and children (see Pomeroy & Parrish, Chapter 4, this volume; Smith, Chapter 8, this volume). After birth, some babies, at least in the short term, appear to suffer no ill effects from prenatal drug exposure, whereas others may be premature or small for gestational age and have resulting complications such as respiratory problems. Some newborns suffer from drug withdrawal and have symptoms such as excessive crying and irritability; hypertonia (stiff muscles); tremors; sleep disturbances; and increased sensitivity to light, sound, and touch. As the child develops, other physiological effects may become evident. These can include developmental delays of various kinds, such as failure to thrive, cognitive deficits, and speech, language, and motor delays. Physical problems, such as asthma, may develop in connection with respiratory deficiencies. During the school years, learning disabilities and behavioral problems such as attention deficit hyperactivity disorder and conduct disorder may become evident (Azmitia, 2001; Floyd et al., 2008; Nadel & Straussner, 2006).

Although there has been some research on the effects of cocaine, marijuana, and tobacco on newborns, it has been difficult to disentangle the unique effects of each substance as polysubstance use, and nutritional deficiencies are prevalent in the populations studied (Floyd et al., 2008). Research has documented that prenatal cocaine and methamphetamine use leads to an increased risk of perinatal death, placenta abruption, low birth weight, prematurity, and small gestational birth weight. Prenatal smoking also increases the chances of sudden infant death syndrome (SIDS) and orofacial clefts (Floyd et al., 2008).

During the 1980s, concern was raised over symptoms displayed by the so-called crack babies. Although many of these concerns were later viewed as a societal overreaction, some of these children have been found to have attention deficit and problems with mental organization as they grew up (Azmitia, 2001). More recently, similar concerns have been voiced about babies exposed in utero to methamphetamines, sometimes referred to as "crank babies." Although the long-term effects of methamphetamine exposure on these children is yet unknown, such babies should be evaluated and observed for birth defects and other problems that may be related to this exposure (Jewett, 2005).

Provision of Services

There is no cure for fetal alcohol disorders, but there are certain interventions that have proven to be helpful when dealing with both mothers and their young children with FASD or other prenatal effects. Preventing such prenatal effects requires a multipronged approach ranging from patient education focusing on abstinence from drugs and alcohol during pregnancy, to provision of proper nutrition and obstetric care during pregnancy. Substitution therapy under medical supervision such as use of methadone or buprenorphine for heroin or other narcotic users can avoid some of the medical complications related to illicit narcotic use.

Although many substance abuse treatment programs, particularly inpatient ones, are reluctant to admit pregnant women, there has been an increase in specialized treatment programs for this population (Wong, 2006). However, some inpatient programs that do admit pregnant women will not allow them to bring their other children, or will accept only women with preschool-age children, forcing some mothers to put their older children into foster care.

In order to be effective, treatment programs for pregnant substance-abusing women and those with newborns must provide both tools for recovery as well as hope for a better life for themselves and their children. Individual counseling, group treatment and peer support, parenting and communication skills, and assertiveness training are essential components of treatment for pregnant substance-abusing women (Wong, 2006). Many substance-abusing pregnant women and mothers of very young children also need help in other areas of their lives such as housing, income support and financial planning, education and vocational training, and understanding the nature of their often problematic relationships with substance-abusing men. Help also needs to be offered to the men to become better fathers.

Interventions for children impacted by prenatal substance use vary depending upon the severity of their problems and their age. They may include medication to help with medical and behavioral symptoms, educational and behavioral therapy (for both children and their caregivers), and play therapy. The use of pediatric occupational therapy may help with body organization and modulation. Older children may need help with self-image, depression, and suicidality (Bertrand, 2009).

Impact of Parental Substance Abuse on School-Aged Children

As indicated above, school-aged children of alcoholics can range from those exhibiting severe emotional and behavioral problems to resilient children who do very well in school and are rarely recognized as having any problems at home.

Nonetheless, growing up with a substance-abusing parent is often a painful experience, with many children being at increased risk for negative outcomes with a variety of emotional, behavioral, physical, cognitive, academic, and social problems (Anda et al., 2006; Peleg-Oren & Teichman, 2006). In her classic 1969 study of 115 Canadian boys and girls between the ages of 10 and 16, Margaret Cork described the life histories, feelings, and problems of children of alcoholics who poignantly talked about their lives as being lonely, scary, and without structure. Another early study of children of alcoholics was conducted by Claudia Black (1981) who was among the first to identify the various roles that children of alcoholic parents take on as a way of coping. These included: the Responsible One—who tries to bring order to the chaos at home; the Adjuster—who adjusts to any situation by detaching emotionally; the Placater—who tries to make others feel better; and the Acting Out Child—who by his or her "bad" behavior may distract attention from the dysfunctional parent. Black (1981) was also the first writer to identify the "Don't Talk, Don't Trust and Don't Feel" as reflecting the core dynamics of young and adult children of alcoholic parents.

More recent studies have focused mainly on the Acting Out Child—often referred to as children with "externalizing behavior problems" (Hill et al., 2008; Schuckit, Smith, Pierson, Trim, & Danko, 2007). Such children, particularly boys, not only exhibit attention deficits, hyperactivity, conduct disorders, and academic problems but also cause difficulties for teachers and other students, at times leading them to become scapegoated by their peers. Consequently, not only do these children lack the basic supports at home but they also may not obtain the support from peers and school personnel that could ameliorate some of the pain experienced by growing up with a dysfunctional alcoholic parent(s). Other children, most commonly girls, are more likely to exhibit what is currently termed "internalizing" behaviors and feelings, such as social withdrawal, low self-esteem, and feelings of loneliness. These behaviors and feelings can predispose the child of a substance-abusing parent toward depression, suicidality, and addictions, which become more noticeable during adolescence.

Provision of Services

For the school-aged child, peer groups are critically important and can serve as the bases for both diagnostic comparison as well as treatment. It is important to assess the child's relationship with peers and look for such dynamics as bullying and other antisocial behaviors, as well as changes and/or difficulties in mood and school performance (Johnson, Gryczynski, & Moe, Chapter 5, this volume).

For elementary school-aged children group intervention can be an important tool in helping them deal with the impact of parental substance abuse. The group can provide a critical source of support and an arena for the development of appropriate social skills (Peleg-Oren & Taichman, 2006). Psychoeducation for both the non–substance-abusing parent and one who is in the process of recovery needs to focus on the basics of child development aimed at helping parents understand what to expect from their child at different ages, and on parenting skills aimed at helping parents understand how to appropriately set limits, and how to reward and discipline their children (Johnson et al., Chapter 5, this volume).

Moreover, as will be discussed later, adolescent children of alcohol-abusing parents are particularly susceptible to developing their own alcohol and other drug abuse problems; therefore, preadolescence is a prime period in which to target family-systems interventions, since this is when they are more open to parenting influences (Lam, Cance, Eke, Fishbein, Hawkins, & Williams, 2007). A number of evidence-based programs, such as the *Strengthening Families Program* (SFP; www.strengtheningfamiliesprogram.org) and *Celebrating Families* (www.celebratingfamilies.net/gettingstarted.htm), use a holistic model to treat the whole family. These programs will be discussed in more detail in the next section.

Services such as Student Assistance Programs focus on identifying troubled students based on cues like deteriorating academic performance, behavioral changes, excessive lateness or absences, sleepiness in class, or neglected appearance. After meeting individually with the child to further assess his/her situation, the practitioner may then refer the student to appropriate school- or community-based services (Morehouse, Chapter 10, this volume).

Since many COSAPs end up in foster care and group homes or are seen in community-based family and mental health clinics for a variety of psychological or behavioral problems, it is critical that all children be assessed regarding parental substance abuse and provided with specialized services that have been developed for this population. Screening instruments such as the Children of Alcoholics Screening Test (CAST) have been found to be useful in identifying such children

(Pilat & Jones, 1985). Books, pamphlets, and videotapes issued by the *National Association for Children of Alcoholics, Al-Anon,* and individual authors offer useful information for children of substance abusers at various age levels and can be easily provided by schools, foster care agencies, and treatment facilities.

Impact of Parental Substance Use on Adolescents

An estimated 10% of adolescent children live with a substance-abusing parent (SAMHSA, 2008). Although less susceptible than younger children to being physically harmed by their parents, adolescents with substance-abusing parents are at high risk for suffering other negative consequences affecting their physical, emotional, and behavioral health. In fact, it has been argued that, compared with younger children, teenage COSAPs are at greater risk, since, on average, they have had more prolonged exposure to their parents' substance use and its consequences (Fenster, Chapter 6, this volume; Peleg-Oren & Taichman, 2006).

It is important to keep in mind the great variability between early (ages 12–14), mid (ages 15–16), and late adolescence (ages 17–18), as well as the differences among adolescents. For example, an early adolescent boy can be as physically developed as an 18 year old but have the cognitive and emotional development of a much younger child. Generally, younger adolescents are more dependent upon peers for a sense of identity, more loyal to their family, and are much more concrete in their thinking (Freshman, 2004; Morehouse, Chapter 10, this volume).

At times, the physical and psychological changes faced by adolescents may play a more critical role in their lives than being a COSAP. Therefore, understanding the developmental issues of adolescents is crucial to effective interventions. Specifically, it is important to remember that the prefrontal cortex of the adolescent brain is not fully developed, so they do not yet have a well-developed capacity to control emotions and make good judgments. Yet the hormonal changes during adolescence impact the amygdala, which controls the emotions, causing emotions to be intensified. It is common for adolescents to experience everything as a crisis, have mood swings, be impulsive, self-absorbed and overly sensitive, and not be able to plan or understand cause and effect (Cozzolino, 2006).

On top of their emotional instability, adolescent COSAPs are likely to confront a constellation of stress factors within and outside their families. Preexisting internalizing and externalizing problems become more evident during adolescence, placing these children at an increased risk for emotional, familial, social, academic, and legal problems. Of particular concern is the increased risk of substance use problems (Saraceno, Munaf, Heron, Craddock, & van den Bree, 2009). According to studies, over half of children who were exposed to parental substance use disorders during adolescence developed their own substance use disorders, compared with 15% of those who were not so exposed (Biederman, Faraone, Monuteaux, & Feighner, 2000; Rothman, Edwards, Heeren, & Hingson, 2008). Moreover, as was found among younger children, adolescents often experience feelings of guilt and shame about their parents' substance use and may be reluctant to discuss it with peers, authority figures, or even helping professionals.

Provision of Services

Assessment of the adolescent with an alcoholic parent needs to be comprehensive and should focus on the previously identified psychological, behavioral, cognitive, social and physical aspects, as well as family dynamics. The clinician also needs to carefully attend to the adolescent's strengths, attitudes, aspirations, and resources.

Two screening tools that have been shown to be appropriate for use with adolescent children of alcoholics are the CAST and the Family Drinking Survey. The CAST (www.coaf.org/professionals/screenCAST .htm) is a 30-item self-report measure that gauges the experiences and feelings of adolescents regarding their parents' drinking behaviors. The Family Drinking Survey (Whitfield, 1991), which assesses the effect of a parent's drinking on an adolescent's physical, emotional, and social health, can help clarify the impact of the parents' substance use. In addition, standardized instruments designed specifically for adolescents can also help determine the existence, extent, and impact of the adolescent's own substance misuse. One such instrument, the CRAFFT, consists of six age-appropriate questions related to alcohol and drug use and has been found to have good reliability and validity (Knight et al., 1999).

School- and community-based individual, group, and family counseling approaches as well as self-help groups are all helpful for this population. One of the most widely available and free community-based programs for teenage children of alcoholic parents are the Alateen self-help groups provided under the auspices of Al-Anon Family Groups. Utilizing the principles of Alcoholics Anonymous and of Al-Anon, Alateen teaches children about the progressive nature of alcoholism and the importance of detaching from the alcoholic parent's pathological behavior and focusing on their own functioning. Another free resource is a Web-based discussion board run by the National Association for Children of Alcoholics (www .nacoa.org), where teens can go online to discuss their experiences of living with substance-abusing parents. In addition, a variety of books, booklets, and movies about COSAPs are readily available and should be used in conjunction with other interventions.

Individual insight-oriented treatment as well as cognitive-behavioral therapies are frequently used approaches for this age group (Eyberg, Nelson & Boggs, 2008; Silverman, Pina, & Viswesvaran, 2008). Regardless of the approach utilized, the overarching goal of treatment is to enhance adolescents' abilities to care for themselves emotionally, physically, and socially. Adolescents also need to be helped to develop coping strategies to deal with negative affects and develop awareness of their own thinking processes and build skills in problem solving, interpersonal communication, conflict resolution, and negotiation. Relaxation techniques, physical exercises, and other strategies for self-soothing can diminish anxiety or other negative mood states. Helping teens set and follow through with educational and vocational goals is also important, since adolescents with clear goals are less likely to use drugs and to become parents during their teenage years (Harden, Brunton, Fletcher, & Oakley, 2009).

As with school-age children, group treatment is a commonly utilized format for intervention with adolescent children of substance abusers (Fenster, Chapter 6, this volume). Treatment is typically short term, although some groups are long lasting. Groups are particularly helpful in teaching adolescents that they are not alone in dealing with the consequences of having a substance-abusing parent, thereby reducing feelings of guilt, and providing opportunities to interact with peers who are engaged in pro-social behaviors (Fenster, Chapter 6, this volume).

The parents of an adolescent need to be helped to establish appropriate and effective discipline and expectations. Of particular value is help in reinstitution of family routines and rituals such as family meals and holiday and religious celebrations, as these help strengthen bonds and restore a sense of normalcy to the family (CASA, 2007; Steinglass, 2009). If needed, a referral for substance abuse treatment for the parent should be made. As mentioned in the previous section, a number of evidence-based family programs are increasingly being used in different settings. One such program is SFP (Kumpfer, Williams, & Baxley, 1997). The SFP is a family skills training program designed to increase resilience and reduce risk factors for behavioral, emotional, academic, and social problems in high-risk families with both younger children (ages 3–5) and teens (ages 12–16). It is designed specifically for parents who have a history of substance abuse but are now in the early stages of recovery. This highly structured intervention teaches parents and teenagers skills in problem solving, interpersonal communication, and conflict resolution. Each week begins with a family group dinner, followed by separate group meetings for parents and youth, and ends with a family session. Both parents and children receive age-appropriate education and experiential learning in 14 weekly, 2-hour sessions with a focus on multiple themes, such as goal setting, health, and communication. This program has shown a great deal of success with multiple ethnic groups and in both rural and urban settings (Kumpfer, Pinyuchon, Teixeira de Melo, & Whiteside, 2008).

Another program evidencing success in treating addicted parents and their adolescent children is *Celebrating Families!*, which was originally developed for parents involved in drug court proceedings, and later adapted for use with alcohol-involved families in which there is a high risk for domestic violence, child abuse, or neglect. The *Celebrating Families!* curriculum, currently distributed by the National Association of Children of Alcoholics (NACoA), is an evidence-based cognitive behavioral support group model that works with every member of the family, from age 3 through adulthood (for more details, see www.celebratingfamilies.net/ gettingstarted.htm).

Finally, it is critically important to help young people in a dysfunctional family with a substance-abusing parent to develop a relationship with a caring adult who can model healthy behaviors. In addition to a caring clinician, community supports, including teachers, sports coaches, and religious leaders, can provide positive role models and growth experiences. Moreover, making teens aware of their increased risk to inherit a substance use problem, and helping them come to terms with that risk, is an essential part of clinical work with COSAPs.

Impact of Parental Substance Use on Young Adult College Students

The age span for young adults, generally between the ages of 20 and 30, encompasses many developmental tasks and preparations for undertaking the responsibilities of adulthood, including the formation of families, obtaining and maintaining jobs, and/or establishing career choices. For many young COSAPs, these tasks are complicated by concerns regarding their parents and their own emotional and social difficulties resulting from growing up in dysfunctional families. Some, particularly those from disenfranchised backgrounds, may wind up in jails and prisons (Begun & Rose, Chapter 12, this volume; Lemieux, 2009), whereas many others who are in their late teens and early 20s, can be found on college campuses across the United States. The focus of this section is on these relatively resilient children, who often wind up being seen in college counseling centers not understanding what brought them there (Wright, Crawford, & Del Castillo, 2009).

During the years 2009–2010, there were an estimated 19 million students enrolled in colleges and universities in the United States (U.S. Census Bureau, 2009), with an approximate 3 million of them impacted by a substance-abusing parent (Venarde & Payton, Chapter 11, this volume). College students in general face a myriad of developmental, academic, social, and health challenges. Those who continue to live at home while attending college must balance family relationships with their new social and academic requirements, whereas those who reside on campus need to adapt to an independent lifestyle and a new pattern of communication with peers and family members. For children of parents with substance-use disorders, these adjustments can be even more complex.

In general, college COSAPs are a heterogeneous group representing a range of socioeconomic and ethnic/racial backgrounds. Although some have been characterized as overachievers, others may begin to manifest a range of negative emotions and behaviors (Venarde & Payton, Chapter 11, this volume). Some of the variability in college students' adjustment may be explained not only by parental substance abuse, but by the quality of parent–child attachment style (Fewell, 2006).

Of special concern for college students who are COSAPs is the wide availability of substances in the college environment. Alcohol remains the substance of choice on college campuses in the United States. However, the use of some illicit drugs and the misuse of prescription medications have risen on college campuses in the past decade (Johnston, O'Malley, Bachman, & Schulenberg, 2006). Thus, adolescents, who, as discussed above, are at greater risk for developing substance use disorders, are pursuing their educations in contexts where alcohol and other substances may be readily available and frequently used by their peers (CASA, 2007).

Provision of Services

Although some college students come to counseling services with parental substance use as their identified concern, most present for other emotional reasons, such as academic problems, stress, relationship problems, eating disorders or depression, and may not even mention parental substance use as an issue. Moreover, some may not consider their home experience as particularly unusual or out of the norm. Thus, it is critically important to obtain a thorough history of substance use by all family members, especially parents. And though some students may not be ready to discuss this topic in treatment, others may be relieved at finally being able to talk about this "family secret" (Venarde & Payton, Chapter 11, this volume).

A variety of programs and treatment approaches are available on many college campuses. These include preventive programs and outreach approaches utilizing a public health education model. These "wellness" or "health promotion" programs can be offered throughout the campus, including classrooms, student centers, and dormitories. Psychoeducational programming can help students to identify the effects of growing up with a substance-abusing parent on their own sense of self, moods, interpersonal relationships, and personal substance use (Venarde & Payton, Chapter 11, this volume).

Many college programs include referrals to individual or group treatment on campus or to community facilities or private practitioners familiar with this population. According to Venarde and Payton (Chapter 11, this volume), individual counseling may be most appropriate for those students who have recently become aware of parental substance abuse, or who are being acutely impacted by a parent's chronic substance use. In addition, it may be indicated for students who react with shame or who fear the judgment of their peers. Group treatment, on the other hand, may be more appropriate for those students who wish to better understand their experiences as COSAPs and those wishing to connect with supportive peers. Such support groups may be the only place where students can feel comfortable voicing their concerns regarding alcohol and other substance use on campus without fear of being judged or rejected. These groups can also provide the opportunity for students to explore their "struggles with the extremes"—of having either a strong aversion to and even repulsion to alcohol or drug use, or their own destructive use of substances, and find a healthy middle ground.

An especially useful tool for college students is the use of Internet resources, including virtual communities and social networks. As an anonymous means of obtaining information and interacting with other COSAPs, the Internet allows young people to absorb and share information and feelings at their own time and place.

Impact of Parental Alcohol Use on Adult Children of Substance Abusers

Much has been written about the impact of parental alcohol abuse on what has been termed "adult children of alcoholics" or ACOAs. As mentioned earlier, the work of Claudia Black (1981) and others, such as Janet Woititz (1983), has led to the formation of the well-known ACOA movement and the identification of a set of symptoms or characteristics of such individuals. Despite the popular and clinical literature regarding personality types or codependency among ACOAs, empirical support for these descriptions is lacking (Doweiko, 2009). Nonetheless, some individuals do find the descriptions of family roles and styles of relating to others helpful in understanding what they are feeling now and what has happened to them in their childhood.

Studies show that multiple adverse childhood experiences such as neglect, abuse, exposure to domestic violence, and parental alcohol or drug use are associated with depression, poor health outcomes, and early mortality in adults (Anda et al., 2006). Over the past decade, a new perspective has developed on the shared dynamics exhibited by ACOAs and other drug abusers: ". . . The Adult Children of Alcoholics (ACOA) syndrome is, in fact, a posttraumatic stress reaction in which unresolved childhood wounds that lay dormant for decades resurface in adulthood as a delayed reaction to childhood trauma" (Dayton, Chapter 7, this volume). Those childhood wounds are often the result of inadequate caretaking by parents who themselves were the victims of dysfunctional attachment patterns. Such intergenerational transmission of dysfunctional attachment behaviors has been demonstrated in a number of longitudinal studies (Cassidy & Shaver, 2008; Fewell, Chapter 2, this volume).

While not all COSAPs develop dysfunctional symptoms or dynamics, and, as indicated previously, many are highly resilient and emotionally strong, some adults who grew up in traumatized and traumatizing families with an alcohol or other drug-abusing parent may present some of the following characteristics (see Dayton, Chapter 7, this volume):

1. Rigid psychological defenses aimed at protecting oneself from emotional pain, including dissociation, denial, and splitting.
2. Development of a "false self" by creating a persona that "looks good" both within the family and outside, at the expense of one's authentic self.
3. Problems with emotional dysregulation, which can be manifested by the lack of ability to regulate feeling states, appetite, sleep, or sex drive, as well as swings between states of emotional intensity and numbing.
4. Hyper-vigilance about potential danger, which can lead to perceptions of problems that do not exist, or to an exaggeration of problems that might have been easily managed.
5. A lack of awareness of one's feelings or discomfort in sharing of feelings.
6. Unresolved grief resulting from actual or psychological losses related to use of substances.
7. Learned helplessness resulting from living in a situation where one feels a lack of control over one's environment, which may lead to adopting a permanent position of being a victim.

8. Somatization of feelings resulting from an inability to experience or act on powerful emotions, which are then converted into bodily symptoms and experienced as back pains, headaches, stomach, or other physical ailments.
9. Shame that has been internalized as a sense of "I am bad" as opposed to "I did something bad." It is then manifested as a lack of energy, a hesitancy to become more self-affirming, or a sense that one does not deserve love and caring from others.
10. Survivor's guilt experience when one has managed to escape an unhealthy family system while a sibling or an abused parent still remains there. This can lead to self-sabotage or becoming overly pre-occupied with fixing one's family and others. It is not unusual for such individuals to become "professional helpers," such as nurses or social workers.
11. Traumatic bonding resulting from early traumatic relationships that can impel people not only to withdraw from close connections but also to seek them desperately. Traumatized adult COSAPs may repeat this type of unhealthy bonding style in relationships throughout their lives, often without their conscious awareness.
12. Tendency to isolate and inability to trust and accept caring from others as a way of avoiding further feelings of being hurt.
13. Loss of faith and hope in life's ability to repair and renew itself.
14. High-risk and compulsive behaviors, which are an attempt to overcome a numbed inner world by overstimulating the nervous system. These may include substance abuse, excessive speeding when driving, sexual acting out, overspending, fighting, or dangerous work.
15. Co-occurring mental health disorders on top of substance use disorders, such as anxiety disorders (including PTSD), depression, and various personality disorders.
16. Desire to self-medicate as an attempt to restore calm and inner "balance," which may lead to substance use disorders.

Provision of Services

Given the potential for growing up in a traumatizing household, it is important that every adult child of a substance-abusing parent be assessed for a history of trauma. However, as pointed out previously, children of traumatizing substance-abusing parents have learned to distrust adults, and fears of disloyalty to the family or being ostracized for "telling the truth" can keep adult COSAPs not only telling lies to the outside world but living lies within themselves, thereby complicating the treatment process. It is the clinicians' task to ensure the establishment of a trustworthy, healthy therapeutic relationship to make their patients curious about what they are feeling, and consequently feel willing to open up and explore their emotions. Clients also need to be helped to mourn the various losses they experienced, as well as things they never had an opportunity to experience (Dayton, Chapter 7, this volume). They also need to learn to trust again, to overcome their feelings of guilt and shame, and to connect to others while still hanging onto their own, autonomous sense of self. Sometimes this may be better accomplished through the use of nonverbal, expressive therapies, including art, music, gestalt, or psychodrama therapy.

Twelve-step programs, such as ACOA, Al-Anon, Co-Anon (for families of cocaine addicts) and Nar-Anon (for families of narcotic addicts), can be wonderful adjuncts or even offer an initial initiation to therapy since they provide a safe and constantly available "holding environment" in which individuals can slowly identify with the stories of others and feel supported and less alone in their pain (Spiegel & Fewell, 2004; Straussner & Spiegel, 1996). There are also a variety of other 12-step programs that address common issues faced by some adult COSAPs, including eating problems (Overeaters Anonymous), spending (Debtors Anonymous), or sexual problems (Sex and Love Addicts Anonymous) (Dayton, Chapter 7, this volume).

CONCLUSION

According to numerous studies, for healthy development a child needs a safe and stable environment and a caring family that provides acceptance, trust, sense of autonomy, and security. Children of parents with alcohol- and drug-use disorders are often unable to experience such an environment and are at an increased risk for lifelong problems, including a relatively high level of depressive symptoms and anxiety, low self-esteem, guilt feelings, difficulties with interpersonal relationships, and their own abuse of substances (Anda et al., 2006).

In assessing and intervening with COSAPs, it is important to note that each child is unique and each has strengths that need to be acknowledged and reinforced. A child's age plays a critical factor in the kind of intervention that needs to be offered. What is appropriate for a preschool child is not the same as that for an adolescent or a young adult. Even seemingly well-functioning adult COSAPs may need help at different times in their lives so that the destructive family scenarios do not continue into the next generations. It is the responsibility of all clinicians to understand the dynamics of young and adult COSAPs and how to best help them lead more productive and happier lives.

REFERENCES

American Psychiatric Association [APA]. (2000). *Diagnostic and statistical manual of mental disorders* (5th ed., text rev). Washington, DC: American Psychiatric Association.

Anda, R., Felitti, V., Bremner, J., Walker, J., Whitfield, C., Perry, B., et al. (2006). The enduring effects of abuse and related adverse experiences in childhood. *European Archives of Psychiatry and Clinical Neuroscience, 256*(3), 174–186.

Azmita, E. C. (2001). Impact of drugs and alcohol on the brain through the life cycle: Knowledge for social workers. *Journal of Social Work Practice in the Addictions, 1*(3), 41–64.

Bertrand, J. (2009). Interventions for children with fetal alcohol spectrum disorders (FASDs): Overview of findings for five innovative research projects. *Research in Developmental Disabilities, 30*(5), 986–1006.

Biederman, J., Faraone, S. V., Monuteaux, M. C., & Feighner, J. A. (2000). Patterns of alcohol and drug use in adolescents can be predicted by parental substance use disorders. *Pediatrics, 106,* 792–797.

Black, C. (1981). *It will never happen to me.* Denver, CO: MAC

Cassidy, J., & Shaver, P. R. (Eds.). (2008). *Handbook of attachment: Theory, research, and clinical applications* (2nd ed.). New York: The Guilford Press.

Centers for Disease Control and Prevention (CDC) (2009). *Alcohol use among pregnant and nonpregnant women of childbearing age—United States 1991–2005.* Retrieved from http://www.cdc.gov/ncbddd/index.html

Cork, M. R. (1969). *The forgotten children.* Toronto, ON: Alcoholism & Drug Addiction Research Foundation.

Cozzolino, L. (2006). *The neuroscience of human relationships.* New York: W.W. Norton & Co., Inc.

Donohue, B., & Romero, V., & Hill, H. H. (2006). Treatment of co-occurring child maltreatment and substance abuse. *Aggression and Violent Behavior, 11,* 636–640.

Doweiko, H. E. (2009). *Concepts of chemical dependency* (7th ed.). Pacific Grove, CA: Brooks/Cole.

Edwards, E., Eiden, R. D., & Leonard, K. (2004). Impact of fathers' alcoholism and associated risk factors on parent-infant attachment stability from 12 to 18 months. *Infant Mental Health Journal, 25,* 556–579.

Eiden, R. D., Colder, C., Edwards, E. P., & Leonard, K. E. (2009). A longitudinal study of social competence among children of alcoholic and nonalcoholic parents: Role of parental psychpathology, parental warmth, and self-regulation. *Psychology of Addictive Behaviors, 23*(1), 36–46.

Eyberg, S. M., Nelson, M. M., & Boggs, S. R. (2008). Evidence-based psychosocial treatments for children and adolescents with disruptive behavior. *Journal of Clinical Child and Adolescent Psychology, 37*(1), 215–237.

Fewell, C. H. (2006). *Attachment, reflective function, family dysfunction, and psychological distress among college students with alcoholic parents.* Unpublished doctoral dissertation, New York: New York University.

Fitzgerald, M. M., Schneider, R. A., Salstrom, S., Zinzow, H. M., Jackson, J., & Fossel, R. V. (2008). Child sexual abuse, early family risk, and childhood parentification: Pathways to current psychosocial adjustment. *Journal of Family Psychology, 22*(2), 320–324.

Floyd, R. L., Jack, B. W., Cefalo, R., Atrash, H., Mahoney, J., Herron, A., et al. (2008). The clinical content of preconception care: Alcohol, tobacco, and illicit drug exposures. *American Journal of Obstetrics & Gynecology, 199*(6), S333–S339.

Freshman, A. (2004). Assessment and treatment of adolescent substance abusers. In S. L. A. Straussner (Ed.), *Clinical work with substance-abusing clients* (2nd ed., pp. 305–329). New York: Guilford.

Friedman, E. G., & Wilson, R. (2004). Treatment of opiate addiction. In S. L. A. Straussner (Ed.), *Clinical work with substance-abusing clients* (2nd ed., pp. 187–208). New York: Guilford.

Greenfield, B., Brooks, A. J., Gordon, S. M., Green, C. A., Kropp, F., McHugh, R. K., et al. (2007). Substance abuse treatment entry, retention, and outcome in women: A review of the literature. *Drug and Alcohol Dependence, 86*(1), 1–21.

Gruber, K. J., & Taylor, M. F. (2006). A family perspective for substance abuse: Implications from the literature. *Journal of Social Work Practice in the Addictions, 6*(1/2), 1–29.

Grucza, R. A., Bucholz, K. K., Rice, J. P., & Bierut, L. J. (2008). Secular trends in the lifetime prevalence of alcohol dependence in the United States: A re-evaluation. *Alcoholism: Clinical and Experimental Research, 32*(5), 1–8.

Harden, A., Brunton, G., Fletcher, A., & Oakley, A. (2009). Teenage pregnancy and social disadvantage: Systematic review integrating controlled trials and qualitative studies. *British Medical Journal, 339*, b4254.

Hill, S. Y., Shen, S., Lowers, L., Locke-Wellman, J., Matthews, A. G., & McDermott, M. (2008). Psychopathology in offspring from multiplex alcohol dependence families and without parental alcohol dependence: A prospective study during childhood and adolescence. *Psychiatric Research, 160*(2), 155–166.

Hussong, A. M., Bauer, D. J., Huang, W., Chassin, L., Sher, K. J., & Zucker, R. A. (2008). Characterizing the life stressors of children of alcoholic parents. *Journal of Family Psychology, 22*(6), 819–832.

Jewett, C. (2005, April 17). New drug wave delivers "crank babies." Earlier alarm over cocaine's effects could limit aid for meth abuse. *Sacramento Bee*, p. A1.

Johnston, L. D., O'Malley, P. M., Bachman, J. G., & Schulenberg, J. E. (2006). *Monitoring the future: National survey results on drug use, 1975–2005: Volume II: College students and adults ages 19–45* (NIH Publication No. 06-5584). Bethesda, MD: National Institute on Drug Abuse.

Kaufman, E. (1994). *Psychotherapy of addicted persons*. New York: Guilford Press.

Klonoff-Cohen, H., & Lam-Kruglick, P. (2001). Maternal and paternal recreational drug use and sudden infant death syndrome. *Archives of Pediatric Adolescence Medicine, 155*, 765–770.

Knight, J. R., Shrier, L. A., Bravender, T. D., Farrell, M., Vander Bilt, J., & Shaffer, H. J. (1999). A new brief screen for adolescent substance abuse. *Archives of Pediatric Adolescent Medicine, 153*, 591–596.

Kumpfer, K. L., Pinyuchon, M., Teixeira de Melo, A., & Whiteside, H. O. (2008). *Cultural adaptation process for international dissemination of the strengthening families program.* Retrieved from http://ehp.sagepub.com/cgi/content/abstract/31/2/226

Kumpfer, K. L., Williams, M. K., & Baxley, G. (1997). *Drug abuse prevention for se-lective groups: The strengthening families program*. Resource Manual, National Institute on Drug Abuse, Technology Transfer Program, NCADI, # BKD201. NTIS BP#98-113103.

Lam, W. K., Cance, J. D., Eke, A. N., Fishbein, D. H., Hawkins, S. R., & Williams, J. C. (2007). Children of African-American mothers who use crack cocaine: Parenting influences on youth substance use. *Journal of Pediatric Psychology, 32*, 877–887.

Lam, W. K., Fals-Stewart, W., & Kelley, M. L. (2008). Effects of parent skills training with behavioral couples therapy for alcoholism on children: A randomized clinical pilot trial. *Addictive Behaviors, 33*, 1076–1080.

Lemieux, C. M. (2009). *Offenders and substance abuse: Bringing the family into focus*. Odenton, MD: Gasch Printing, LLC. (American Correctional Association).

Lester, P. E., Weiss, R. E., Comulada, W. S., Lord, L., Alber, S., & Rotheram-Borus, M. J. (2009). The longitudinal impact of HIV + parents' drug use on their adolescent children. *American Journal of Orthopsychiatry, 79*(1), 51–59.

Nadel, M., & Straussner, S. L. A. (2006). Children in substance-abusing families. In N. Phillips & S. L. A. Straussner (Eds.), *Children in the urban environment: Linking social policy and clinical practice* (2nd ed., pp. 169–190). Springfield, IL: Charles C. Thomas.

National Institute on Drug Abuse. (2006). *Research report series: HIV/AIDS*. Retrieved from http://www.drugabuse.gov/ResearchReports/hiv/hiv.html

Nichols, M. P. (2011). *The essentials of family therapy* (5th ed.). Boston: Allyn & Bacon.

Ockert, D., Baier, A., & Coons, E. (2004). Treatment with clients abusing cocaine, crack and other stimulants. In S. L. A. Straussner (Ed.), *Clinical work with substance-abusing clients* (2nd ed., pp. 209–234). New York: Guilford Press.

O'Farrell, T. J., & Fals-Stewart, W. (2006). *Behavioral couples therapy for alcoholism and drug abuse*. New York: Guilford Press.

Pederson, C. L., Vanhorn, D. R., Wilson, J. F., Martorano, L. M., Venema, J. M., & Kennedy, S. M. (2008). Childhood abuse related to nicotine, illicit and prescription drug use by women: Pilot study. *Psychological Reports, 103*(2), 459–466.

Peleg-Oren, N., & Teichman, M. (2006). Young children of parents with Substance Use Disorders (SUD): A review of the literature and implication for social work practice. *Journal of Social Work Practice in the Addictions, 6*(1/2),49–61.

Pilat, J. M., & Jones, J. W. (1985). A comprehensive treatment program for children of alcoholics. In E. M. Freeman (Ed.),*Social work practice with clients who have alcohol problems* (pp. 141–159). Springfield, IL: Charles C. Thomas.

Rothman, E. F., Edwards, E. M., Heeren, T., & Hingson, R. W. (2008). Adverse childhood experiences predict earlier age drinking onset: Results from a representative US sample of current or former drinkers. *Pediatrics, 122*(2), e298–e304.

Saraceno, L., Munaf, M., Heron, J., Craddock, N., & van den Bree, M. B. M. (2009). Genetic and non-genetic influences on the development of co-occurring alcohol problem use and internalizing symptomatology in adolescence: A review. *Addiction, 104*(7), 1100–1121.

Schuckit, M. A., Smith, T. L., Pierson, J., Trim, R., & Danko, G. P. (2007). Externalizing disorders in the offspring from the San Diego prospective study of alcoholism. *Psychiatric Research, 42*(8),644–652.

Senreich, E., & Vairo, E. (2004). Treatment of gay, lesbian and bisexual substance abusers. In S. L. A. Straussner (Ed.), *Clinical work with substance-abusing clients* (2nd ed., pp. 392–422). New York: Guilford.

Silverman, W. K., Pina, A. A., & Visesvaran, C. (2008). Evidence-based psychosocial treatments for phobic and anxiety disorders in children and adolescents. *Journal of Clinical Child and Adolescent Psychology, 37*(1), 105–130.

Spiegel, B. R., & Fewell, C. H. (2004). Twelve-step programs as a treatment modality. In S. L. A. Straussner (Ed.), *Clinical work with substance-abusing clients* (2nd ed., pp. 125–145). New York: Guilford Press.

Steinglass, P. (2009). Systemic-motivational therapy for substance abuse disorders: An integrative model. *Journal of Family Therapy, 31*(2), 155–174.

Straussner, S. L. A. (1994). The impact of alcohol and other drug abuse on the American family. *Drug and Alcohol Review, 13,* 393–399.

Straussner, S. L. A. (2001). *Ethnocultural factors in substance abuse treatment.* New York: Guilford Press.

Straussner, S. L. A. (2004). Assessment and treatment of clients with alcohol and other drug abuse problems: An overview. In S. L. A. Straussner (Ed.), *Clinical work with substance-abusing clients* (2nd ed., pp. 3–36). New York: Guilford.

Straussner, S. L. A., & Brown, S. (Eds.). (2002). *The handbook of addiction treatment for women: Theory and practice.* San Francisco, CA: Jossey-Bass.

Straussner, S. L. A., & Spiegel, B. R. (1996). An analysis of 12-step programs for substance abusers from a developmental perspective. *Clinical Social Work Journal, 24*(3), 299–309.

Substance Abuse and Mental Health Services Administration [SAMHSA] (2008). *The NSDUH Report: Children living with substance-dependent or substance-abusing parents: 2002 to 2007.* Rockville, MD: Office of Applied Studies.

The National Center on Addiction and Substance Abuse at Columbia University (CASA) (2005). *Family matters: Substance abuse and the American family.* Retrieved from http://www.casacolumbia.org/templates/publications_ reports.aspx.

The National Center on Addiction and Substance Abuse at Columbia University CASA (2007). *Wasting the best and the brightest: Substance abuse at America's colleges and universities.* New York: CASA.

U.S. Census Bureau (2009). *Facts for features: Back to school: 2009–2010.* Retrieved from http://www.census.gov/Press-Release/www/releases/archives/ facts_for_features_special_editions/013847.html

van der Kolk, B. (2003). Posttraumatic stress disorder and the nature of trauma. In M. F. Solomon & D. J. Siegel (Eds.), *Healing trauma: Attachment, mind, body, and brain* (pp. 168–195). New York: W.W. Norton.

Werner, E. E., & Johnson, J. L. (2004). The role of caring adults in the lives of children of alcoholics. *Substance Use and Misuse, 39*(5), 699–720.

Whitfield, C. (1991). *Co-dependence: Healing the human condition.* Deerfield Beach, FL: Health Communications, Inc.

Woititz, J. (1983). *Adult children of alcoholics*. Orlando, FL: Health Communications.

Wong, J. (2006). Social support: A key to positive parenting outcomes for mothers in residential drug treatment with their children. *Journal of Social Work Practice in the Addictions, 6*(1/2), 113–137.

Wright, M. O., Crawford, E., & Del Castillo, D. (2009). Childhood emotional maltreatment and later psychological distress among college students: The mediating role of maladaptive schemas. *Child Abuse & Neglect, 33*(1), 59–68.

Zelvin, E. (2004). Treating the partners of substance abusers. In S. L. A. Straussner (Eds.), Clinical work with substance-abusing clients (2nd ed., pp. 264–283). New York: Guilford Press.

RESOURCES

National Association for Children of
   Alcoholics (NACoA)
11426 Rockville Pike, Suite 100
Rockville, MD 20852
(888) 554-COAS
Web site: www.nacoa.net

National Association for Native American
   Children of Alcoholics (NANACoA)
6145 Lehman Drive Suite 200
Colorado Springs, CO 80918
(719) 548-1000
Web site: www.whitebison.org/nanacoa

National Black Alcoholism and Addictions
   Council (NBAC)
5104 N. Orange Blossom Trail, Suite 207
Orlando, FL 32810
(877) 622-2674
Web site: www.nbacinc.org

National Clearinghouse for Alcohol and
   Drug Information (NCADI)
11420 Rockville Pike
Rockville, MD 20852
(800) 729-6686
Web site: ncadi.samhsa.gov

National Council on Alcoholism and Drug
   Dependence (NCADD)
20 Exchange Place, Suite 2902
New York, NY 10005
(800) NCA-CALL
Web site: www.ncadd.org

Children's Program at the Betty Ford
   Center
39000 Bob Hope Drive
Rancho Mirage, CA 92270
Phone: 760/773-4291; 800/854-9211 x4191
Web site: www.bettyfordcenter.org

Hazelden Center for Youth and Families
11505 36th Avenue North
Plymouth, MN 55441
Phone: 800/257-7810
Fax: 763/559-0149
Web site: www.hazelden.org

National Student Assistance Association
4200 Wisconsin Avenue, NW
Suite 106-118
Washington, DC 20016
Web site: www.nasap.org

Strengthening Families Program
Department of Health Promotion and
   Education
University of Utah
1901 E. South Campus Drive, Room 2142
Phone: 801/581-8498
Fax: 801/581-5872
Web site: www.strengtheningfamilies
   program.org

SAMHSA's Children's Program Kit
Available free through the National
  Clearinghouse for Alcohol and Drug
  Information
Phone: 800/729-6686
Web site: http://ncadi.samhsa.gov/
  promos/coa/

College-Specific Sites

Binghamton University, State University
  of New York
Web site: www2.binghamton.edu/smart-
  choices/but-is-it-a-problem/when-i-
  was-kid.html

Georgetown University
Web site: www3.georgetown.edu/be/
  article.cfm?ObjectID=906
University of California, Los Angeles
Web site: http://www.counseling.ucla.edu/

University of Illinois at Urbana-Champaign
Web site: www.counselingcenter.illinois.
  edu/?page_id=144

Vanderbilt University
Web site: www.vanderbilt.edu/alcohol/
  students_acoas.html

Self-Help Groups for COSAPs

Al-Anon Family Group Headquarters, Inc.,
1600 Corporate Landing Parkway
Virginia Beach, VA 23454-5617
(888) 425-2666
Web site: www.al-anon.org

Adult Children of Alcoholics (ACA/ACoA)
P.O. Box 3216
Torrance, CA 90510
(310) 534-1815
Web site: www.adultchildren.org

Co-Anon Family Groups World Services
P.O. Box 12722
Tucson, AZ 85732-2722
800-898-9985
Web site: www.co-anon.org

Families Anonymous
P.O. Box 3475
Culver City, CA 90231-3475
(800) 736-9805
Web site: www.familiesanonymous.org

Nar-Anon Family Group Headquarters, Inc.
22527 Crenshaw Blvd. Suite 200B
Torrance, CA 90505
(800) 477-6291
Web site: www.nar-anon.org/Nar-Anon/
  Nar-Anon_Home.html

2

An Attachment and Mentalizing Perspective on Children of Substance-Abusing Parents

Christine Huff Fewell

INTRODUCTION

A college student who participated in a study on attachment, reflective function, family dysfunction, and psychological distress in children of alcoholics was asked to write an essay about why her alcohol-abusing mother acted the way she did during her childhood and what affect it had on her (Fewell, 2006). She wrote:

> *My mother was lonely and desperate. She always looked outside herself for satisfaction and happiness. Her parents are alcoholics, so she learned to cope with life by drinking. She wanted to feel loved, so she looked to men. As a single mother, she dated. Sometimes I had to fill her in on "what happened.". . . She acted sexually in front of us kids. But when I wanted love and attention and touching and caring from her, I was always too needy, a pain to deal with. Obviously, in her mind, I wasn't the answer to her loneliness. I was more like a cute decoration. . . . Alcohol gives her permission to act like the adult child that she really is. Even when she's sober I've found that it's best to talk to her like a child—she likes it. I am affected in that I'm also an addict. I want to control everything—my weight is a repetitive thought. If I eat well, no comment. If not, I torture myself. I'm not sure how that's related. I'm an alcoholic. At 14 years old I started doing the same behaviors as her. I was lonely. I had sex and I tried to drink. I wanted to rescue my mother for a long time. Sometimes I think I'm lucky. My suffering led me to question life instead of just letting*

it pass me by. . . . It is awkward being awake sometimes. I'm angry with
my mother. I don't know how to love her with compassion. . . . It's so sad to
see. (pp. 143–144)

For this 20-year-old college student, the conflicting feelings generated
by growing up with an alcohol-abusing mother are poignantly evident.
Although she recognizes the intergenerational aspects of the problems her
mother faced, and that she now also faces, she has not been able to interrupt them. The need to be a caretaker to her mother and the loneliness she
feels because of it have caused her to be unsure of how to self soothe, and
she uses sexual encounters, alcohol, and food to fill the inner emptiness.

One way of understanding the dynamics reflected by this young
woman is through the lens of attachment theory. Attachment patterns in
families with parental substance abuse have assumed increasing importance as a research variable and studies indicate that growing up with
alcohol- and drug-abusing parents may impair the child's ability to become
securely attached (Das Eiden & Leonard, 1996; O'Connor, Sigman, & Brill,
1987). Neuroscience studies have repeatedly shown the importance of
attachment relationship as an organizer of physiological and brain regulation, effecting both cognitive and emotional development (Schore,
2003). Children who grow up with substance-abusing parents are often
faced with the need to adapt to a cycle of intermittent availability and
responsiveness on the part of caregivers whose moods and behaviors are
influenced by the physical, neurological, and emotional consequences of
intoxication and its aftermath. This lack of consistency has been described
as a chronic trauma (Brown & Schmid, 1999; Cermack, 1986).

Mentalization is another concept that has gained importance in the
literature as a means of explaining the pathways to acquiring emotional
regulation. Mentalization is the capacity for understanding behavior in
light of underlying mental states and intentions. It is acquired within
the context of social interaction with a caregiver who is able to give the
child the experience of being understood as an individual with a mind
that experiences beliefs, desires, feelings and wishes (Fonagy & Target,
2005). Based on this ability to understand others' minds, the child is
able to learn to regulate emotions, which is the foundation for healthy,
symptom-free development. This ability is developed in children between
the ages of 2 and 3, and continues to develop throughout life. Recent
research indicates that mentalizing is the means by which attachment security is transmitted intergenerationally (Slade, Grienenberger, Bernbach,
Levy, & Locker, 2005).

This chapter explores the contributions of attachment theory and the
related development of mentalizing as concepts that provide the theoretical
cornerstones for clinical interventions with children of substance-abusing

parents (COSAPs) of all ages as well as for substance-abusing parents of infants. It describes attachment and mentalization-based treatment programs that have been developed to help people who have difficulty with affect regulation, resulting from insecure attachment with their substance-abusing parents.

ATTACHMENT THEORY

John Bowlby formulated attachment theory (1969/1982) as a consequence of his observations of infants and young children. According to Bowlby (1977), attachment behavior is aimed at seeking to be near another person from whom one can seek protection and emotional support. The attachment system is activated when the child experiences a need, such as illness, fatigue, hunger or pain, or when the environment produces a threatening situation, such as the mother's absence, rejection, or withdrawal (Bowlby, 1969/1982). The infant uses the attachment figure as "a secure base from which to explore" (Ainsworth, 1963; Bowlby, 1969/1982). When children are satisfied that there is an attachment figure nearby who will be available if needed, they feel free to investigate their environment.

According to Bowlby (1977), the actual experiences with caregivers become organized into an internal working model or mental representation that contains an image of who the attachment figures are, how emotionally available they are, and how supportive they are of exploratory activities. At the same time, the model contains a complementary view of how acceptable or unacceptable the child is in the eyes of his or her attachment figure. The child develops a working model of the self as being valued and competent when parents are both emotionally available and supportive of exploration. On the other hand, the child whose parents are rejecting or ignoring of attachment behavior develops a model of the self as devalued and incompetent (Bretherton & Munholland, 1999). These working models are established by age 4. Research has supported the continuity of attachment patterns from infancy to young adulthood, as well as the fact that attachment representations may be altered, in both positive and negative ways, by real life experiences (Waters, Merrick, Treboux, Crowell, & Albersheim, 2000).

During early adolescence, attachment undergoes a fundamental transformation as the youngster makes tremendous efforts to become less dependent upon early caregiving figures and gradually develops the capacity to become a potential romantic partner and a caregiver to his/her own children. In addition, this period brings about an enormous increase in differentiation of the self and others, which allows the adolescent to have a view of himself or herself that is more internally based and less dependent upon a particular relationship. However, while the attachment-related developmental goal of adolescence is to become less dependent upon parents, the enduring relationship with parents is of utmost importance in this process, as it provides the anchor against which the changes can be negotiated (J. P. Allen & Land, 1999).

These behaviors continue in the adult's need to form intimate bonds with others. Similar to the mother–infant relationship, pair bonds in adulthood contain intimate physical contact, which serves to establish and maintain the connection, and likewise, involves reactions of grief and loss when the bond is disrupted (Bowlby, 1988).

Attachment patterns in adults play a key role in the type of parenting they provide, and consequently, the type of attachment patterns their infants develop. The predictability of intergenerational transmission of attachment behaviors has been demonstrated in a number of studies, including longitudinal studies that have shown that attachment security can be stable from infancy through early adulthood (Waters et al., 2000; Weinfield, Stroufe, & Egelund, 2000).

Attachment Patterns in Childhood

During the first year of life, most children develop an organized strategy for dealing with the stresses and threats of their environments, which have been categorized as *secure attachment, insecure avoidant attachment, insecure ambivalent attachment, or disorganized attachment* (Ainsworth, Blehar, Waters, & Wall, 1978). Children classified as having *secure attachment* have learned that when they are in distress the caretaker will respond in a way that quickly soothes them. Knowing that this help is readily available, these children feel free to explore the environment on their own. On the other hand, children with *insecure avoidant attachment* have received parenting that fostered the view that people are not likely to be available to help when they are distressed and it is best to manage on their own. Parenting of these children has been less emotionally supportive and helpful, and in many instances has been cold, remote, and controlling (Belsky, 1999; Hesse & Main, 2000). Children who are viewed as having *insecure ambivalent attachment* are likely to have had parents who responded to expressions of fear in their babies, but not to expressions of exuberance (Belsky, 1999; Hesse & Main, 2000). These children have not had their affect contained and soothed and may be overwhelmed when in distress and continue to search for cues about whether help will be forthcoming. This preoccupation interferes with a sense of confidence about managing in their environment.

Unlike the other three groups of children who demonstrate well-organized strategies for dealing with attachment stress, which were adaptive in their environments, children with *disorganized attachment* do not have an organized pattern. This classification is strongly associated with children who are maltreated or whose parents have a history of unresolved loss (Adam, Keller, & West, 1995). These children show fear but are unable to determine where they can find help and thus are unable to act on their own behalf. They may be hypervigilant and highly sensitive to their parents' mental states and, as they get older, often show patterns such as feeling afraid and unable to do anything about it, describe catastrophic fantasies, are unable to speak or whisper, may be too upset to continue the task at hand, or become disorganized in language and behavior, so that they say or do contradictory things without acknowledging the contradiction. The implications of these dynamics for COSAPs will be described later.

Attachment Through the Life Span

Data from two longitudinal studies of attachment have demonstrated that infants with secure attachments to their mothers have more supportive and satisfying relationships with siblings, friends, peers, and romantic partners as much as 20 years later (Berlin, Zeanah, & Lieberman, 2008). On the other hand, disorganized attachment in childhood has been found to be a predictor of later psychopathology (Lyons-Ruth & Jacobvitz, 2008). As the child grows, the disorganized attachment pattern undergoes changes in how it is manifested behaviorally. Studies have linked the disorganized attachment pattern of infancy to disruptive, aggressive behavior in middle childhood and adolescence (Hesse & Main, 1999). Studies of 6-year-old children rated as disorganized at 1 year of age have shown that after separation from their parents, they used controlling or role-inverting behaviors, which could either take the form of being punitively controlling or, conversely, caregiving and overly solicitous (Lyons-Ruth & Jacobvitz, 2008).

Attachment classifications in adolescence and adulthood, which are measured by the Adult Attachment Interview (George, Kaplan, & Main, 1985), tend to have different labels, which nonetheless resemble those of early childhood. The term "autonomous" corresponds to the childhood secure category; "dismissing" resembles the childhood insecure avoidant classification; "preoccupied" corresponds to the childhood category of insecure ambivalent; and "unresolved/disorganized," to the childhood disorganized category.

As adolescents develop cognitive structures that allow reflection on their own states of mind apart from attachment figures, they have less need to be dependent upon them. Adolescents with secure attachment may have intense or heated disagreements with parents, but they are able to engage them in a way that fosters constructive problem solving and balances the need for autonomy with the need to preserve the relationship (J. P. Allen, 2008). Dismissing adolescents tend to use strategies associated with externalizing symptoms and to have substance abuse and conduct disorders (J. P. Allen, 2008). Preoccupied adolescents have been shown to use strategies linked to internalizing behaviors manifested by symptoms such as anxiety and depression. However, under some circumstances, when preoccupied teens had mothers who were not responsive, they also developed externalizing symptoms, had high levels of drug use, and engaged in precocious sexual activity and higher levels of delinquent behavior (J. P. Allen, Moore, Kuperminc, & Bell, 1998).

In adulthood, attachment strategies influence the formation of intimate relationships in both heterosexual and same-sex relationships. The issues of anxiety, fear, loneliness, and grief are played out based on the kinds of expectations that partners have of each other (Feeney, 2008). In particular, ways of handling conflict through distance or closeness in both healthy and unhealthy ways are influenced by expectations of availability of the other. However, research has also shown that changes in internal working models of attachment can occur when parenting becomes more responsive or when an adult forms a romantic relationship that is meeting his or her attachment needs (Berlin et al., 2008).

Attachment and Mentalization

Although attachment patterns have been shown to pass from one generation to another, until recently, attachment research had not answered the question of how this happened (Fonagy, H. Steele, & M. Steele, 1991; Fonagy, M. Steele, Moran, H. Steele, & Higgitt, 1992). A meta-analysis of attachment transmission revealed that maternal sensitivity to the child accounted for 23% of the variance in association between maternal attachment and infant attachment (Van IJzendoorn, 1995). Moreover, recent studies have linked a mother's capacity to mentalize about or regard her child as an intentional agent with a mind of his or her own as the process by which attachment patterns are transferred intergenerationally and through which it is believed they can be altered (Fonagy, Gergely, Jurist, & Target, 2002; Slade, 2008).

The Role of Parenting in Mentalization

As indicated previously, the capacity for mentalization is acquired through the process of the child's mental states being reflected on accurately by the mother or primary caretaker (Fonagy & Target, 1997). This process of dyadic regulation begins at birth (Beebe, Lachmann, & Jaffe, 1997). The caregiver's attuned responses to the infant serve to reflect back to the infant what he or she is feeling at the same time that these feelings are contained. When the mother is able to reflect on both her own and her child's mental states and to appropriately mirror the reality of the child's internal experience, it provides a representation of the inner self which is then internalized by the child.

The child learns through this process of mirroring what he or she is feeling, how to name feelings, and how to manage feelings. Reponses of caregivers must reflect the child's mental state and provide some form of soothing at the same time. In this process, the parent demonstrates to the child a person who is considering the child's mind, while also reflecting that the parent has his or her own feelings, thoughts, and motivations. This eventually results in the child's being able to understand the affects displayed by others, as well as to regulate his or her own emotions. If the mother is not able to mirror her child's feelings accurately, or is preoccupied by her own feelings, the child is not able to develop a coherent image of the self as a separate person with his or her own feelings and thoughts (Fonagy et al., 2002).

Trauma and Mentalization

The most difficult situations for a child are those where emotional distress is experienced. Since mentalization, or the capacity to reflect, arises from the process of the child's having his or her mental states reflected on accurately by the parents, children who are maltreated have been found to be impaired in their reflective capacities (Fonagy & Target, 1997). Authoritarian parenting that demands obedience has been found to inhibit the development of mentalization, while parenting that reasons with the child and explains why rules must take into account others' points of view tends to facilitate it (Baumrind, 1971). In abusive families, the meaning of people's behavior is frequently denied or distorted and abusive parents are unable to help their children reflect on the feelings and intentions behind their abusive behavior. This prevents the child from testing out the true meaning of the mental states of themselves and others. In addition, if the child tries to understand the thoughts and feelings of an abusive parent through the use of mentalization, he or she will be confronted by painful feelings about the self (Fonagy et al., 2002; Fonagy & Target, 1997). For example, contemplating why parents are abusive or neglectful may lead children to speculate that that they themselves are bad or unworthy of being treated better. Thus, they would interpret the abuse as inevitable, rather than being able to understand that it was a result of the parent's emotionally dysregulated mental state.

For the maltreated child, having limited mentalization or reflective functioning within the family context can be then seen as adaptive. However, this lack of ability to understand mental states will cause difficulties with later interpersonal relationships (Fonagy et al., 2002). People who have been traumatized by their family environments are frequently left with the feelings related to the trauma, in addition to the difficulty in developing a mentalizing stance to help them understand the minds of others.

Research on Attachment and Mentalization in Alcohol- and Drug-Abusing Families

There are a growing number of studies on attachment-related variables in substance-abusing families and efforts to apply this framework to treatment programs and interventions. Insecure attachment has been found in 1-year-old infants of heavy drinking mothers (O'Connor et al., 1987) and in families where the father, but not the mother, was alcohol dependent (Das Eiden & Leonard, 1996). The fact that these insecure attachments had already developed at the early age of one, and that the father's alcoholism also had an impact on insecure attachment, suggests the need to work with the entire family system in order to prevent later difficulties. Alcoholic parents have been found to have differences in their ability to be attuned to their children's needs compared to nonalcoholic parents, with alcoholic families expressing less positive affect and making more demands on their children to be self-reliant (Whipple, Fitzgerald, & Zucker, 1995). Longitudinal research has shown mothers with alcoholic partners to be less warm and sensitive during play interactions with their toddlers, which was predictive of lower social competence in kindergarten (Eiden, Colder, Edwards, & Leonard, 2009). As Eiden et al. (2009) point out, this may be because having an alcoholic partner makes it difficult for the mother to be consistently warm and supportive in her interactions with the child. They conclude that the findings "also suggest an additional avenue for prevention beyond treating the alcoholic, specifically providing parent training and coping skills to women with alcoholic partners" (p. 42).

Research on attachment and mentalization in drug-abusing families is just beginning to appear in the literature. A study on the effects of prenatal cocaine exposure on mother–infant interaction in a low-income sample of African American mothers found very little difference in interactive behaviors in the cocaine-using mothers compared to non–drug-using mothers (Ukeje, Bendersky, & Lewis, 2001). A longitudinal study of low-income prenatally exposed infants and their primary caretakers found that although prenatal cocaine exposure was not directly related to insecure or disorganized attachment status, when other risk factors were considered there was a higher incidence of disorganized behavior (Beeghly, Frank, Rose-Jacobs, Cabral, & Tronick, 2003). Subtle differences were also found when comparing a large sample of cocaine-exposed, opiate-exposed, and non-exposed infants and their interactions with their mothers. Although differences were small, heavy cocaine exposure was associated with negative interchanges with the mother, which may have a cumulative impact on later development. Mothers on methadone treatment have been shown to be more likely to have children with disorganized attachment (Finger, 2006).

There has been little research to date on mentalization or reflective function in children of substance-abusing parents. School-aged children in foster care exposed to parental methamphetamine abuse who had high reflective function were found to have fewer mental health problems and be rated higher on social competence by their foster parents (Ostler, Bahar, & Jessee, 2010). College students with alcoholic parents were found to have significantly less secure attachment to both parents but to have high reflective function toward their mothers, who were generally not the substance abuser (Fewell, 2006). A major finding of the study was that insecure attachment explained psychological distress, which was also significantly higher in the ACOAs. It may be that these college students were drawn to try to understand the motivations and minds of their nonalcoholic mothers, although it did not protect them from high psychological distress.

ATTACHMENT- AND MENTALIZATION-BASED PREVENTION AND INTERVENTION PROGRAMS

A review of prevention programs for children of alcoholics delineates social support, information, skills training, and coping with emotional problems as common components, while pointing out that there is no evidence to support their effectiveness (Cuijpers, 2005). As described above, attachment theory provides a way of understanding the internal world of individuals, their experiences and affects, and their experience of the treatment relationship (Slade, 2000). However, reflective functioning provides an important pathway for intervening with internalized attachment schema. Fonagy and Target (2005) point out that while attachment theory can inform the understanding of interpersonal difficulties, it does not provide a means for intervention or prevention.

Previously it was thought that the way attachment patterns were transmitted from mother to child was directly through the type of caregiving behaviors provided (Main, Kaplan, & Cassidy, 1985). Research has begun to demonstrate, however, that the transfer of attachment patterns is through the ability of the mother to regard her child has having a mind with his or her own needs, thoughts, and feelings that are motivating behavior and to see these within a developmental framework. This has been called parental reflective functioning (Slade et al., 2005). An important implication of this research is that efforts to modify parental behavior need to be geared to enhancing reflective functioning rather than to changing behavior per se (Slade et al., 2005). Changing the focus in a parenting program from simply changing parenting behaviors to focusing on thinking about what the child is thinking is an example of this shift. This change in thinking, or increasing the ability to mentalize, would most likely eventually lead to a change in behavior. However, the change would stem from an altered internalized means of interpreting thoughts and feelings. Consequently, a number of treatment protocols have been established which use mentalization-based models specifically designed to enhance reflective functioning in parents (Grienenberger et al., 2004; Slade, 2002). Treatment interventions based on attachment constructs, including mentalization-based treatment that assists in enhancing reflective functioning, may provide a useful way of intervening with the chronic trauma COSAPs may have experienced and internalized. Following is an overview of programs that have been developed to promote reflective functioning or mentalizing.

Mentalization-Based Treatment

Mentalization-based treatment (MBT) has received empirical validation as a way to help people regulate their affects by maintaining a mentalizing stance in the face of intense affect arousal and has been used specifically to help individuals with borderline personality disorder (J. G. Allen & Fonagy, 2006). It combines an attachment-based psychodynamic understanding with elements of cognitive behavioral therapy, including a focus on psychoeducation. The development of a secure and safe therapeutic relationship is important for promoting mentalizing, just as the secure attachment to early caregivers is important in the development of the child's mentalizing capacities (J. G. Allen & Fonagy, 2006). While mentalizing is a part of all therapy, mentalization-based treatment focuses specifically on the process of fostering the client's capacity to generate multiple perspectives and can be used as part of any theoretical construct. Allen, Fonagy, and Bateman (2008) describe the aims of mentalization-based treatment as promoting mentalizing about oneself, about others, and about relationships.

Mentalization-Based Programs for Parents

Based on an attachment- and mentalization-based framework, Suchman and colleagues have developed a pilot program called Mothers and Toddlers Program (MTP), which is an individual therapy intervention for mothers in outpatient drug abuse treatment caring for children aged 18–36 months (Suchman, Pajulo, DeCoste, & Mayes, 2006). The program aims at helping mothers develop a more balanced mental representation of their children; a better capacity for understanding their own and their children's intentions; and a better understanding of these intentions and behaviors within a developmental framework. Mothers who were clients at an outpatient drug abuse treatment for cocaine, heroin, marijuana and/ or alcohol abuse or dependence enrolled for a period of up to 20 weeks. Initially attention was placed on forming a therapeutic alliance, which sometimes included concrete assistance with paperwork and resources. Early interventions focused on identifying strengths of the mother–child relationship and identifying "shining moments." Efforts were made to understand the mothers' feelings and concerns about their children and parenting. Later sessions focused on becoming realistically attuned to what the child was experiencing and teasing out the mother's own distress from what the child might be feeling. When mothers became more invested in and curious about their children's behavior, the therapists assisted them in understanding their children's developmental needs. The MTP will be evaluated in a randomized clinical trial to test its efficacy compared to the more traditional behavioral parent skills training.

"Minding the Baby" is a community-based, home visiting program for high-risk, first-time parents living in poverty, that was developed at the Yale Child Study Center (Sadler, Slade, & Mayes, 2006). A multidisciplinary team provides in-home interventions from pregnancy to the child's second birthday. The interventions often begin with providing concrete services and information in the process of developing a relationship. They then move to helping the mother with the development of the capacity to acknowledge, label, and tolerate mental states, and then to mentalize both her own and the baby's feelings. This is done by giving continual attention to the baby's states by such techniques as speaking for the baby to help the mother consider what might be going in the baby's mind. They also wonder aloud about what the mother is feeling, what the baby is feeling, and what might be the meaning and intention of behaviors. Other techniques involve guiding mothers in play, using visual aids, and videotaping to help the mother envision possible reasons for behaviors. Ongoing longitudinal research is being conducted to evaluate the results of this program.

Another reflective parenting program called Parents First was developed to be delivered in normal educational and childcare settings (Goyette-Ewing et al., 2003). This is a 12-week group intervention with parents of infants, toddlers, and preschoolers designed to provide parents with a series of progressive reflective exercises. Parents are asked to participate in such simple family activities as blowing bubbles or having a tea party between meetings. The goal is to be able to work at a level of relating to the parent that is comfortable for them, model reflectiveness, facilitate wondering, elicit affect, and hold the parents in mind.

A pilot group program developed at the Narcotic Treatment Program (NTP) at Acadia Hospital in Bangor, Maine, was designed to intervene with women in the methadone treatment who were pregnant or who were parenting preschool children (Jenkins & Williams, 2008). Based on the goal of enhancing maternal reflective-function, the group lasted 6 weeks, followed a structured curriculum, and included brief meditation to help with relaxation and give time to process feelings. Programs to enhance reflective functioning in substance-abusing pregnant women and mothers of infants in residential treatment have also been developed in Finland (Pajulo, Suchman, Kalland, & Mayes, 2006).

Mentalization-Based Family Therapy for Children and Adolescents

Short-term mentalization and relational therapy (SMART) has been developed to apply mentalization-based interventions to clinical work with children and adolescents and their families (Fearon et al., 2006). The underlying philosophy is to promote longer-term resilience in the family by promoting healthy means of coping. Incorporating psychodynamic principles, cognitive behavioral principles, and systemic therapy, the focus of interventions is to promote mentalizing by family members about what each of the others is thinking and feeling. The therapeutic relationship is emphasized as a way to help family members reduce emotional arousal, which interferes with mentalizing. A working hypothesis of the family's strengths and difficulties in mentalizing serves as a basis for the therapist's understanding of how these difficulties are contributing to the family's inability to resolve emotional conflict. Interventions include identifying skillful examples of mentalizing, sharing and provoking curiosity, and identifying and labeling hidden feeling states. Examples of the theory behind Mentalization-Based Treatment for Families (MBT-F), sequences of interactions, psychoeducational material about mentalization, and specific interventive techniques can be accessed at http://tiddlymanuals.tiddlyspace.com/.

Mentalization-Based Interventions With Adolescents

An innovative approach to mentalization-based treatment for adolescents developed at the Anna Freud Centre in London is called Adolescent Mentalization-Based Integrative Therapy (AMBIT). It provides community-based services to high risk adolescents with psychiatric and substance use disorders, who are involved with multiple social systems and are often estranged from their families. The Stages of Change Model (Prochaska, DiClemente, & Norcross, 1992) is used to guide the types of mentalizing interventions used. A single team member handles each client in order to foster an attachment relationship in which interventions can be used to enhance mentalizing. However, team members work in close connection to each other to support and foster mentalizing in the individual worker who is often dealing with chaotic events alone in the community. This is done through such means as the use of telephone conferencing from the field to assist in critical decisions that need to be made immediately, in addition to team meetings in the agency. A comprehensive manualized protocol that is under continual development is available online at http://tiddlymanuals.tiddlyspace.com/. It contains specific interventions used by the team as well as role-played training videos. This site is available to any program using mentalization-based treatment anywhere in the world to post their experiences with implementation and evolving best practices.

Mentalization-Based Interventions With Adults in Individual Treatment

Mentalization-based interventions can also be used to help adult COSAPs in individual treatment to deepen their abilities to understand their own minds and those of others (Allen et al., 2008). As indicated previously, mentalization-based treatment promotes a spirit of inquisitiveness and focuses on process rather than content. Many theoretical models, including psychodynamic psychotherapy, cognitive behavioral therapy, and dialectical behavioral therapy promote mentalizing. Dayton (Chapter 7, this volume) describes therapeutic interventions using psychodrama, which can be said to promote mentalizing. Psychodrama helps group members to view problematic situations from the multiple perspectives of the self and others in order to gain mastery over traumatic affect arousal and foster alternative solutions.

Using Mentalizing Interventions in Individual Treatment: Case of Sarah

The following case example describes the use of mentalizing interventions in individual treatment with an adult COSAP.

> *Sarah was a single woman in her mid-fifties who was very accomplished in her work life. She struggled in treatment with her need to continue a relationship with a married man named Sam whom she saw in person infrequently, although she spoke to him on the telephone several times a day. He often stood her up, making a date for which she would prepare and then he would fail to show up or even to contact her for days afterwards. On other occasions, he would offer to help her out with fixing things and would exceed her expectations of helpfulness. He attended social events with her friends and endeared himself to them by his helpfulness and charm. She often remarked how important it was to her to know that she was not alone in case of an emergency. Simply knowing in her mind that he was there was a comfort to her. After Sam declared that he would divorce his wife and marry her, Sarah purchased a large diamond engagement ring for herself and enjoyed fantasizing about the day she would be able to wear it public.*
>
> *Eventually Sam borrowed a huge sum of money from her and then disappeared, leaving her in a very difficult financial situation and feeling enraged and betrayed. As Sarah gradually came to see that he had lied and manipulated her and her friends, she struggled with her rage and desire for revenge and began to realize that his behavior resembled that of her alcoholic father and that her attraction, connection, and inability to let go of him were similar to the conflicting feelings she felt toward her father.*
>
> *One day she came to a session especially perturbed by the remark of a friend, who, after criticizing her for not being able to see that her boyfriend was no good, said to her in an authoritative tone, "Sarah, why do you still need to go to therapy? What can you tell her that you can't tell me?" Sarah asked the therapist directly for help in understanding and dealing with her strong feelings of distress, stating, "I can't get it out of my head. It really bothers me because my mother said the same thing to me when I was in my twenties and wanted to go to therapy. I wanted to scream at my friend, 'Who do you think you are? You're not my mother.'"*
>
> *As it was clear that Sarah was very upset and making efforts to mentalize about her friend's remark, the therapist attempted to encourage this by asking, "Let's see if we can think about what your friend's motives for saying that might be. What do you think might be going on in her mind?" With a look of great concentration, Sarah responded that her friend had also been involved with a man who deceived her and that she had resisted her sister's urging to go to therapy. She was able to spend some time processing why her friend was confusing what was on her mind with what she thought should be on Sarah's.*

The therapist went on to ask Sarah why she thought her mother had said that about going to therapy when she was in her twenties. Sarah responded that she thought her mother was afraid that Sarah hated her and it was true that she had hated her for a long time. The therapist reflected that it seemed that her mother feared Sarah might blame her or leave her. Sarah then responded, "You know, I always think about my father and all the terrible things he did because of his drinking. But he actually did some very nice things for me. He often drove me places. He drove me to therapy and picked me up. And I felt sorry for him because he did have to live in that tiny house with my grandmother who was very nasty."

The therapist encouraged Sarah to mentalize further by asking why she thought her mother's and father's reactions to her going to therapy were different. After thinking very hard, Sarah replied, "Well, I think he felt stuck in the house with my mother and grandmother and didn't want me to be stuck there also. My mother wanted me to stay there. But my mother also contributed to the problem, because her way of handling the times my father came home drunk to our tiny house was to have my brother and I sit on the couch so there would be nowhere for him to sit. We weren't allowed to say a word. She thought he would then go to bed. But we were very angry that we had no choice in the matter, that we were manipulated and there was no way to talk about it."

Discussion of the Case of Sarah

Sarah spent considerable time in treatment, certain that her lover would truly leave his wife to marry her. She allowed his helpful and charming behavior to reinforce her pretend mode of thinking and ignored his dismissive and cruel actions. Thinking in pretend mode is an earlier form of thought used before mentalization has developed and is similar to precontemplation in the stages of change model (Fewell, 2010; Prochaska et al., 1992). It was important that the therapist did not challenge her need for this pretend mode of thinking until she was ready to mentalize. Sarah and the therapist had explored a number of other relationships with women friends, her brother, and her boss in the context of a secure therapeutic attachment relationship, and there had been considerable improvement in Sarah's ability to understand their intensions and motivations and to separate them from hers, which helped her diminish painful feelings of humiliation and bring a measure of stability to her functioning.

In this session, the therapist perceived Sarah's question about why her friend had acted as she did as a message that she could not regulate her distress, but was in a position where she could mentalize with help. Beginning with understanding her distress over her friend's comment allowed Sarah to generate an alternative hypothesis about why her friend had acted as she did. Sarah was then able to feel secure enough in her ability to mentalize that she could extend this to her long unresolved feelings toward her father and mother with the therapist's encouragement. Sarah was able to mentalize about why her parents acted as they did and to see the situation from each of their perspectives, including her own. Interestingly, the subject of the distress was over the friend's current and mother's past efforts to keep Sarah from having a secure therapeutic relationship where she could gain relief for painful feelings.

CONCLUSION

Attachment patterns developed early in life provide a template through which people approach their interpersonal relationships and regulate their feelings of pleasure and distress. Families with substance-abusing parents often suffer from inconsistency and difficulty in communication that can lead to insecure attachment, and even more importantly, to disorganized attachment, which has implications for later psychopathology. Being unable to regulate feelings is a primary difficulty of people who develop substance-abuse disorders for which COSAPs are at high risk. Mentalization-based treatment is providing a promising means to alter internalized difficulties with self-esteem and through increasing parental reflective-functioning, thereby halting the intergenerational transfer of insecure attachment patterns. There is a growing interest in investigating the role that mentalization might play in resilience, although this has not yet been proven. In a number of studies that are using mentalization-based treatment, research on efficacy is an important component. Mentalization-based treatment holds the promise of providing a way to prevent and ameliorate emotional disturbance in children and adolescents from substance-abusing families and to teach new ways to regulate emotional distress in adult COSAPs.

REFERENCES

Adam, K. S., Keller, A. E. S., & West, M. (1995). Attachment organization and vulnerability to loss, separation, and abuse in disturbed adolescents. In S. Goldberg, R. Muir, & J. Kerr (Eds.), *Attachment theory: Social, developmental, and clinical perspectives* (pp. 309–341). Hillsdale, NJ: The Analytic Press.

Ainsworth, M. (1963). The development of infant-mother interaction among the Ganda. In B. M. Foss (Ed.), *Determinants of infant behavior* (Vol. 2, pp. 67–112). New York: Wiley & Sons.

Ainsworth, M., Blehar, M. C., Waters, E., & Wall, S. (1978). *Patterns of attachment.* Hillsdale, NJ: Lawrence Erlbaum Associates.

Allen, J. G., & Fonagy, P. (2006). *Handbook of mentalization-based treatment.* Chichester, England: John Wiley & Sons.

Allen, J. G., Fonagy, P., & Bateman, A.W. (2008). Mentalizing in clinical practice. Washington, DC: American Psychiatric Publishing.

Allen, J. P. (2008). The attachment system in adolescence. In J. Cassidy & P. R. Shaver (Eds.), *Handbook of attachment: Theory, research, and clinical application* (2nd ed., pp. 410–435). New York: Guilford Press.

Allen, J. P., & Land, D. (1999). Attachment in adolescence. In J. Cassidy & P. R. Shaver (Eds.), *Handbook of attachment: Theory, research, and clinical applications* (pp. 319–335). New York: Guilford Press.

Allen, J. P., Moore, C., Kuperminc, G., & Bell, K. (1998). Attachment and adolescent psychosocial functioning. *Child Development, 69*(5), 1406–1419.

Baumrind, D. (1971). Current patterns of parental authority. *Developmental Psychology Monographs, 4*, 1–103.

Beebe, B., Lachmann, F., & Jaffe, J. (1997). Mother-infant interaction structures and presymbolic self- and object-representations. *Psychoanalytic Dialogues, 7*, 133–182.

Beeghly, M., Frank, D. A., Rose-Jacobs, R., Cabral, H., & Tronick, E. (2003). Level of prenatal cocaine exposure and infant-caregiver attachment behavior. *Neurotoxicology and Teratology, 25*, 23–38.

Belsky, J. (1999). Modern evolutionary theory and patterns of attachment. In J. Cassidy & P. Shaver (Eds.), *Handbook of attachment: Theory, research, and clinical applications* (pp. 141–161). New York: Guilford Press.

Berlin, L. J., Zeanah, C. H., & Lieberman, A. F. (2008). Prevention and intervention programs for supporting early attachment security. In J. Cassidy & P. R. Shaver (Eds.), *Handbook of attachment: Theory, research, and clinical applications* (2nd ed., pp. 745–761). New York: Guilford Press.

Bowlby, J. (1969/82). *Attachment and loss: Vol. 1. Attachment.* New York: Basic Books.

Bowlby, J. (1977). The making and breaking of affectional bonds: I. Aetiology and psychopathology in the light of attachment theory. *British Journal of Psychiatry, 130*, 201–210.

Bowlby, J. (1988). Developmental psychiatry comes of age. *The American Journal of Psychiatry, 145*(1), 1–10.

Bretherton, I., & Munholland, K. A. (1999). Internal working models in attachment relationships. In J. Cassidy & P. R. Shaver (Eds.), *Handbook of attachment: Theory, research, and clinical applications* (pp. 89–111). New York: Guilford Press.

Brown, S., & Schmid, J. (1999). Adult children of alcoholics. In P. Ott, R. Tarter & R. Ammerman (Eds.), *Sourcebook on substance abuse: Etiology, epidemiology, assessment, and treatment* (pp. 416–429). Boston: Allyn and Bacon.

Cermack, T. L. (1986). *Diagnosing and treating co-dependence.* Minneapolis, MN: Johnson Institute Books.

Cuijpers, P. (2005). Prevention programmes for children of problem drinkers: A review. *Drugs: Education, Prevention and Policy, 12*(6), 465–475.

Das Eiden, R., & Leonard, K. E. (1996). Paternal alcohol use and the mother-infant relationship. *Development and Psychopathology, 8*, 307–323.

Eiden, R. D., Colder, C., Edwards, E. P., & Leonard, K. E. (2009). A longitudinal study of social competence among children of alcoholic and nonalcoholic parents: Role of parental psychpathology, parental warmth, and self-regulation. *Psychology of Addictive Behaviors, 23*(1), 36–46.

Fearon, P., Target, M., Sargent, J., Williams, L. L., McGregor, J., Bleiberg, E., et al. (2006). Short-term mentalization and relational therapy (SMART): An integrative family therapy for children and adolescents. In J. G. Allen & P. Fonagy (Eds.), *Handbook of mentalization-based treatment* (pp. 201–222). Chichester, England: John Wiley & Sons.

Feeney, J. A. (2008). Adult romantic attachment: Developments in the study of couple relationships. In J. Cassidy & P. R. Shaver (Eds.), *Handbook of attachment: Theory, research, and clinical applications* (2nd ed., pp. 456–481). New York: Guilford Press.

Fewell, C. H. (2006). *Attachment, reflective function, family dysfunction, and psychological distress among college students with alcoholic parents.* Unpublished doctoral dissertation, New York University School of Social Work, New York, NY.

Fewell, C. H. (2010). Using a mentalization-based framework to assist hard-to-reach clients in individual treatment. In S. Bennett & J. K. Nelson (Eds.), *Adult attachment in clinical social work* (pp. 113–126). New York: Springer Publishing Company.

Finger, B. (2006). *Exploring the intergenerational transmission of attachment disorganization.* Unpublished doctoral dissertation. University of Chicago, Chicago, IL.

Fonagy, P., Gergely, G., Jurist, E., & Target, M. (2002). *Affect regulation, mentalization, and the development of the self.* New York: Other Press.

Fonagy, P., Steele, H., & Steele, M. (1991). Maternal representations of attachment during pregnancy predict the organization of infant-mother attachment at one year of age. *Child Development, 62,* 891–905.

Fonagy, P., Steele, M., Moran, G., Steele, H., & Higgitt, A. (1992). Measuring the ghost in the nursery: An empirical study of the relation between parents' mental representations of their childhood experiences and their infants' security of attachment. *Journal of American Psychoanalytic Association, 41*(4), 957–989.

Fonagy, P., & Target, M. (1997). Attachment and reflective function: Their role in self-organization. *Development and Psychopathology, 9,* 679–700.

Fonagy, P., & Target, M. (2005). Bridging the transmission gap: An end to an important mystery of attachment research? *Attachment & Human Development, 7,* 333–343.

George, C., Kaplan, N., & Main, M. (1985). *The adult attachment interview.* Unpublished manuscript, Berkeley, CA: University of California at Berkeley, Department of Psychology.

Goyette-Ewing, M., Slade, A., Knoebber, K., Gilliam, W., Truman, S., & Mayes, L. (2003). *Parents first: A developmental parenting program. Yale Child Study Center.* Presented at the National Association for the Education of Young Children, New York.

Grienenberger, J., Popek, P., Stein, S., Solow, J., Morrow, M., & Levine, N., et al. (2004). *The Wright Institute reflective parenting program workshop parenting manual* (Unpublished manual). Los Angeles, CA: The Wright Institute.

Hesse, E., & Main, M. (1999). Second-generation effects of unresolved trauma in nonmaltreating parents: Dissociated, frightened, and threatening parental behavior. *Psychoanalytic Inquiry, 19*(4), 481–540.

Hesse, E., & Main, M. (2000). Disorganized infant, child, and adult attachment: Collapse in behavioral and attentional strategies. *Journal of the American Psychoanalytic Association, 48*(4), 1097–1127.

Jenkins, C., & Williams, A. (2008). The mother-baby prenatal group: Nurturing reflective functioning in a methadone-maintenance clinic. *Journal of Prenatal & Perinatal Psychology & Health, 22*(3), 163–181.

Lyons-Ruth, K., & Jacobvitz, D. (2008). Attachment disorganization: Genetic factors, parenting contexts, and developmental transformation from infancy to adulthood. In J. Cassidy & P. R. Shaver (Eds.), *Handbook of attachment: Theory, research, and clinical applications* (Vol. 2, pp. 666–697). New York: The Guilford Press.

Main, M., Kaplan, N., & Cassidy, J. (1985). Security in infancy and adulthood: A move to the level of representation. In I. Bretherton & E. Waters (Eds.), *Growing points of attachment theory and research* (Vol. 50, pp. 66–104).

O'Connor, M. J., Sigman, M., & Brill, N. (1987). Disorganization of attachment in relation to maternal alcohol consumption. *Journal of Counseling and Clinical Psychology, 55,* 831–836.

Ostler, T., Bahar, O. S., & Jessee, A. (2010). Mentalization in children exposed to parental methamphetamine abuse: Relations to children's mental health and behavioral outcomes. *Attachment and Human Development, 12*(5), 193–207.

Pajulo, M., Suchman, N., Kalland, M., & Mayes, L. (2006). Enhancing the effectiveness of residential treatment for substance abusing pregnant and parenting women: Focus on maternal reflective functioning and mother-child relationship. *Infant Mental Health Journal, 27*(5), 448–465.

Prochaska, J. O., DiClemente, C. C., & Norcross, J. C. (1992). In search of how people change: Application to addictive disorders. *American Psychologist, 47*(9), 1102–1114.

Sadler, L. S., Slade, A., & Mayes, L. C. (2006). Minding the baby: A mentalization-based parenting program. In J. G. Allen & P. Fonagy (Eds.), *Handbook of mentalization-based treatment* (pp. 271–288). Chichester, UK: John Wiley & Sons.

Schore, A. N. (2003). *Affect regulation and the repair of the self.* New York: W. W. Norton.

Slade, A. (2000). The development and organization of attachment: Implications for psychoanalysis. *Journal of the American Psychoanalytic Association, 48*(4), 1147–1174.

Slade, A. (2002). Keeping the baby in mind: A critical factor in perinatal mental health. *Zero to Three, 22*(6), 10–16.

Slade, A. (2008). The implications of attachment theory and research for adult psychotherapy: Research and clinical perspectives. In J. Cassidy & P. Shaver (Eds.), *Handbook of attachment: Theory, research, and clinical applications* (2nd ed., pp. 762–782). New York: Guilford Press.

Slade, A., Grienenberger, J., Bernbach, E., Levy, D., & Locker, A. (2005). Maternal reflective functioning, attachment, and the transmission gap: A preliminary study. *Attachment and Human Development, 7,* 282–298.

Suchman, N., Pajulo, M., DeCoste, C., & Mayes, L. (2006). Parenting interventions for drug-dependent mothers and their young children: The case for an attachment-based approach. *Family Relations, 55,* 211–226.

Ukeje, I., Bendersky, M., & Lewis, M. (2001). Mother-infant interaction at 12 months in prenatally cocaine-exposed children. *American Journal of Drug and Alcohol Abuse, 27*(2), 203–224.

Van IJzendoorn, M. H. (1995). Adult attachment representations, parental responsiveness, and infant attachment: A meta-analysis on the predictive validity of the Adult Attachment Interview. *Psychological Bulletin, 117,* 387–403.

Waters, E., Merrick, S., Treboux, D., Crowell, J., & Albersheim, L. (2000). Attachment security in infancy and early adulthood: A twenty-year longitudinal study. *Child Development, 71,* 684–689.

Weinfield, N. S., Stroufe, L. A., & Egelund, B. (2000). Attachment from infancy to early adulthood in a high-risk sample: Continuity, discontinuity, and their correlates. *Child Development, 71,* 695–702.

Whipple, E. E., Fitzgerald, H. E., & Zucker, R. A. (1995). Parent-child interactions in alcoholic and nonalcoholic families. *American Journal of Orthopsychiatry, 65*(1), 153–159.

3

Dynamics of Substance-Abusing Families and Implications for Treatment

Wendy K. K. Lam and Timothy J. O'Farrell

INTRODUCTION

Over the past three decades, substance abuse has become widely acknowledged to be a disorder that affects not only the afflicted individual, but also affects and is substantively influenced by family members with whom the individual lives and interacts. Although some continue to view and treat substance abuse as largely an individual problem, the clinical and historical literature across disciplines have converged in recognition of the systemic impact of alcohol, and more recently, other substances, on the family (O'Farrell & Fals-Stewart, 2006; Stanton & Shadish, 1997; Steinglass, Bennett, Wolin, & Reiss, 1993; Straussner & Fewell, 2006). Understanding the role family members may play in the development, maintenance, and treatment of alcoholism and drug abuse has not been limited to researchers or even the broader professional community. To wit, in the popular press, the sheer volume of texts which has appeared on the topics of codependency, adult children of alcoholics, addictive personality, enabling, and so forth, is voluminous. For example, an Internet search of a large on-line book retailer revealed that over 400 books were currently available for purchase on the topic of codependency alone. Moreover, self-help support groups for family members of alcoholics and drugs abusers (e.g., Al-Anon) are available in virtually every community. Because relationship problems and substance use disorders so frequently co-occur, it would be very difficult to find clinicians who specialize in the treatment of substance use disorders or relationship problems that have not had to address both sets of issues concurrently for many clients seeking help (either with the client individually or in the context of the client's larger family system).

Although the effects of substance use by a spouse or parent vary considerably from family to family, fairly common patterns of familial interaction and behavior have been recognized and described by treatment providers. For example, it is not uncommon for family members to engage in behaviors that maintain and perpetuate addictive behaviors by protecting the substance abuser from negative consequences of drinking or drug taking. Calling in sick for a partner's hangover or assuming greater responsibility for household chores are typical responses stemming from a partner's substance misuse. Although these actions are an effort at caretaking, such patterns have the effect of inadvertently reinforcing continued substance use. Other family problems may also co-occur with or be exacerbated by parental substance abuse. Families of individuals with substance use disorders are often characterized by conflict, chaos, communication problems, unpredictability, inconsistencies in messages to children, breakdown in rituals and traditional family rules, and emotional and physical abuse (Connors, Donovan, & DiClemente, 2001).

In many respects, substance use by a parent and its effects on the family can be best understood as dynamic and reciprocally causal antecedents and consequences that tend to repeat themselves over time. More specifically, parental drinking and drug use, along with concomitant behavior, serves to create a dysfunctional family environment, which negatively affects children and other family members. These problems can affect relationships between parents and their children, which can contribute further to the poor psychosocial adjustment of children of substance-abusing parents (COSAPs). In turn, such unhealthful and dysfunctional environments become self-perpetuating by increasing the likelihood for ongoing substance use or relapse. Clinicians who understand these behavioral patterns and the familial environments in which they occur may be able to modify members' interactions to make for a more healthful system that is conducive not only for sobriety, but also for improved adjustment for all family members, including children.

If we accept the close connections between family interaction and substance abuse, it comes as no surprise that treatment approaches that focus on family and relationship processes have been shown in multiple studies to be highly effective in reducing and eliminating substance abuse (Liddle & Dakof, 1995; Powers, Vedel, & Emmelkamp, 2008; Stanton, 1979). As importantly, such interventions have very powerful and positive effects on the children of substance-abusing parents, suggesting these methods pay dividends not only in the short term but also for subsequent generations.

In this chapter, we will draw from existing literature to review what we know about how substance abuse affects relationships and family processes of parents and children, identify assessment issues for substance abuse from a family perspective, and describe current evidence-based treatment approaches for parental substance abuse. The chapter concludes with a discussion of future directions, highlighting the important gaps between current empirical and clinical literatures.

CURRENT STATE OF KNOWLEDGE

Prevalence of Parental Substance Abuse

With the potentially negative consequences and stigma surrounding disclosure of parental substance use, it is difficult to fully know how many families face these challenges. However, information from national household surveys coupled with targeted studies of individuals with substance use disorders can offer some rough estimates of how many children are exposed to parental substance misuse. Results from the 2007 National Survey on Drug Use and Health estimated that approximately 22.3 million persons 12 years or older, or nearly 1 in 10 persons (9%) in the population, met diagnostic criteria for substance dependence or abuse in the past year (Substance Abuse Mental Health Service Administration [SAMHSA], 2008). Of these, most (15.5 million) were dependent upon or abused alcohol, but not illicit drugs. An additional 3.7 million were dependent upon or abused illicit drugs but not alcohol, and 3.2 million were classified with dependence or abuse of both alcohol and illicit drugs.

These startling figures become even more striking when considering the other family members, such as children, who are exposed to an individual's substance abuse. It is estimated that more than 8.3 million children in the United States live with a parent who abuses or is dependent upon illegal substances (U.S. Department of Health and Human Services, 2005). Some, but far from all, of these parents are receiving professional help through substance abuse treatment services. Although precise statistics are not available, research studies with substance-abusing populations find that between 66% and 85% of parents who are entering substance abuse treatment are caring for a dependent child in the home (Hohman, Shillington, & Baxter, 2003; Tyler, Howard, Espinosa, & Doakes, 1997), and that 37% to 57% of mothers or fathers who are not receiving substance abuse treatment services have retained custody and primary caregiving responsibility for their children (Lam, Wechsberg, & Zule, 2004; Pilowsky et al., 2001). Thus, many children continue to live with substance-abusing parents, only some of whom are receiving treatment for their alcohol and/or drug use.

Children of Substance Abusers

Research has consistently found that children who reside with substance-abusing parents are at greater risk for a myriad of problems, including depression and anxiety (Stanger et al., 1999), poor self-concept (Drucker & Greco-Vigorito, 2002), externalizing symptoms (Catalano, Haggerty, Fleming, Brewer, & Gainey, 2002), academic difficulties (Blanchard, Sexton, & Morganstern, 2005), and alcohol and drug use (King, Vidourek, & Wagner, 2003). Additionally, these children may suffer from child abuse, and especially neglect (Walsh, MacMillan, & Jamieson, 2003), and are often removed from the home (McNichol & Tash, 2001).

Comparatively, our understanding of the developmental processes of COSAPs is far less evolved than what we know about typically developing children. However, across studies, a general picture has emerged of how children may be affected by their exposure to parental substance abuse at different developmental ages. During infancy and preschool years, some areas of disturbance, such as problems with attention, have been identified, but there is little evidence of global psychiatric impairment (Mayes & Truman, 2002). By late childhood and early adolescence, however, a number of problems may become evident. Prior to adolescence, COSAPs exhibit increased emotional problems (e.g., low self-esteem, depression, anxiety), behavioral problems (e.g., conduct disorder, impulsivity), and learning problems compared with children of non-addicted parents (Liepman, Keller, Botelho, Monroe, & Sloane, 1998). Lifetime behavioral disorders, such as conduct disorder, appear to be more common among school-age children living with drug-dependent mothers compared with children of non–substance-abusing mothers, although elevated prevalence rates of such psychiatric disturbances may be comparable with offspring of mothers with other psychiatric dysfunctions (Luthar, Cushing, Merikangas, & Roundsaville, 1998). Of notable concern is the specific heightened risk of intergenerational substance use itself during the adolescent years. Over half of the children who were exposed to parental substance use disorders during adolescence had substance use disorders themselves, compared with 15% of those who were not exposed to substance-abusing parents during adolescence (Biederman, Faraone, Monuteaux, & Feighner, 2000). Indeed, adolescent COSAPs are one of the groups at highest risk for increased drug use problems (Rowe, Liddle, Greenbaum, & Henderson, 2004). Thus, preadolescence is a prime period in which to target COSAPs for family-systems interventions, since this is when they are particularly susceptible to parenting influences (e.g., Lam et al., 2007).

How Does Parental Substance Abuse Affect Child Adjustment?

Although COSAPs often display emotional and behavioral difficulties, and parental substance abuse is a significant risk factor for these problems, far less is known about how these problems come about. Available literature assumes that factors associated with parental substance use, rather than his or her substance use behaviors in isolation, present the most serious risks to children in their care (e.g., Merikangas, Dierker, & Szatmari, 1998). These factors range from biological (e.g., temperament, genetic heritability) through psychosocial (e.g., stress, family conflict, parenting) to socio-environment factors (e.g., socio-economic status). Some investigators have argued that psychosocial problems observed in COSAPs are largely a consequence of prenatal chemical exposure, which results in growth deficits and neurodevelopmental problems (e.g., Householder, Hatcher, Burns, & Chasnoff, 1982). Others, however, have failed to find this link, particularly when other risk factors, such as poverty and less optimal caregiving environments, are taken into account (Eyler & Behnke, 1999). More recent investigations have focused on these postnatal caregiving and psychosocial environments associated with parental drug use, such as poor parenting and high interparental conflict, as primary contributing factors in the emotional and behavioral problems observed in COSAPs (Smith, Johnson, Pears, Fisher, & DeGarmo, 2007). Clearly, the multiple environmental risks associated with substance use disorders suggest a large number of factors that may link parental substance abuse with adverse outcomes for their children directly or through cumulative effects. Although very few studies have been able to formally test these possible mediating mechanisms, research has begun to identify key elements in families affected by substance abuse which may be malleable for clinical intervention and treatment, including interparental conflict and parenting (Kelley et al., 2010).

Interparental Conflict

Couples in which one of the partners abuses drugs or alcohol usually have extensive relationship problems, often characterized by comparatively high levels of relationship dissatisfaction, distress, and instability (i.e., partners taking significant steps toward separation or divorce), and by high prevalence and frequency of verbal aggression (e.g., Fals-Stewart, Birchler, & O'Farrell, 1996). The effects of interparental conflict on children are well established. Children's exposure to parental conflict increase risks of fear and anxiety (Yates, Dodd, Sroufe, & Egeland, 2003). These negative effects on children's emotional well-being may be hindering their trust in the emotional security of the family, further increasing youth risk for adjustment problems and prone-ness to bullying, aggressive, violent, and delinquent behavior, adding more stress to the family system (e.g., Moretti, Obsuth, Odgers, & Reebye, 2006).

Interparental conflict may take on a variety of forms. In its most cor-rosive form, relationship conflict can include physical aggression between partners, which can vary greatly along such dimensions as (a) type and severity of aggression (e.g., a push versus a severe beating), (b) frequency (e.g., a single push versus repeated pushing over an extended time frame), and (c) psychological and physical impact (i.e., aggression that induces fear; O'Leary, 2002). Johnson (2004) identified two types of IPV that appear con-ceptually and etiologically distinct. *Patriarchal terrorism* is characterized by severe male-to-female physical aggression (e.g., punching, threatening with weapons), with less severe female-to-male violence occurring during the course of these episodes primarily as self-defense. Family members in these homes experience fear and high likelihood of physical injury. The distinctive feature of patriarchal terrorism is that the aggression serves the purpose of dominating and controlling the partner. In contrast, *common couple violence*, the most frequent pattern of couple violence (Vivian & Langhinrichsen-Rohling, 1994), is bi-directional, often arises from arguments, relationship dissatisfaction, or past behavior, and is typically mild to moderate in severity.

These patterns hold true for substance-abusing couples. Among cou-ples entering substance abuse treatment, approximately 60% report at least one episode of IPV. The vast majority of these couples (i.e., more than 95%) reported episodes of partner aggression analogous to descriptions of com-mon couple violence (Klostermann & Fals-Stewart, 2006). That is, relation-ship violence was mutual and reciprocal in nature rather than necessarily done for power or control. For instance, over a 15-month period, detailed diary information revealed that the odds of domestic violence were 11 times higher on days when men drank (Fals-Stewart, 2003). Among men entering outpatient treatment for drug use, Fals-Stewart, Leonard, and Birchler (2005) showed that after controlling for Antisocial Personality Disorder and dyadic satisfaction, the odds of severe male-to-female physical aggression were over three times higher on days of cocaine use. Using data from the National Family Violence Survey and the National Survey of Families and Households, O'Leary and Schumacher (2003) also found that the odds of severe male-to-female physical aggression were higher on days of cocaine use.

Partner Violence and Child Abuse

The co-occurrence of IPV and physical child abuse has been well docu-mented, with a commonly cited prevalence estimate of about 40% (Appel & Holden, 1998). Studies linking specific episodes of parental substance abuse with child maltreatment are limited. However, Hartley (2002) found that, among families identified by the child welfare system as having mal-treated a minor child, fathers who also were identified as having battered their wives were significantly more likely to report using drugs or alcohol at the time of physical maltreatment (18.4% vs. 4.2%) than those identi-fied as only physically abusing their children. Thus, father's drug use may increase the likelihood of co-occurring partner, as well as child, abuse.

Parenting

Parental substance abuse may also affect parenting through "spillover" effects, in which negative interactions between parents are intrinsically related to family and parenting processes (Bradford & Barber, 2005; Cummings, Goeke-Morey, & Graham, 2002; Krishnakumar & Buehler, 2000). Conflicted interactions within the couple dyad may reflect a style of how parents communicate and work through everyday disagreements, which "spillover" into interactions between the parent and child, and children's functioning. Within family systems that involve parents with substance problems, negative communications that are highly critical and involve considerable amounts of nagging, judgments, blame, complaints, and guilt affect not only the parental relationship, but relationships with their children.

Studies of parenting and substance abuse (e.g., Mayes & Truman, 2002) have begun to identify the types of parenting practices that have been closely associated with the development of child problems including inconsistent, irritable, explosive, or inflexible discipline; low supervision and involvement; little nurturance; and lack of disapproval of youth sub-stance use (Lam et al., 2007; Stanger, Dumenci, Kamon, & Burstein, 2004). A recent review suggests that among families with a substance-abusing parent, both poor parenting and interparental conflict may have unique effects on children's outcomes (Kelley et al., 2010). Thus, attention to both relationship and parenting interactions is important in interventions with parental substance abusers to benefit the family system.

Comorbid Parental Psychopathology

Studies indicate that COSAPs are, indeed, at very high risk to manifest psychosocial adjustment problems due to parental psychopathology that contributes even further to deleterious family contexts (e.g., alcohol and drug use, parental violence), which then lead to ineffective parenting prac-tices (poor discipline, low supervision) and subsequent child psychosocial difficulties (Capaldi, DeGarmo, Patterson, & Forgatch, 2002). In particular, parental antisocial personality and psychological distress (i.e., depression and stress), both of which are common in parents of drug abusing families (e.g., Miller, 1993), covary significantly with emotional and behavioral problems in children (e.g., Patterson, 1999). Depression, particularly in mothers, is associated with less responsiveness to children and less engagement in cooperative problem-solving with their children (Radke-Yarrow, 1998), yet is common among non–substance-abusing partners. Within substance using populations, comorbid maternal psychopathology is linked to whether children remain in maternal care (Nair et al., 1997), as well as parenting and children's developmental outcomes (Hans, Bernstein, & Henson, 1999). The presence of such comorbidities may exacerbate the effects of parental substance abuse on children, and is critical when considering strengths and resource limitations of families during treatment.

Dynamics Among Parental Substance Abuse, Relationships, and Child Behavior

Most professionals would agree that the relationships among parental substance abuse, interparental conflict, and child functioning are not unidirectional, with any one factor consistently causing the other. Rather, each can serve as a precursor to the other, creating a vicious cycle from which parents who abuse drugs or alcohol often have difficulty escaping (O'Farrell & Fals-Stewart, 2006). Chronic substance use is correlated with reduced marital satisfaction for both spouses. Conversely, relationship dysfunction is associated with increased problematic substance use and is related to relapse after treatment (Maisto, O'Farrell, McKay, Connors, & Pelcovitz, 1988). Negative interactions within the parental dyad may spillover to impair parenting interactions with children, leading to children's problem behaviors. Children's problem behaviors may, in turn, contribute to parental conflict and substance abuse problems (Pelham & Lang, 1993). This sequence of family dynamics creates a vicious cycle that serves to maintain parental substance abuse within the family system. Only by understanding parental substance abuse in this broader perspective can treatment interventions be effective.

ASSESSMENT ISSUES

Parental substance abuse is perhaps best understood within a larger couple- and family-context. As such, evaluations of these disorders and concomitant behavior are best conducted within this context. The following section presents an overview of assessment methods often used in partner- and family-involved therapy approaches with additional assessments for parenting and child functioning (Fals-Stewart, Lam, & Kelley, 2010). It should be noted that these issues rest on the assumption that the parental substance abuser is the identified patient in psychosocial or substance abuse treatment settings, that the parent's substance abuse disorder has been diagnosed, and that the patient is sober at the time of assessment. Although young COSAPs quite often enter the service system for their own presenting symptoms, their providers are typically constrained from addressing parental substance abuse directly for reasons such as confidentiality, and focus instead on the immediate presenting needs of the child.

Couple therapy for substance abuse, particularly when based on a social-learning, cognitive-behavioral approach, has a fairly distinct tradition of beginning the evaluation of the relationship by employing three interrelated methods of gathering information in order to understand the problems and strengths of relationships within the family.

First, there are a series of semi-structured and unstructured clinical interviews, typically conducted over the course of 2–4 sessions, which often include separate interviews with each partner and child, as well as meeting the partners together in a conjoint format. Very often, in the first meeting, the therapist will help the parents to develop a problem list, which indicates each person's perception of the problems in the relationship. Problems can be categorized into *matters of content* and *process*. Problematic content areas often include specific stresses that adversely affect the marriage and family, such as unemployment, finances, sex, in-laws, children-rearing problems, and mental or physical illnesses. Process concerns have to do with parent and family adaptive processes, or *how* each parent interacts with the other, with their child(ren), and among siblings if appropriate.

Second, a fairly common assessment procedure used to gather diagnostic information about the family is the administration of various paper-and-pencil questionnaires and inventories to learn more about specific strengths and problem areas, such as relationship functioning and conflict, communication, and parenting. Table 3.1 presents a list of recommended domains for assessment and paper-and-pencil measures. Whenever possible, obtaining child self-report of behaviors, especially internalizing symptoms, perceptions of interparental conflict, and parenting, offers a multi-rater perspective that may be critical in these families in which parental report may not be the most valid (Treutler & Epkins, 2003). In clinic settings, practitioners typically ask the parents to complete a selected set of instruments either before or at the very beginning of the evaluation process. In most cases, feedback and interpretation of results are given to the parents and older children regarding their responses.

TABLE 3.1
Assessment Domains and Paper-and-Pencil Questionnaires
for Couple- and Family-Functioning for Parental Substance Abusers

Domain	Measure		Reference
Psychopathology	SCL-R 90	SCL-90-R	Derogatis (1983)
Relationship functioning	Dyadic Adjustment Scale	DAS	Spanier (1976)
	Marital Status Inventory	MSI	Weiss & Cerreto (1980)
Communication / conflict resolution	Communication Patterns Questionnaire	CPQ	Christensen & Sullaway (1984); Hahlweg et al. (2000)
	Areas of Change Questionnaire	ACQ	Weiss & Birchler (1975)
	Conflict Tactics Scale-2	CTS-2	Straus et al. (1996)
	Response to Conflict	RTC	Birchler & Fals-Stewart (1994)
Family	Family Environment Scale	FES	Moos & Moos (1981)
Parenting	Parenting Scale	PS	Arnold, O'Leary, Wolff, & Acker (1993)
	Children's Report of Parent Behavior Inventory	CRPBI	Schluderman & Schluderman (1970)
Child functioning	Pediatric Symptom Checklist	PSC	Jellinek et al. (1999)
	Child Behavior Checklist	CBCL	Achenbach & Rescorla (2001)
	Children's Depression Inventory	CDI	
	Revised Manifest Anxiety Scale for Children	RMASC	Kovacs (1992) Reynolds & Paget (1983)

Notes:
1. Measures in *italics* are child report; all others are parent report.
2. For further information about these assessments, see Fals-Stewart, W., Lam, W. K., & Kelley, M. L. (2010). Marital dyads. In D. L. Segal & M. Hersen (Eds.), *Diagnostic interviewing,* (4th ed., pp. 392–421). New York: Springer Publishing.

The third assessment procedure that is routinely conducted is direct observation and analysis of a sample of in vivo marital conflict resolution and of parent–child interactions. Couples are helped to identify an existing issue about which they have disagreement and then they are asked to spend 10–15 minutes in the session talking together in a demonstration of just how they go about attempting to resolve the problem. Structured parent–child interactions offer a 5–15 minute situation (e.g., developmentally appropriate play activity or joint task), in which to demonstrate the parenting and discipline styles, behaviors, affective tone, and observe the child's responses, behaviorally and affectively. If both parents are available, pairing the child with each parent, and both parents jointly, may further identify potential buffering or avoidant behaviors that arise in the presence or absence of the substance-abusing parent. The communication and interaction sample provides important information regarding the level of problem-solving skill the parents possess to resolve relationship conflicts and the extent to which improvement in these adaptive processes will become treatment goals.

The multi-method assessment procedures employed by many couple and family therapists provide a solid basis for describing presenting problems of a parental substance abuser, how parental substance abuse is maintained and contributes to family processes, and strengths within the family. The procedures provide converging and diverging information that may be used to conceptualize relationship (dys)function, to formulate an initial treatment plan, and identify other possible areas of concern that may require more in-depth assessment.

INTERVENTIONS

The dynamic interrelationships among parental substance use, couple relationships, and child and family functioning suggest that interventions addressing the behavior of only one family member, in isolation from the larger family system, may be less than optimal. Despite the challenges created by involving family members in treatment, the importance placed on their role is reflected in how substance abuse treatment is conceptualized and delivered in contemporary practice. For example, the Joint Commission on Accreditation of Health Care Organization standard for accrediting substance abuse treatment programs in the United States requires that an adult family member who lives with an identified substance-abusing patient be included in at least the initial assessment (Brown, O'Farrell, Maisto, Boies, & Suchinsky, 1997). As noted in the beginning of this chapter, use of partner-involved interventions, as well as family-based treatments for substance abuse, has been on the rise. Two primary objectives have evolved from recognition of the interrelationship between substance use and family adjustment: (1) eliminate abusive drinking and drug use and harness the support of the couple and family relationships to encourage the patients' efforts to change and relatedly; and (2) promote a home environment that is more conducive to long-term stable abstinence. That is, treatments need to comprehensively target all aspects of the "vicious cycle" among substance abuse, parental relationships, and child functioning, in order to effect and sustain parental abstinence and healthy family functioning within a "virtuous cycle."

Family Therapy

Meta-analytic reviews have consistently concluded family therapy results in superior substance use and psychosocial outcomes compared to individual therapy approaches (e.g., O'Farrell & Fals-Stewart, 2001; Stanton & Shadish,

1997). Although specific assumptions may vary, most family therapy approaches assume that substance abuse behaviors are influenced by inter-actions and subsystems within the family (e.g., Steinglass, Bennett, Wolin, & Reiss, 1993; Stanton & Heath, 1997). As such, these approaches attempt to involve family members in the treatment process. Importantly, family-involved approaches to treat substance-abusing adults appear to have beneficial, secondary effects on children (Kumpfer & Alvarado, 2003). It appears reasonable to assume that improving family regulatory mecha-nisms (e.g., family problem-solving style, daily routines) benefits not only the substance-abusing parent, but children as well.

No single treatment model has dominated family therapy for parental substance abuse. In fact, it is uncommon that an individual would present his or her substance use disorder in the context of the parenting role due to custodial threats or stigma. As such, two family therapy approaches that have developed a strong evidence base have been developed for substance-abusing adolescents and their families. These are: (1) Brief Strategic Family Therapy and (2) Multidimensional Family Therapy. Although not designed specifically for parental sub-stance abuse, these family-systems treatments often reach higher risk families in which youth substance abuse has developed from parental substance abuse and other co-occurring risk factors.

Brief Strategic Family Therapy (BSFT; Szapocznik, Hervis, & Schwartz, 2003) is based on the theory that substance-abusing behavior develops in response to unsuccessful attempts at dealing with developmental chal-lenges. Rigid family structures, such as those potentially created by paren-tal substance abusers, are also believed to contribute to the development of adolescent substance abuse. The therapist attempts to intervene in the system through the parents by changing parenting practices, improving the parent–adolescent relationship, and teaching conflict resolution skills.

Multidimensional Family Therapy (MDFT; Liddle & Hogue, 2001) views adolescent substance abuse as a result of multiple interacting fac-tors, which may include failure to meet developmental challenges, as well as other forms of abuse or trauma, including parental substance abuse or children's exposure to violence. The primary goals of treatment are to improve adolescent, parental, and overall family functioning, which in turn will impact the substance-abusing and other problematic behav-ior. MDFT is a very flexible approach; treatment length is determined by the treatment provider, setting, and family and may include a combina-tion of individual and family sessions. MDFT begins with a thorough multi-system assessment of both developmental and ecological risks and protective factors. This information is then used to create a MDFT case conceptualization, which identifies the strengths and weaknesses in the adolescent's multiple systems and becomes the basis of treatment.

Despite the positive effects of family therapy mentioned previously, there are very substantial barriers to the inclusion of children as participants. First, whether due to complicated scheduling logistics or reluctance by parents, it is often very difficult to convene all family members of a substance abuser for therapy (Stanton & Heath, 1997). More importantly, a survey of several substance abuse treatment programs found that the vast majority (80%) of patients who are parents did not want their custodial school-aged children involved in their treatment, nor did they want their children to receive other mental health services (Fals-Stewart, Fincham, & Kelley, 2004). Furthermore, children in homes in which parents did not want their children to be involved in treatment had significantly greater emotional and behavioral problems (as reported by both parents) than children in homes in which parents were willing to let their children engage in some form of psychosocial intervention. This suggests that children who may have the most need for intervention are the very ones who are effectively cut off from receiving services. This reluctance can be viewed as therapeutic resistance, but it may also reflect some awareness of the negative stereotyping that occurs for children of substance users among peers and professionals. For example, teenagers view children of alcoholics as more deviant than typical teenagers and similar to "mentally ill" teenagers (Burk & Sher, 1990). Thus, interventions for substance-abusing parents that do not directly involve children, but nonetheless are designed to improve the family environment as a whole, may hold the most potential for promoting family health.

Behavioral Couples Therapy

Working with couples provides an opportunity to have positive effects on their children's adjustment without involving them directly as participants. Although many different types of couple-based interventions are available and have been used with alcohol- and drug-abusing patients, an approach developed for this population that has garnered the most empirical support to date is Behavioral Couples Therapy (BCT; see Fals-Stewart, Lam, & Kelley, 2009).

BCT includes interventions that focus exclusively on the substance-abusing patient or parent (e.g., individual counseling, self-help support groups) and those that involve the patient and his or her partner. The partner-involved BCT sessions, which are founded on behavioral therapy with couples are used to: (a) help the substance-abusing partner remain abstinent from alcohol and other drugs by reviewing and reinforcing commitment to a verbal *Recovery Contract* negotiated by the partners during the first two conjoint sessions, in which the partners discuss and support the using partners' abstinence from alcohol on a daily basis; (b) teach more effective communication skills, such as active listening and expressing feelings directly; and (c) enhance relationship satisfaction and increase positive behavioral exchanges between partners by encouraging them to acknowledge pleasing behaviors and engage in shared recreational activities. A recently developed manual describing this approach with alcohol and drug abusing patients is available (O'Farrell & Fals-Stewart, 2006).

Findings from several investigations conducted during the last three decades indicate that participation in BCT is associated with robust positive outcomes for couples in which a partner has a psychoactive substance use disorder. More specifically, the results of multiple randomized clinical trials have demonstrated consistently that, among substance-abusing patients and their partners, those who received BCT reported significantly (a) fewer days of alcohol and drug use; (b) longer periods of abstinence; (c) fewer arrests; (d) fewer alcohol- or drug-related hospitalizations; (e) lower levels of intimate partner violence; and (f) higher relationship satisfaction at posttreatment and through 12-month follow-up than substance-abusing patients receiving treatment-as-usual or those receiving a partner-involved attention control intervention (Fals-Stewart et al., 2005). A recent meta-analysis of 12 controlled studies showed a medium effect size favoring BCT over individual treatment (Powers et al., 2008); BCT has also been identified as an evidence-based program by SAMHSA and the National Institute of Clinical Excellence in the United Kingdom. Preliminary investigations with married or cohabiting female clients and their non–substance-abusing male partners also have yielded similarly positive results on substance use, relationship satisfaction, and intimate partner violence (e.g., Winters, Fals-Stewart, O'Farrell, Birchler, & Kelley, 2002).

With these positive effects on not only substance abuse, but the parental relationship, it is not surprising that we observe improvements in number of other areas as well. Of most relevance here is that BCT also appears to have very positive benefits for children. In a seminal study, Kelley and Fals-Stewart (2002) found children whose substance-abusing fathers and non–substance-abusing mothers participated in BCT displayed higher psychosocial adjustment at posttreatment and during a 1-year follow-up than children whose substance-abusing fathers participated in treatment-as-usual or whose parents participated in a couples-based attention control treatment. Further examination of BCT effects on children of alcohol abusing fathers entering treatment found that preadolescent children (8–12 years old) experienced greater benefits than adolescents (13–17 years old), suggesting that preadolescence may be a critical developmental period for intervening with these children's parents (Kelley & Fals-Stewart, 2007). These encouraging findings indicate BCT has effects on the family that extend beyond the couple to their children, even though (a) the children themselves were not actively involved in treatment, (b) parent skills training was not a component of the treatment, and (c) parenting issues were not discussed during the course of BCT. Thus, couples-based interventions may provide an entry point into the family system from which to improve the psychosocial adjustment of children living in the homes of substance-abusing parents under the very common circumstance in which parents refuse to involve their children in treatment. Along with reduction in alcohol use, which evidence suggests has a positive impact on children even in individual-based treatment (Andreas, O'Farrell, & Fals-Stewart, 2006), many of the skills developed in BCT, such as better communication, reduced partner conflict, and improved problem-solving, are likely to "spillover" into the larger family system and parenting roles as well (Bradford & Barber, 2005; Cummings et al., 2002; Krishanakumur & Buehler, 2000). In turn, this leads to psychosocial improvement for the children in these families.

Substance Abuse Treatment and Parent Training

Researchers have called for integrative interventions that address not only interparental conflict, but also parenting skills to more directly impact children's functioning (Bradford & Barber, 2005). As indicated previously, parental substance use is associated with such parenting practices as inconsistent and explosive discipline, low supervision and involvement, and poor nurturance, which can lead to the development of child behavior problems. These child behavior problems, in turn, may exacerbate stress in parents, thereby increasing the risk of continued substance use or relapse (see Pelham et al., 1997). Therefore, it is somewhat surprising that parent training has been only rarely incorporated into treatments for substance abuse. Perhaps this reflects the belief held by many providers that substance-abusing parents must first address their addiction before being able to positively influence their children. However, Brook and colleagues (2002) showed that even when fathers are substance abusers, positive father–child relationships may still have a positive influence on developmental outcomes for children. Alternatively, some believe that parent training necessarily involves the child's attendance at treatment sessions which, as noted, substance-abusing parents often resist. Although this is certainly one way to operationalize parent training, child attendance is, in fact, not a necessary component for many parent skills training systems. Parent training is defined as an approach to treating child behavior problems by using "procedures by which parents are trained to alter their child's behavior in the home. The parents meet with a therapist or trainer who teaches them to use specific procedures to alter interactions with their child, to promote prosocial behavior, and to decrease deviant behavior . . ." (Kazdin, 1995, p. 82). Perhaps Bowen's (1985) comment about including children in parent skills training is most telling: "Some of the best results have come when the symptomatic child was never seen by the therapist . . . The child's symptoms subside faster when the child is not present in the therapy . . ." (p. 309).

In the past 30 years, numerous studies have examined the effects of parent training and there is an extensive body of literature to show that teaching parents to change their children's behavior can be a highly effective intervention procedure (e.g., Jones, Olson, Forehand, Gaffney, Zens, & Bau, 2005; McMahon & Forehand, 2003; Serketich & Dumas, 1996). There are now dozens of parent-training interventions that, as noted by several researchers (e.g., Kazdin, 1995), share a number of commonalities, including: (a) the intervention is conducted primarily with the parents; (b) there is a refocusing from a preoccupation with problem behavior to an emphasis on prosocial goals; (c) the content of these programs typically includes instruction in the social learning principles underlying the parenting techniques (e.g., training in positive reinforcement procedures, including praise and other forms of positive parent attention and token or point systems; training in extinction and mild punishment procedures such as ignoring, response cost, and time out in lieu of physical punishment; training in giving clear instructions or commands; and training in problem-solving); and (d) extensive use of didactic instruction, modeling, role playing, and structured homework exercises. In particular, behaviorally oriented parenting programs and family-skills approaches have been shown to be effective in changing non-optimal parenting behaviors (Center for Substance Abuse Prevention [CSAP], 1998).

What remains to be seen is whether providing a treatment component that specifically addresses some of the parenting practices thought to be problematic among substance users can effect significant and positive changes on parenting behaviors as well as on their children's functioning, above and beyond the "trickle-down" or "spillover" effects of BCT. There is evidence that including a couple component to enhance communication, problem-solving skills, and pleasant activities engaged in by spouses increased the effectiveness of parent training (Griest, Forehand, Rogers, Breiner, Fury, & Williams, 1982). More recently, Sanders and colleagues (2000) obtained similar findings when they included a component on marital conflict and partner support in their parenting program. With the conclusions of these studies taken together, a "spillover" and even dynamic interplay between interparental conflict and parenting behavior becomes clear, with both of these factors ultimately influencing child adjustment.

Therefore, current evidence indicates that including modules in BCT aimed at improving parenting skills or otherwise addressing parenting problems may be a useful way to intervene with COSAPs. This possibility appears to be viable as BCT has shown itself to be a flexible treatment and has been modified over the years to address drug problems (e.g., Fals-Stewart, Birchler, & O'Farrell, 1999), female substance abuse (Fals-Stewart, Birchler, & Kelley, 2006; Winters et al., 2002), and spousal violence (Fals-Stewart, Kashdan, O'Farrell, & Birchler, 2002).

Indeed, results of a recent pilot study suggest that integrating parent skills training with behavioral couples therapy (PSBCT) may be quite promising. Results strongly suggest that the addition of parent skills training to such partner-involved therapy for fathers' alcohol abuse is feasible and may enhance the effects of BCT alone on both child functioning (Lam, Fals-Stewart, & Kelley, 2008) and parenting practices (Lam, Fals-Stewart, & Kelley, 2009). Early evidence from a large clinical trial by Fals-Stewart and colleagues suggests similarly positive effects of parent skills with BCT among drug using parents. Moreover, the PSBCT treatment for fathers' alcoholism further shows evidence of reducing child maltreatment risk, with PSBCT participants reporting meaningful reductions in involvement with Child Protective Services after treatment and throughout a 1-year follow-up period (Lam et al., 2009).

CASE EXAMPLE: JOE AND SYLVIA

The following brief vignette illustrates the interactive corrosive effects of substance misuse on the couple, child, and family and the interventions that might be used to mitigate them.

> *Joe, a 39-year-old Caucasian man, and his wife Sylvia, a 36-year-old Caucasian woman, presented for therapy 12 years into their marriage. The couple had one son, 11-year-old Kyle. Joe was a factory worker, who was recently laid off. Sylvia started working part-time at a local department store to help with the bills. Despite an increase in tension around family relationships, Joe's drinking, parenting, and finances, Joe and Sylvia expressed a strong desire to strengthen their marriage and improve the home environment for the sake of their child. As part of this effort, Joe had sought intervention for alcohol dependence and, as part of the overall treatment plan, was referred to 12 sessions of couples-based treatment.*

Presenting Complaints

> *When they attended a conjoint assessment, Joe and Sylvia reported that there had been an increase in conflict since Joe's drinking had, according to Sylvia, gotten "out of control." These fights typically escalated quickly from disagreeing to the partners' yelling and cursing at each other. The last time this*

happened, each partner reported that Sylvia pushed Joe to where he lost his balance; according to the partners, it was the first and only time any of the conflicts had become physical. Sylvia became tearful describing how she felt caught in the middle between the needs of her husband and her family, and sometimes felt hopeless about her family's future. Joe, who lamented that "I am always the one in the wrong," felt like Sylvia never stopped nagging him. Sylvia and Joe also reported an ongoing disagreement about Joe's parenting behaviors. Sylvia found Joe unpredictable and explosive, adding that he rarely spent time with their son. Kyle was described by both parents as a "good boy," who kept mostly to himself in his room. Sylvia encouraged Kyle to not bother his father. Joe said he missed his boy and blamed Sylvia for "putting a mommy wall" between him and Kyle.

Course of Treatment

Joe and Sylvia completed 15 sessions of behavior couple therapy for alcohol misuse (O'Farrell & Fals-Stewart, 2006) over the course of 4 months. The initial conjoint sessions focused on assessment of the couple's relationship difficulties and strengths, as well as on each partner's individual history. Because an episode of physical aggression was reported, the therapist asked the couple to agree to "no angry touching" during the course of treatment. Core BCT components (e.g., sobriety trust discussion, communication skills training) were taught and practiced over the course of treatment through in-session and homework assignments. By mid-treatment, both partners reported Joe had greatly reduced his drinking and that the partners' frequency of verbal conflict had dramatically decreased. Reports of Kyle's behavior indicated that he continued to show symptoms of anxiety and withdrawal. However, when interviewed, Kyle said things were different, that his dad didn't drink as much now. Kyle reported that his dad talked to him now. For example, Kyle noted that "Dad would ask me how my day was, which was weird but good."

As treatment progressed, the therapists encouraged the couple to use communication skills (e.g., paraphrasing, validating) to address topics of disagreement, including encouraging a stance of curiosity about the other person's position rather than trying to disprove it or finding blame in the other partner for problems. Several sessions were devoted to helping Sylvia ask Joe for what she wanted, rather than demanding or nagging, and helping him to agree to hear her out rather than immediately dismissing her concerns. Finally, Joe was assigned to spend more time with Kyle (to which Sylvia agreed) and was able to use the more constructive communication skills with his son.

As communications and family interactions became less corrosive and more rewarding, the family began to engage in more mutually rewarding activities together. Both partners stated that it was helpful to make deliberate choices about their behaviors toward each other, rather than simply reacting. These behavior changes were further generalized to and reinforced with their son. Joe and Sylvia reported that Kyle started bringing friends over to the house. Although the couple continued to have fundamental disagreements in certain areas, they were increasingly able to tolerate these differences and to find compromises. As treatment neared completion, both reported that Joe's alcohol use had ceased and that the frequency of conflict between the partners had been reduced dramatically. Joe and Sylvia were engaging in more shared rewarding activities (e.g., watching television, going to sporting events, eating dinner together), both with each other and with Kyle.

Although only a brief glimpse of this family is presented, this case underscores the importance of understanding and intervening with the parent's relationship with a partner, or other adult family members as appropriate. By harnessing the power of the couple's relationship, children in the home can also benefit, even if they are not active parts of the treatment process.

FUTURE DIRECTIONS

Considerations of Feasibility and Effectiveness in Practice

To date, BCT and PSBCT clearly offer some of the strongest benefits for addressing parental substance abuse and the concurrent problems in family dynamics and child functioning. That these treatments appear to have broad positive effects that reach both the family and children is promising, since most parents are reluctant to involve their children in the treatment process (Fals-Stewart et al., 2004). However, despite BCT's strong evidence base, treatment programs have been slow to adopt such couples-based approaches. A survey of treatment programs who had participated as recruitment sites for full BCT trials found that only one of five programs continued to use BCT after federal research support was gone. Program respondents cited other intractable, non-financial obstacles to using couples therapy in routine substance abuse services, including patient-, counselor-, supervisor-, and administration-level barriers (e.g., patient resistance to including family members; third-party reimbursement problems; staff turnover) (Fals-Stewart, Logsdon, & Birchler, 2004). These represent important barriers for integration of BCT into community practice that need to be addressed.

Certainly, one approach is to use different sorts of engagement strategies to increase participation. These might include incentives for family members and for providers, among others (O'Farrell & Fals-Stewart, 2006). However, for those substance-abusing parents who are unable or unwilling to involve their partners in treatment, a promising approach in both effectiveness and acceptability among treatment programs may be to add to the standard individual-based modality a relationship-focused treatment component that addresses relationships with partners and with children that only requires the participation of the identified patient (and no other family members). A pilot trial of such an approach, called *Getting Along*, suggests that providing family- and relationship-focused treatment with one person may be both feasible and effective (Morgan-Lopez & Fals-Stewart, 2007). Logistically, such an approach eschews all of the scheduling issues for families and providers, making *Getting Along* particularly attractive if future research continues to support its benefits.

CONCLUSION

Couple- and family-based approaches have demonstrated robust and broad positive effects in the treatment of the corrosive effects of substance abuse on the family. Reductions in substance use, partner violence, and relationship conflict serve to benefit parenting and communication patterns within the family environment, which are, in turn, linked to more positive child adjustment. As with all family therapy approaches, however, engaging family members in the treatment process is challenging. Development of alternative modalities of couples-based treatment, such as one-person family approaches (e.g., *Getting Along*), may offer comparable benefits within a more flexible and acceptable treatment modality. By working to accommodate both providers and families, we may better engage families in evidence-based treatments that will most aptly meet their complex needs.

ACKNOWLEDGMENTS

This project was supported, in part, by grants from the National Institute on Drug Abuse (R01DA12189, R01DA014402, R01DA014402-SUPL, R01DA015937, R01DA016236), and by the Department of Veterans Affairs. Our sincere thanks go to Bill Fals-Stewart, for his comments on earlier versions of this chapter, and the research team, clinic partners, and families who have participated in our trials.

REFERENCES

Achenbach, T. M., & Rescorla, L. A. (2001). *Manual for the ASEBA school-age forms & profiles*. Burlington, VT: University of Vermont, Research Center for Children, Youth, & Families.

Andreas, J. B., O'Farrell, T. J., & Fals-Stewart, W. (2006). Does individual treatment for alcoholic fathers benefit their children? A longitudinal assessment. *Journal of Consulting and Clinical Psychology, 74*, 191–198.

Appel, A. E., & Holden, G. W. (1998). The co-occurrence of spouse and physical child abuse: A review and appraisal. *Journal of Family Psychology, 12*, 578–599.

Arnold, D., O'Leary, S., Wolff, L., & Acker, M. (1993). The parenting scale: A measure of dysfunctional parenting in discipline situations. *Psychological Assessment, 5*, 137–144.

Biederman, J., Faraone, S. V., Monuteaux, M. C., & Feighner, J. A. (2000). Patterns of alcohol and drug use in adolescents can be predicted by parental substance use disorders. *Pediatrics, 106,* 792–797.

Birchler, G. R., & Fals-Stewart, W. (1994). The response to conflict scale: Psychometric properties. *Assessment, 1,* 335–344.

Blanchard, K. A., Sexton, C. C., & Morgenstern, J. (2005). Children of substance-abusing women on federal welfare: Implications for child well-being and TANF policy. *Journal of Human Behavior in the Social Environment, 12,* 89–110.

Bowen, M. (1985). *Family therapy in clinical practice.* Northvale, NJ: Jason Aronson.

Bradford, K., & Barber, B. K. (2005). Interparental conflict as intrusive family process. *Journal of Emotional Abuse, 5,* 143–167.

Brook, D. W., Brook, J. S., & Whiteman, M. (2002). Coping in adolescent children of HIV-positive and HIV-negative substance-abusing fathers. *Journal of Genetic Psychology, 163,* 5–23.

Brown, E. D., O'Farrell, T. J., Maisto, S. A., Boies, K., & Suchinsky, R. (Eds.). (1997). *Accreditation guide for substance abuse treatment programs.* Newbury Park, CA: Sage.

Burk, J. P., & Sher, K. J. (1990). Labeling the child of an alcoholic: Negative stereotyping by mental health professionals and peers. *Journal of Studies on Alcohol, 51,* 156–163.

Capaldi, D., DeGarmo, D., Patterson, G. R., & Forgatch, M. (2002). Context risk across the early life span and association with antisocial behavior. In J. B. Reid, G. R. Patterson, & J. Snyder (Eds.), *Antisocial behavior in children and adolescents* (pp. 123–146). Washington, DC: American Psychological Association.

Catalano, R. F., Haggerty, K. P., Fleming, C. B., Brewer, D. D., & Gainey, R. R. (2002). Children of substance-abusing parents: Current findings from the focus on families project. In R. J. McMahon & R. D. V. Peters (Eds.), *The effects of parental dysfunction on children* (pp. 179–204). New York: Kluwer Academic Press/ Plenum Publishers.

Center for Substance Abuse Prevention. (1998). *Family centered approaches to prevent substance abuse among children and adolescents.* Bethesda, MD: Author.

Christensen, A., & Sullaway, M. (1984). *Communication Patterns Questionnaire (CPQ).* Unpublished manuscript, University of California at Los Angeles.

Connors, G. J., Donovan, D. M., & DiClemente, C. C. (2001). *Substance abuse treatment and the stages of change: Selecting and planning interventions.* New York: Guilford.

Cummings, E. M., Goeke-Morey, M. C., & Graham, M. A. (2002). Interparental relations as a dimension of parenting. In J. G. Borkowski, S. L. Ramey, & M. Bristol-Power (Eds.), *Parenting and the child's world: Influences on academic, intellectual, and social-emotional development* (pp. 251–263). Mahwah, NJ: Lawrence Erlbaum.

Derogatis, R. L. (1983). *SCL-90-R: Administration, scoring and procedures manual - II.* Towson, MD: Clinical Psychometric Research.

Drucker, P. M., & Greco-Vigorito, C. (2002). An exploratory factor analysis of children's depression inventory scores in young children of substance abusers. *Psychological Reports, 91,* 131–141.

Eyler, F. D., & Behnke, M. (1999). Early development of infants exposed to drugs prenatally. *Clinics in Perinatology, 26,* 107–150.

Fals-Stewart, W. (2003). The occurrence of partner physical aggression on days of alcohol consumption: A longitudinal diary study. *Journal of Consulting and Clinical Psychology, 71,* 41–52.

Fals-Stewart, W., Birchler, G. R., & Kelley, M. L. (2006). Learning sobriety together: A randomized clinical trial examining behavioral couples therapy with alcoholic female patients. *Journal of Consulting and Clinical Psychology, 74,* 579–591.

Fals-Stewart, W., Birchler, G. R., & O'Farrell, T. J. (1996). Behavioral couples therapy for male substance-abusing patients: Effects on relationship adjustment and drug-using behavior. *Journal of Consulting and Clinical Psychology, 64,* 959–972.

Fals-Stewart, W., Birchler, G. R., & O'Farrell, T. (1999). Drug-abusing patients and their intimate partners: Dyadic adjustment, relationship stability, and substance use. *Journal of Abnormal Psychology, 108,* 11–23.

Fals-Stewart, W., Fincham, F., & Kelley, M. L. (2004). Substance-abusing parents' attitudes toward allowing their custodial children to participate in treatment: A comparison of mothers versus fathers. *Journal of Family Psychology, 18,* 666–671.

Fals-Stewart, W., Kashdan, T. B., O'Farrell, T. J., & Birchler, G. R. (2002). Behavioral couples therapy for drug-abusing patients: Effects on partner violence. *Journal of Substance Abuse Treatment, 22,* 87–96.

Fals-Stewart, W., Lam, W. K., & Kelley, M. L. (2009). Learning sobriety together: Behavioral couples therapy for alcoholism and drug abuse. *Journal of Family Therapy, 31,* 115–125.

Fals-Stewart, W., Lam, W. K., & Kelley, M. L. (2010). Marital dyads. In D. L. Segal & M. Hersen (Eds.), *Diagnostic interviewing* (4th ed., pp. 397–421). New York: Springer Publishing.

Fals-Stewart, W., Leonard, K. E., & Birchler, G. R. (2005). The occurrence of male-to-female intimate partner violence on days of men's drinking: The moderating effects of antisocial personality disorder. *Journal of Consulting and Clinical Psychology, 73,* 239–248.

Fals-Stewart, W., Logsdon, T., & Birchler, G. R. (2004). Diffusion of an empirically-supported treatment for substance abuse: An organizational autopsy of technology transfer success and failure. *Clinical Psychology: Science and Practice, 11,* 177–182.

Fals-Stewart, W., O'Farrell, T. J., Birchler, G. R., Cordova, J., & Kelley, M. L. (2005). Behavioral couples therapy for alcoholism and drug abuse: Where we've been, where we are, and where we're going. *Journal of Cognitive Psychotherapy, 30,* 1479–1495.

Griest, D. L., Forehand, R., Rogers, T., Breiner, J., Fury, W., & Williams, C. A. (1982). The effects of parent enhancement therapy on treatment outcome and generalization of a parent training program. *Behaviour Research and Therapy, 20,* 429–436.

Hahlweg, K., Kaiser, A., Christensen, A., Fehm-Wolfsdorf, G., & Groth, T. (2000). Self-report and observational assessment of couples' conflict: The concordance between the communication patterns questionnaire and the KPI observation system. *Journal of Marriage and Family, 62,* 61–67.

Hans, S. L., Bernstein, V. J., & Henson, L. G. (1999). The role of psychopathology in the parenting of drug-dependent women. *Development and Psychopathology, 11,* 957–977.

Hartley, C. C. (2002). The co-occurrence of child maltreatment and domestic violence: Examining both neglect and child physical abuse. *Child Maltreatment, 7,* 349–358.

Hohman, M. M., Shillington, A. M., & Baxter, H. G. (2003). A comparison of pregnant women presenting for alcohol and other drug treatment by CPS status. *Child Abuse and Neglect, 27,* 303–317.

Householder, J., Hatcher, R., Burns, W., & Chasnoff, I. (1982). Infants born to narcotic-addicted mothers. *Psychology Bulletin, 92,* 453–458.

Jellinek M. S., Murphy, J. M., Little, M., Pagano, M. E., Comer, D. M., Kelleher, K. J., et al. (1999). Use of the Pediatric Symptom Checklist (PSC) to screen for psychosocial problems in pediatric primary care: A national feasibility study. *Archives of Pediatric and Adolescent Medicine, 153,* 254–260.

Johnson, M. P. (2004). Patriarchal terrorism and common couple violence: Two forms of violence against women in U.S. families (pp. 471–482). In H. T. Reis & C. E. Rusbult (Eds.), *Close relationships: Key readings.* Philadelphia: Taylor & Francis Publishing.

Jones, D. J., Olson, A. L., Forehand, R., Gaffney, C. A., Zens, M. S., & Bau, J. J. (2005). A family-focused randomized controlled trial to prevent adolescent alcohol and tobacco use: The moderating roles of positive parenting and adolescent gender. *Behavior Therapy, 36,* 247–355.

Kazdin, A. E. (1995). *Conduct disorders in childhood and adolescence* (2nd ed.). Thousand Oaks, CA: Sage.

Kelley, M. L., & Fals-Stewart, W. (2002). Couples- versus individual-based therapy for alcholism and drug abuse: Effects on children's psychosocial functioning. *Journal of Consulting and Clinical Psychology, 70,* 417–427.

Kelley, M. L., & Fals-Stewart, W. (2007). Treating paternal alcoholism using learning sobriety together: Effects on adolescents versus preadolescents. *Journal of Family Psychology, 21,* 435–444.

Kelley, M. L., Klostermann, K., Doane, A. N., Mignone, T., Lam, W. K., & Fals-Stewart, W. (2010). The case for examining and treating the combined effects of parental drug use and interparental violence on children in their homes. *Aggression and Violent Behavior: A Review Journal, 15,* 76–82.

King, K. A., Vidourek, R. A., & Wagner, D. I. (2003). Effect of parent drug use and parent–child time spent together on adolescent involvement in alcohol, tobacco, and other drugs. *Adolescent Family Health, 3,* 171–176.

Klostermann, K. C., & Fals-Stewart, W. (2006). Intimate partner violence and alcohol use: Exploring the role of drinking in partner violence and its implications for intervention. *Aggression and Violent Behavior, 11,* 587–597.

Kovacs, M. (1992). *Children's depression inventory.* New York: Multi-Health Systems.

Krishnakumar, A., & Buehler, C. (2000). Interparental conflict and parenting behaviors: A meta-analytic review. *Family Relations, 49,* 25–44.

Kumpfer, K. L., & Alvarado, R. (2003). Family-strengthening approaches for the prevention of youth problem behaviors. *American Psychologist, 58,* 457–465.

Lam, W. K., Cance, J. D., Eke, A. N., Fishbein, D. H., Hawkins, S. R., & Williams, J. C. (2007). Children of African-American mothers who use crack cocaine: Parenting influences on youth substance use. *Journal of Pediatric Psychology, 32,* 877–887.

Lam, W. K., Fals-Stewart, W., & Kelley, M. L. (2008). Effects of parent skills training with behavioral couples therapy for alcoholism on children: A randomized clinical pilot trial. *Addictive Behaviors, 33,* 1076–1080.

Lam, W. K., Fals-Stewart, W., & Kelley, M. L. (2009). Parent training with behavioral couples therapy for paternal substance abuse: Effects on substance abuse, parental relationship, parenting, and CPS involvement. *Child Maltreatment, 14,* 243–254.

Lam, W. K., Wechsberg, W., & Zule, W. (2004). African-American women who use crack cocaine: A comparison of mothers who live with and have been separated from their children. *Child Abuse & Neglect, 28,* 1229–1247.

Liddle, H. A., & Dakof, G. A. (1995). Efficacy of family therapy for drug abuse: Promising but not definitive. *Journal of Marital and Family Therapy, 21,* 511–543.

Liddle, H. A., & Hogue, A. (2001). Multidimensional family therapy for adolescent substance abuse. In E. F. Wagner & H. B. Waldron (Eds.), *Innovations in adolescent substance abuse interventions* (pp. 229–261). New York: Pergamon.

Liepman, M. R., Keller, D. M., Botelho, R. J., Monroe, A. D., & Sloane, M. A. (1998). Understanding and preventing substance abuse by adolescents: A guide for primary care clinicians. *Primary Care, 25,* 137–162.

Luthar, S. S., Cushing, G., Merikangas, K. R., & Roundsaville, B. J. (1998). Multiple jeopardy: Risk/protective factors among addicted mothers' offspring. *Development and Psychopathology, 11,* 117–136.

Maisto, S. A., O'Farrell, T. J., McKay, J., Connors, G. J., & Pelcovitz, M. A. (1988). Alcoholics' attributions of factors affecting their relapse to drinking and reasons for terminating relapse events. *Addictive Behaviors, 13,* 79–82.

Mayes, L., & Truman, S. (2002). Substance abuse and parenting. In M. H. Bornstein (Ed.), *Handbook of parenting* (pp 329–350). Mahwah, NJ: Lawrence Erlbaum.

McMahon, R. J., & Forehand, R. (2003). *Helping the noncompliant child: A clinician's guide to effective parent training* (2nd ed.). New York: Guilford.

McNichol, T., & Tash, C. (2001). Parental substance abuse and the development of children in foster care. *Child Welfare, 80,* 239–256.

Merikangas, K. R., Dierker, L. C., & Szatmari, P. (1998). Psychopathology among offspring of parents with substance abuse and/or anxiety disorders: A high-risk study. *Journal of Child Psychology and Psychiatry, 39,* 711–720.

Miller, W. R. (1993). Behavioral treatments for drug problems: Lessons from the alcohol treatment literature. In L. S. Onken, J. D. Blaine, & J. Boren, (Eds.), *Behavioral treatments for drug abuse and dependence* (pp. 303–321) (NIDA Research Monograph Series no. 137). Rockville, MD: National Institute on Drug Abuse.

Moos, R. H., & Moos, B. S. (1981). Family environment scale manual. Palo Alto, CA: Consulting Psychologists Press.

Moretti, M. M., Obsuth, I., Odgers, C. L., & Reebye, P. (2006). Exposure to maternal vs. patneral partner violence, PTSD, and aggression in adolescent girls and boys. *Aggressive Behavior, 32,* 385–395.

Morgan-Lopez, A., & Fals-Stewart, W. (2007). Analytic methods for modeling longitudinal data from rolling therapy groups with membership turnover. *Journal of Consulting and Clinical Psychology, 75,* 580–593.

Nair, P., Black, M. M., Schuler, M., Keane, V., Snow, L., Rigney, B. A., et al. (1997). Risk factors for disruption in primary caregiving among infants of substance-abusing women. *Child Abuse & Neglect, 21,* 1039–1051.

O'Farrell, T. J., & Fals-Stewart, W. (2001). Family-involved alcoholism treatment: An update. In M. Galanter (Ed.), *Recent developments in alcoholism: Vol. 15. Services research in the era of managed care* (pp. 329–365). New York: Plenum.

O'Farrell, T. J., & Fals-Stewart, W. (2006). *Behavioral couples therapy for alcoholism and drug abuse*. New York: Guilford Press.

O'Leary, K. D. (2002). Conjoint therapy for partners who engage in physically aggressive behavior. *Journal of Aggression, Maltreatment, and Trauma, 5*, 145–164.

O'Leary, K. D., & Schumacher, J. A. (2003). The association between alcohol use and intimate partner violence: Linear effect, threshold effect, or both? *Addictive Behaviors, 28*, 1575–1585.

Patterson, G. R. (1999). A proposal relating a theory of delinquency to societal rates of juvenile crime: Putting humpty dumpty together again. In M. J. Cox & J. Brooks-Gunn (Eds.), *Conflict and cohesion in families: Causes and consequences* (pp. 11–35). Mahwah, NJ: Lawrence Erlbaum.

Pelham, W. E., & Lang, A. R. (1993). Parental alcohol consumption and deviant child behavior: Laboratory studies of reciprocal effects. *Clinical Psychology Review, 13*, 763–784.

Pelham, W. E., Lang, A. R., Atkeson, B., Murphy, D. A., Gnagy, E. M., Greiner, A. R., et al. (1997). Effects of deviant child behavior on parental distress and alcohol consumption in laboratory interactions. *Journal of Abnormal Child Psychology, 25*, 413–424.

Pilowsky, D. J., Lyles, C. M., Cross, S. I., Celentano, D., Nelson, K. E., & Vlahov, D. (2001). Characteristics of injection drug using parents who retain their children. *Drug and Alcohol Dependence, 61*, 113–122.

Powers, M. B., Vedel, E., & Emmelkamp, P. M. G. (2008). Behavioral Couples Therapy (BCT) for alcohol and drug use disorders: A meta-analysis. *Clinical Psychology Review, 28*, 952–962.

Radke-Yarrow, M. (1998). *Children of depressed mothers: From early childhood to maturity*. New York: Cambridge University Press, xv, 216.

Reynolds, C. R., & Paget, K. D. (1983). National normative and reliability data for the revised Children's Manifest Anxiety Scale. *School Psychology Review, 12*, 324–333.

Rowe, C. L., Liddle, H. A., Greenbaum P. E., & Henderson, C. E. (2004). Impact of psychiatric comorbidity on treatment of adolescent drug abusers. *Journal of Substance Abuse Treatment, 26*, 129–140.

Sanders, M., Markie-Dads, C., Tully, L., & Bor, W. (2000). The triple P-positive parenting program: A comparison of enhanced, standard, and self-directed behavioral family intervention for parents of children with early onset conduct problems. *Journal of Consulting and Clinical Psychology, 68*, 624–640.

Schluderman, E., & Schluderman, S. (1970). Replicability of factors in children's report of parental behavior (CRPBI). *Journal of Psychology, 76*, 239–249.

Serketich, W., & Dumas, J. (1996). The effectiveness of behavioral training to modify antisocial behavior in children: A meta-analysis. *Behavior Therapy, 27*, 171–186.

Smith, D. K., Johnson, A. B., Pears, K. C., Fisher, P. A., & DeGarmo, D. S. (2007). Child maltreatment and foster care: Unpacking the effects of prenatal and postnatal parental substance use. *Child Maltreatment, 12*, 150–160.

Spanier, G. B. (1976). Measuring dyadic adjustment: New scales for assessing the quality of marriage and similar dyads. *Journal of Marriage and the Family, 38*, 15–28.

Stanger, C., Dumenci, L., Kamon, J., & Burstein, M. (2004). Parenting and children's externalizing problems in substance-abusing families. *Journal of Clinical Child and Adolescent Psychology, 33*, 590–600.

Stanger, C., Higgins, S. T., Bickel, W. K., Elk, R., Grabowski, J., Schmitz, J., et al. (1999). Behavioral and emotional problems among children of cocaine- and opiate dependent opiate dependent parents. *Journal of the American Academy of Child & Adolescent Psychiatry, 38,* 421–428.

Stanton, M. D. (1979). Family treatment approaches to drug abuse problems: A review. *Family Process, 18,* 251–280.

Stanton, M. D., & Heath, A. W. (1997). Family and marital therapy. In J. H. Lowinson, P. Ruiz, R. B. Millman & J. G. Langrod (Eds.), *Substance abuse: A comprehensive textbook* (pp. 448–454). Philadelphia: Williams & Wilkins.

Stanton, M. D., & Shadish, W. R. (1997). Outcome, attrition, and family-couple treatment for drug abuse: A meta-analysis and review of the controlled, comparative studies. *Psychological Bulletin, 122,* 170–191.

Steinglass, P., Bennett, L. A., Wolin, S. J., & Reiss, D. (1993). *The alcoholic family.* New York: Basic Books.

Straus, M. A., Hamby, S. L., Boney-McCoy, S., & Sugarman, D. B. (1996). The revised Conflict Tactics Scale (CTS2). Development and preliminary psychometric data. *Journal of Family Issues, 17,* 283–316.

Straussner, S. L., & Fewell, C. H. (Eds). (2006). *Impact of substance abuse on children and families: Research and practice implications.* New York: Haworth Press.

Substance Abuse and Mental Health Services Administration. (2008). *Results from the 2007 National Survey on Drug Use and Health: National Findings* (NSDUH Series H-34, DHHS Publication No. SMA 08-4343). Rockville, MD: Substance Abuse and Mental Health Services Administration.

Szapocznik, J., Hervis, O., & Schwartz, S. (2003). *Therapy manuals for drug addiction: Brief strategic family therapy for adolescent drug abuse* (NIH Publication No. 03-4751). Bethesda, MD: National Institute on Drug Abuse.

Treutler, C. M., & Epkins, C. C. (2003). Are discrepancies among child, mother, and father reports on children's behavior related to parents' psychological symptoms and aspects of parent-child relationships? *Journal of Abnormal Child Psychology, 31,* 13–27.

Tyler, R., Howard, J., Espinosa, M., & Doakes, S. S. (1997). Placement with substance-abusing mothers vs. placement with other relatives: Infant outcomes. *Child Abuse and Neglect, 21,* 337–349.

U.S. Department of Health and Human Services. (2005). *Results from the 2004 national survey on drug use and health. National findings.* Retrieved November 1, 2006, from http://www.drugabusestatistics.samhsa.gov/NSDUH/2k4NSDUH/2k4results/2k4results.htm#ch3

Vivian, D., & Langhinrichsen-Rohling, J. (1994). Are bi-directionally violent couples mutually victimized? A gender-sensitive comparison. *Violence and Victims, 9,* 107–123.

Walsh, C., MacMillan, H. L., & Jamieson, E. (2003). The relationship between parental substance abuse and child maltreatment: Findings from the Ontario Health Supplement. *Child Abuse & Neglect, 27,* 1409–1425.

Weiss, R. L., & Birchler, G. R. (1975). *Areas of change questionnaire.* Unpublished manuscript, University of Oregon at Eugene.

Weiss, R. L., & Cerreto, M. C. (1980). The marital status inventory: Development of a measure of dissolution potential. *The American Journal of Family Therapy, 8,* 80–85.

Winters, J., Fals-Stewart, W., O'Farrell, T. J., Birchler, G. R., & Kelley, M. L. (2002). Behavioral couples therapy for female substance-abusing patients: Effects on substance use and relationship adjustment. *Journal of Consulting and Clinical Psychology, 70,* 344–355.

Yates, T. M., Dodds, M. F., Sroufe, L. A., & Egeland, B. (2003). Exposure to partner violence and child behavior problems: A prospective study controlling for child physical abuse and neglect, child cognitive ability, socioeconomic status, and life stress. *Developmental Psychopathology, 15,* 199–218.

4

Prenatal Impact of Alcohol and Drugs on Young Children: Implications for Interventions With Children and Parents

Elizabeth C. Pomeroy and Danielle E. Parrish

INTRODUCTION

Alcohol, tobacco, and illicit drug use are among the most common causes of disease and mortality in the United States (Floyd et al., 2008; Mokdad, Marks, Stroup, & Gerberding, 2004). Substantial numbers of women of childbearing age (15–44) consume one or more of these substances, putting themselves at risk for deleterious health outcomes (Floyd et al., 2008). Women of childbearing age who become pregnant while using such substances are more likely to have adverse pregnancy outcomes that can impact both the mother and the child. Prenatal alcohol use can result in birth defects and developmental disabilities, and has been found to be especially harmful during the first trimester when many women have not yet realized they are pregnant (Floyd et al., 2008). Data from a recent national survey indicate that as many as 19% of pregnant women (who actually knew they were pregnant at the time of the survey) reported using alcohol during their first trimester (Substance Abuse and Mental Health Services Administration [SAMHSA], 2009).

Similarly, while more recent data indicate that fewer women smoke while pregnant than in previous years, it continues to remain a substantial problem with as many as 22% of women reporting smoking during their pregnancies and 14% during the last 3 months of their pregnancies (Centers for Disease Control and Prevention [CDC], 2007; SAMHSA, 2009). Smoking during pregnancy can lead to several problematic complications during pregnancy such as placenta previa, abruption, premature rupture of membranes, preterm delivery, fetal growth restriction, and low birth weight (Floyd et al., 2008, U.S. Department of Health and Human Services, 2001). Prenatal smoking also increases the chances of sudden infant death syndrome (SIDS) and orofacial clefts (Floyd et al., 2008). Finally, prenatal use of illicit drugs can lead to a greater chance of stillbirth, prematurity, low birth weight, and intrauterine growth restriction (Floyd et al., 2008).

Needless to say, the use of alcohol, nicotine, or illicit drugs during pregnancy can significantly impact the future growth and functioning of young children. Moreover, the cost of medical care related to prenatal substance exposure is staggering (Phibbs, 1991). Women who have used substances during pregnancy are much more likely to have a low birth weight baby and need intensive neonatal care for their child. There are also long-term costs associated with prenatal substance use, as exposed children often require subsequent medical care and educational and developmental assistance through special education and social services (Phibbs, 1991).

The purpose of this chapter is to provide a concise description of the prevalence of prenatal alcohol, tobacco, and illicit drug exposure and to present guidelines for assessing and intervening with children who are dealing with the consequences of such exposure. A systems/strengths approach for intervening with prenatally exposed children will be presented.

PRENATAL USE OF ALCOHOL AND DRUGS: PREVALENCE, CONSEQUENCES, AND RISK FACTORS

Alcohol Use During Pregnancy

According to the 2006 National Survey on Drug Use and Health (NSDUH), more than half (53%) of women of childbearing age reported using alcohol in the previous month and nearly a quarter of women (23.6%) reported binge drinking (>5 drinks on the same occasion) (SAMHSA, 2007a).

Likewise, 11.8% of pregnant women reported current alcohol use, while nearly 3% reported binge drinking (SAMHSA, 2007a). Of the nearly 8% of women of childbearing age who are sexually active and do not use birth control, more than half report alcohol use and 13% binge drinking, putting them at risk for an alcohol-exposed pregnancy (AEP) (CDC, 2004). A recent study found that women at-risk for an AEP were most likely to have past or current drug use, a history of inpatient treatment for drugs or alcohol, a history of physical abuse, a history of smoking, and prior inpatient mental health treatment (Project CHOICES Research Group, 2002).

Alcohol is a known teratogen that can have a negative impact on the development of the central nervous system of the fetus throughout pregnancy (Streissguth & O'Malley, 2000). The consequences of alcohol use during pregnancy can include spontaneous abortion, prenatal and postnatal growth restriction, birth defects, and neurodevelopmental deficits, including mental retardation (Kesmodel, Wisbong, Olsen, Henricksen, & Secher, 2002; Sokol, Delaney-Blac, & Nordstrom, 2003; Stratton, Howe, & Battaglia, 1996; Windham, Von Behren, Fenster, Schaefer, & Swan, 1997). These complications, if caused by prenatal alcohol use, are referred to as *fetal alcohol spectrum disorders* (FASD). FASD is a term that was coined to describe the range of effects that can occur in a person whose mother drank during pregnancy. Multiple diagnostic categories are subsumed under FASD: fetal alcohol syndrome (FAS), fetal alcohol effects (FAE), alcohol-related birth defects (ARBD), and alcohol-related neurodevelopmental disorder (ARND) (Bertrand, Floyd, & Weber, 2005). FASDs include a range of possible physical, mental, behavioral, and learning disabilities that have lifelong implications (Bertrand et al., 2005).

May and Gossage (2001) reviewed FASD estimates from a variety of existing studies and suggested a prevalence of 0.5–2 cases of FASD per 1,000 live births. The cost of FASD for each individual over their lifetime has most recently been estimated to be $2 million (Lupton, Burd, & Harwood, 2004). Many children with FASD are not being accurately identified and assessed (Bertrand et al., 2005). Such children are often diagnosed as having learning disabilities or attention deficit hyperactivity disorder (ADHD) and other behavioral problems, but then lack the integrated support and services at home, school, and other settings that address their specific needs and optimize their future functioning and development. Consequently, there is an urgent need to more accurately assess and assist children with FASD.

Tobacco Use During Pregnancy

Nearly a third of women of childbearing age report tobacco use (SAMHSA, 2007a). While these women are at risk for a myriad of health-related concerns (e.g., many kinds of cancer and cardiovascular disease), smoking can also cause several aforementioned pregnancy-related complications for both the mother and the child. In a recent national survey, 22% of pregnant women reported smoking (SAMHSA, 2009). Women who smoke cigarettes during pregnancy are most likely to be White, non-Hispanic with limited education and income (SAMHSA, 2007a).

Infants prenatally exposed to tobacco are more likely to have sudden infant death syndrome (SIDS) and be born prematurely with low birth weight (U.S. Department of Health and Human Services, 2004a). In fact, estimates suggest that if women stopped smoking during pregnancy, infant deaths would decrease by 5% and low birth weight singleton births would be reduced by 10% (Salihu, Aliyu, Pierre-Louis, & Alexander, 2003; Ventura, Hamilton, Mathews, & Chandra, 2003). Moreover, many women either resume or continue to smoke following the birth of their children, exposing their children to secondhand smoke, which is highly associated with the development of asthma, ear infections, bronchitis, and other respiratory illnesses (Gold et al., 1999; U.S. Department of Health and Human Resources, 2006; SAMHSA, 2009). For this reason, the most recent Surgeon General's Report (2004) on the health consequences of smoking emphasizes that ". . . smoking during pregnancy and after the child's birth should be a target for forceful and effective interventions" (p. 600).

Illicit Drug Use During Pregnancy

According to the 2006 NSDUH, 10% of women of childbearing age and 4% of pregnant women used illicit drugs in the past month (SAMHSA, 2007b). The most commonly used illicit drugs for all respondents included marijuana (6%), cocaine (1%), inhalants (1.3%), hallucinogens (0.7%), and heroin (0.14%) (SAMHSA, 2007b). Similarly, the most commonly reported illicit drug used by pregnant women was marijuana (past month self-reported use ranging from 4.6% of women in the first trimester to 1.4% in the third trimester), while pregnant women entering drug treatment were most likely to report cocaine/crack (17%), amphetamine/methamphetamine (13%), or marijuana (13%) use (SAMHSA, 2002, 2004, 2009). Younger pregnant women (18–25 years of age) were most likely to use an illicit drug during the past month (SAMHSA, 2001).

Women who use illicit drugs are at a greater risk of several social, psychological, and health risk factors, including higher rates of sexually transmitted diseases, HIV, hepatitis, domestic violence, and depression (ACOG Committee on Ethics, 2004). The use of illicit drugs is also associated with maternal complications and adverse outcomes for infants and children. While the effects of cocaine and marijuana have been more thoroughly studied than other illicit drugs, it has been difficult to disentangle the unique effects of each substance (or other substances) as polysubstance use is so prevalent (Floyd et al., 2008). Prior research has found that prenatal cocaine use leads to an increased risk of low birth weight, prematurity, perinatal death, placenta, abruption, and small gestational birth weight (Floyd et al., 2008). Marijuana use during pregnancy, on the other hand, is associated with lower intellectual functioning among exposed children, but fewer complications during pregnancy than is associated with other substances (Day et al., 1994; Goldschmidt, Richardson, Wilford, & Day, 2008; Shiono et al., 1995).

As noted earlier, the use of one substance often co-occurs with the use of another substance (SAMHSA, 2008a). A recent study found that among women who report consuming alcohol and cigarettes, 20.4% also used marijuana and 9.5% used cocaine (SAMHSA, 2008a). When combined, these substances have a multiplicative effect on the health of the mother during pregnancy and her child's behavior (Frank, Augustyn, Knight, Pell, & Zuckerman, 2001).

IDENTIFICATION AND ASSESSMENT OF THE ALCOHOL- OR OTHER DRUG-EXPOSED CHILD

While some substance-exposed infants will exhibit serious medical issues at birth that require immediate attention, many of the long-term developmental and behavioral problems that young children experience are not as obvious. Some children, for example, who were prenatally exposed to alcohol, tobacco, or other drugs (ATOD) may not show any clearly identifiable symptoms until they reach preschool or kindergarten. Often, young children will be identified by pediatricians, family physicians, Head Start or WIC workers, social workers, or preschool teachers as having potential developmental, behavioral, or emotional issues that are atypical for the age group. Assessment and diagnosis of ATOD-exposed children must be ongoing and can change as the child grows and develops. Since many drug-exposed infants are at risk for child abuse and neglect if the parents are known addicts, there is an increased chance that these infants and children will be placed in foster care, respite care, or crisis care nurseries. Therefore, it is important for both biological and foster caregivers as well as professional case workers to be aware of the factors that increase the risk of medical, developmental, and behavioral problems with these high risk children. In addition, research studies indicate that it can be difficult to ascertain the specific cause of the problem due to the interplay of parental polysubstance abuse and environmental conditions that can place children at risk for developmental delays and behavioral problems (Kronstadt, 1991).

Characteristics of Newborns and Infants Prenatally Exposed to Alcohol, Tobacco, or Other Drugs

Newborn infants prenatally exposed to ATOD may present with health-related conditions that include low birth weight (under 5.5 pounds), prematurity (less than 37 weeks), small size for gestational age (weight is less than 97% of infants at the same age), failure to thrive syndrome, neurobehavioral symptoms, infectious diseases, sudden infant death syndrome, and FAS (Kronstadt, 1991). In addition, children born to substance-using mothers may have a variety of dysmorphic features with facial dysmorphia being a common feature of children with FAS. Other features may include cleft lip, protruding ears, short neck, short bones, and other physical abnormalities.

Newborn infants may display sleeping and eating problems, irritability and tremors, fever or seizure activity, excessive vomiting or diarrhea, and inability to be soothed. Infants between 12 months and 2 years of age may exhibit significant language delays, poor or unusual social interactions, lack of typical play skills, and delays in motor development (Kronstadt, 1991). Young children between 3 and 5 years of age may be hyperactive, easily distracted, and unable to control their emotions (Kronstadt, 1991).

Characteristics of School-Aged Children Prenatally Exposed to Alcohol, Tobacco, or Other Drugs

As ATOD-exposed children enter school, they may experience learning difficulties, behavioral problems, and social interaction deficits that draw concern from teachers and other school personnel. While some medical problems may dissipate as the child matures, other behavioral and learning issues may surface. The Miami Prenatal Cocaine Study (2007), a longitudinal research project of 219 cocaine-exposed and 196 non-cocaine-exposed children from birth through 7 years old, indicated that at age 7 cocaine-exposed children had deficits in attention processing and response inhibition as compared to the non-cocaine-exposed

7-year-old children. Another longitudinal study of children prenatally exposed to cocaine conducted at Case Western Reserve University found that these children had poorer performance scores on receptive, expressive, and total language scores and that children prenatally exposed to tobacco had lower receptive language scores. In addition, environmental factors were associated with language delays (Lewis et al., 2007). Finally, a third longitudinal study followed cocaine- and alcohol-exposed children from birth to 8 years old. Findings indicated that cocaine- and alcohol-exposed children were more likely to have lower birth weights, shorter body lengths, and smaller head circumference at birth. However, for cocaine-exposed infants this growth discrepancy was insignificant by school age (Lumeng, Cabral, Gannon, Heeren, & Frank, 2007).

There are subtle impacts of maternal cannabis use during pregnancy on the neurocognitive development of school-aged children (Porath-Waller, 2009). Among 6-year-old children whose mothers reported smoking one or more marijuana cigarettes a day, there was impaired verbal and quantitative reasoning and short-term memory, after controlling for significant covariates (Goldschmidt, Richardson, Willford, & Day, 2008).

Characteristics of school-aged children prenatally exposed to alcohol are well documented. Often, parents and teachers may be alerted to possible problems for the first time when a child enters the classroom environment. Children's learning and behavioral problems may or may not be linked to prenatal alcohol exposure. Nevertheless, children with FAS are more likely to have learning disabilities and require special educational resources (Burd, Klug, Martsolf, & Kerbeshian, 2003). These children often have poor school performance and come to the attention of the teacher before a clear diagnosis has been made. Children with FAS may display symptoms such as lack of attention, distractibility, social skills deficits, and poor impulse control behaviors. It should be noted that many of the issues that affect an FASD child are also seen in children with ADHD and obtaining a thorough assessment is an important component for accurately diagnosing the problem.

Characteristics of Adolescents Prenatally Exposed to Alcohol, Tobacco, or Other Drugs (ATOD)

Individuals who develop FASD deal with lifelong difficulties and challenges. Problematic behavior for adolescents with FASD can increase as the child enters puberty and is faced with social pressures that heretofore were absent in the child's life. For example, adolescents with FASD may have difficulties with social perceptions, physical boundaries, and appropriate sexual behaviors. One major research study found that 58% of adolescents with FASD had peer relationship problems, 48% had engaged in inappropriate sexual conduct, and 53% had been suspended from school (Streissguth et al., 2004). In addition, adolescents with FASD are more likely to either drop out or be expelled from school. Unfortunately, many adolescents have gone through elementary school plagued by poor school performance and remonstrations from teachers and have reached high school without an accurate diagnosis to assist them in obtaining the help they need. By receiving a thorough assessment from a qualified professional who has knowledge of FASD, the adolescent may be perceived as a child with a disability rather than simply a behavior problem.

Heavy maternal cannabis use has been found to result in problems in a child's visual-cognitive functioning into early adolescence (Fried, Watkinson, & Gray, 2003), while maternal cannabis use has also been found to negatively impact the neural circuitry associated with executive functioning, including response inhibition and visuospacial working memory among young adults aged 18–22 (Smith, Fried, Hogan, & Cameron, 2004; 2006).

Legal and Ethical Issues Related to Prenatal Substance Exposure

There has been a great deal of debate regarding the legal and ethical issues related to maternal substance abuse during pregnancy (Murray, 1991). It is not uncommon to feel moral anger at the thought of a woman using alcohol, tobacco, or other drugs during pregnancy, knowing that it will damage the development of the fetus and the child the fetus will become (Murray, 1991). However, it may be helpful to imagine the complex lives that many women lead who use substances during their pregnancies. Many of these women are poor, dealing with violent or abusive relationships that may encourage or even coerce women to smoke or use alcohol or drugs, and they may not have access to proper health care where messages can be communicated regarding the harm of such substances (Murray, 1991). In fact, many women continue to be uninformed about the harm of drinking during pregnancy or receive messages from their physician that "drinking in moderation" will not harm the fetus. Moreover, if a woman is addicted to one more of these substances, she may be ashamed of her use and is afraid to ask for help.

For these and other societal reasons, the "carrot is preferred over the stick" (Murray, 1991, p. 111). First, the cost of policies that would police or monitor the behavior of pregnant women is not only expensive, but restrictive of a woman's personal freedoms (Murray, 1991). Second, a "stick" approach is believed to be even more harmful to the not-yet-born child. Punishing women for substance use during pregnancy is likely to keep women away from essential prenatal care (due to fear that their doctor may initiate legal action) and from seeking substance abuse treatment. Moreover, sending pregnant women who use substances to jail or some other detention facility is only likely to exacerbate maternal stress or other emotional or financial issues, which may impact the woman's ability to successfully bond with and/or provide for her child after birth. The "carrot" approach, on the other hand, increases the availability of high quality and voluntary prenatal care for all pregnant women and access to drug and alcohol rehabilitative programs to assist pregnant women in reducing their drug or alcohol use (Murray, 1991). It also includes, as mentioned previously, sensitive and consistent screening for alcohol, tobacco, and drug use in medical settings and appropriate referral as needed.

ASSESSMENT OF CHILDREN WITH PRENATAL SUBSTANCE EXPOSURE

As with any concern regarding a child, an assessment of the family with a prenatally substance-exposed child includes a description of the presenting problem, a developmental history, a history of the biological parents and their relationship prior to the birth (if available), previous medical and psychiatric history, school history and social history. In addition, an assessment of family dynamics, parenting behavior, and socioeconomic issues are relevant in evaluating the child. If possible, information about prenatal exposure to alcohol or other drugs should be obtained. Finally the family's cultural background should be taken into consideration in order to develop a comprehensive treatment plan. The above information is obtained from the parents or caregiver preferably in a separate session from the child interview.

The clinical interview with the child is often conducted in a play therapy or activity room in which the practitioner has the opportunity to observe the child's behavior and interact with the child while engaging in an activity. While many of these behavioral observations are basic to any evaluation, they are necessary components to an evaluation of a prenatally substance-exposed child. The following observations would be important to note in an assessment: appearance; ability to separate from caregiver; activity level; attention and distractibility levels; impulsive behaviors; ability to interact and relate socially; mood state; emotional regulation; motivational level; response to frustration; response to consequence; developmental level of play activity; speech and use of language; motor functioning; and problem-solving abilities. In addition, the child should be assessed for overall strengths and weaknesses that may become apparent during a play activity (CDC, 2008).

FIGURE 4.1
Children's Assessment Instruments by Development Phase

Age	History	Physical	Visual Spatial/ Fine Motor	Memory	Cognitive	Executive	Attention	Behavioral/ Emotional/ Social	Language	Achievement	Adaptive
Infancy-Toddlerhood (0–3 Years)	• Parent Interview • Records Review	Dysmorphology & Medical Exam	• BSID-III • Beery VMI-5	• BSID-III	• BSID-III	N/A	• BSID-III	• CBCL (≥1.5 yrs) & C-TRF • FABS (≥2 yrs)	• BSID-III • PLS-4	N/A	Vineland II
Preschool (3–4 Years)	• Parent Interview • Records Review	Dysmorphology & Medical Exam	• Beery VMI-5 • NEPSY II	• NEPSY II	• BSID-III OR • WPPSI-III	• NEPSY II	• NEPSY II • CRS-R • K-CPT	• CBCL & C-TRF • CRS-R • PDS (≥4yrs) • FABS	• BSID-III (≥3.5yrs) • PLS-4 • NEPSY II	WIAT-II (≥ 4 yrs)	Vineland II
5–12 Years	• Parent Interview • Patient Inteview (as appropriate) • Records Review	Dysmorphology & Medical Exam	• Beery VMI-5 • NEPSY II • FTT • GPT	• CMS • CVLT-C • WISC-III PI Spatial Span and Digit Span	• WPPSI-III OR • WISC-IV	• BRIEF • CCTT (≥8 yrs) • D-KEFS (≥8 yrs) • NEPSY II • WCST (≥8 yrs)	• NEPSY II • CRS-R • K-CPT or CPT-II • WISC-III PI Spatial Span and Digit Span	• CBCL & TRF (YSR ≥11 yrs) • CRS-R • PDS (4-8 yrs) or CDI (≥8 yrs) • FABS • ASPD • NIMH DISC-IV	• CELF-4 (≥6 yrs) • TLC • NEPSY II	WIAT-II	Vineland II
Adolescence	• Parent Interview • Records Review	Dysmorphology & Medical Exam	• Beery VMI-5 • FTT • GPT (≤14 yrs)	• CMS (≤16 yrs) • CVLT-C or CVLT-II • WISC-III PI Spatial Span and Digit Span	• WISC-IV OR • WAIS III	• BRIEF • CCTT (≤16 yrs) • D-KEFS • WCST	• CRS-R • CPT-II • WISC-III PI Spatial Span and Digit Span	• CBCL, TRF, & YSR • CRS-R • CDI • FABS • NIMH DISC-IV	• CELF-4 • TLC • D-KEFS Verbal Fluency	WIAT-II	Vineland II

ASPD = Antisocial Process Screening Device; BDI-II = Beck Depression Inventory-II; Beery VMI-5: Beery-Buktenica Developmental Test of Visual Motor Integration–5th Edition; BRIEF: Behavior Rating Inventory of Executive Function: Parent and Teacher Forms; BSID-III = Bayley Scales of Infant Development–3rd Edition; CBCL = Child Behavior Checklist; CCTT = Children's Color Trails Test; CDI: Children's Depression Inventory; CELF-4 = Clinical Evaluation of Language Fundamentals, 4th Edition; CMS = Children's Memory Scale: Stories, Dot Locations, Family Pictures Subtest; CPT-II = Continuous Performance Test-II; CRS-R = Conner's Rating Scales – Revised; C-TRF = Caregiver-Teacher Report Form; CVLT-C = California Verbal Learning Test – Children's Version; CVLT-II = California Verbal Learning Test–2nd Edition; D-KEFS = Delis-Kaplan Executive Function System: Twenty Questions Test, Color Word Inference Test, Verbal Fluency, Tower subtests; FABS = Fetal Alcohol Behavior Scale; FTT = Finger Tapping Test; HPT = Grooved Pegboard Test; K-CPT = Kiddie Continuous Performance Test; NEPSY II = NEPSY – 2nd Edition; NIMH DISC-IV = NIMH Diagnostic Interview Schedule for Children, Version IV; PDS = Pictorial Depression Scale; PLS-4 = Preschool Language Scale–4th Edition; TLC = Test of Language Competence–Expanded Edition; TRF = Teacher Report Form; Vineland II = Vineland Adaptive Behavior Scales, 2nd Edition; WAIS III = Wechsler Adult Intelligence Scale–3rd Edition; WISC IV = Wechsler Intelligence Scale for Children–4th Edition; WCST = Wisconsin Card Sorting Test; WIAT-II = Wechsler Individual Achievement Test–2nd Edition; WISC-III PI = Wechsler Intelligence Scale for Children–3rd Edition as a Process Instrument; Digit Span and Spatial Span Subtests; WPPSI-III = Wechsler Preschool and Primary Scale of Intelligence–3rd Edition; YSR = Youth Self-Report.

Source: Centers for Disease Control and Prevention Task Force. (2008). *Fetal alcohol spectrum disorders: Competency based curriculum development guide for medical and allied health education and practice.* Atlanta, GA: Centers for Disease Control and Prevention.

Assessment Using Standardized Instruments

In addition to the psychosocial clinical interview with the caregiver and child, a battery of standardized tests is used to measure cognitive, psychological, intellectual, academic, social, behavioral, and adaptive functioning. Standardized instruments designed for the caregiver/parent to complete are also used if the caregiver/parent is available and knowledgeable about the child's current situation and history. For example, in the case of the potential prenatally alcohol-exposed child, the Fetal Alcohol Behavior Scale (FABS; Streissguth, Bookstein, Barr, Press, & Sampson, 1998) was developed to assess a variety of areas of the child's functioning and is completed by the caregiver/parent. A chart containing the standardized instruments that have been found to be most useful in assessing individuals with FASD by development is provided in Figure 4.1. Given the general orientation of the majority of scales described in this chart, many of these instruments are also useful for assessing the effects of other kinds of prenatal substance exposure.

Finally, a thorough assessment would not be complete without a physical and medical exam, preferably by a developmental pediatrician who is an expert in potential physical abnormalities, growth deficiencies, and medical problems that may be present in a prenatally substance-exposed child. If a developmental pediatric specialist is not available, a pediatrician with knowledge of FASD and prenatal exposure to other substances in children should be utilized for a comprehensive medical evaluation.

Diagnostic Criteria for FAS

Although it is difficult to disentangle the effects of alcohol on children from those of other drugs including cigarettes, there has been definitive research on the development of diagnostic criteria for FAS. The diagnostic criteria for the effects of other illicit drugs, such as cocaine, methamphetamine, and heroin, are not as well developed and may be highly individualized depending upon the drug or drugs used by the mother, the developmental stage of the child, and environmental conditions. For children with FAS or other alcohol-related disorders, the effects are life long, whereas exposure to other substances may dissipate over time. Individuals with a FASD are more likely to have co-morbid psychiatric conditions, experience school and occupational difficulties, be in need of dependent living supports, have an increased risk of criminal acts, and have an arrest history (CDC, 2008). The criteria for FAS are included in Box 4.1.

BOX 4.1
FAS Diagnostic Criteria

1. Smooth or Flattened Upper Lip
2. Thin Upper Lip
3. Small Eye Lid Openings

Other facial features may include (but are not necessary for diagnosis):

Skin folds at the corner of the eye
Low nasal bridge
Short nose
Small midface

In addition, children with FAS have growth abnormalities and central nervous system deficits.

Source: Warren, K. R., & Foudin, L. L. (2001). Alcohol related birth defects: The past, present and future. *Alcohol Research and Health, 25*(3), 153–158.

IMPLICATIONS FOR PRACTICE WITH CHILDREN AFFECTED BY PRENATAL SUBSTANCE EXPOSURE

While the research on intervention with children affected by prenatal substance exposure is still in its early development, there are several multi-systems practice approaches to both medical treatment and psychosocial intervention that have been developed and disseminated. This section will briefly discuss each of the systems of care that may be employed to support children who have been prenatally exposed to substances.

Medical Interventions

A necessary first step in the treatment of a prenatally substance-exposed child is a referral to a physician, specifically a developmental pediatrician, for a complete medical evaluation. A variety of medical professionals may be involved in the child's care depending upon the type and severity of their symptoms. Some common medical providers involved in such care include neurologists, audiologists, dysmorphologists, otolaryngologists, ophthalmologists, and plastic surgeons. Allied medical professionals who may be involved in the child's care are nutritionists, speech therapists, occupational therapists, physical therapists, and recreational therapists (U.S. Department of Health and Human Services, 2004b). Ideally, these services are coordinated and communicated with all medical providers in the form of a single intervention plan. Social workers are essential with regard to helping provide case management and resources, as well as ensuring that the intervention plan is implemented in a seamless manner across various settings (e.g., the school, home, and medical).

Mental Health and Psychopharmacological Interventions

As stated earlier, children with prenatal substance exposure may experience a variety of mood disorders, as well as behavioral and learning disabilities. In order to appropriately assess the potential benefits of psychopharmacological medication, the practitioner should refer the child and their parent/caregiver for a psychiatric evaluation. There are several classes of psychotropic medication that may be useful. The most common classes of drugs used with ATOD-exposed children include stimulant medications, antidepressants, and neuroleptics. Stimulant medications, such as Ritalin, Adderall, Strattera, Concerta, and Dexedrine, can be useful for symptoms associated with ADHD. Antidepressants that may be prescribed include Zoloft, Paxil, Luvox, Clonidine, and Wellbutrin (CDC, 2008). In addition, research has shown that while children with FASDs do not typically display psychotic symptoms, they may be prescribed neuroleptic medication for the management of aggressive behavior and anxiety related to developmental disabilities. These medications include such drugs as Risperdal and Clozarile, which can be used in combination with antidepressants (CDC, 2008). If a child is taking these medications, the social worker should closely collaborate with the prescribing physician and make sure that the parents or guardians are aware of any possible negative side effects.

Behavioral and Educational Services

It has only been in recent years that behavioral and educational services for children with FASDs have been developed that specifically take into account the unique challenges that these children must face in school, at home, and in relationships. Previously, interventions were based on what appeared to be helpful to children with other developmental and learning disabilities. Evidence-based interventions specifically for children with FASDs had yet to be developed. Currently, however, there is research to support the efficacy of some specific educational and behavioral treatment plans for children with FASDs.

Children under the age of 3 years who are diagnosed with a developmental problem can be referred to an early intervention program which provides specialized services in speech, physical, and occupational therapy as well as special education (CDC, 2008). These programs are available in all 50 states and are of invaluable assistance to children prior to entering the school system. There are a variety of funding sources, so social workers should specifically research these programs in their state and local community.

When a child with a FASD enters school, they may be eligible for special education services due to their learning or developmental disabilities. While having a FASD is not a diagnosis per se and, alone, does not necessarily qualify a child for special education, the symptoms of the disorder may qualify the child. On the other hand, a child with a FAS diagnosis does have a right to an Individualized Education Plan (IEP), which is designed to outline an educational program that will meet the child's learning needs and functional capacities.

In addition, research has shown the effectiveness of a 12-week social skills training program to enhance peer relationships (O'Connor et al., 2007), a math tutoring program to improve math skills for children with FASD (Kable, Coles, & Taddeo, 2007), and a program to improve behavioral regulation and executive functioning (Bertrand et al., 2009). While these programs are only available in certain areas of the country, they have yielded promising results that may lead to wider dissemination in the future. Finally, the University of Seattle has examined the effectiveness of a parent training program to teach parents how to work with their children who have FASDs. This program has been shown to significantly improve the problematic behavior difficulties of children with FASDs (CDC, 2008).

Parenting and Family-Based Interventions

Many families with prenatally substance-exposed children are living in impoverished and environmentally challenging conditions where survival is a priority. Due to their circumstances, many of these families must have their basic needs addressed before focusing on parenting or other supportive issues for their children. It is essential that the practitioner form a strong and mutually respectful, collaborative relationship when working with the parent/caregiver in order to ensure the implementation and sustainability of this unique set of parenting skills. Moreover, given the demanding and challenging nature of parenting a child with prenatal substance exposure, a supportive professional relationship can have a positive, long-term effect on both the parent/caregiver and child.

A multi-system, strength-based approach to intervening with children who were prenatally exposed to substances includes the careful consideration of family culture, strengths, and dynamics, as well as the use of family-based interventions. It is ideal to intervene as early as possible with the infant or child, as such immediate intervention can support the development and maintenance of more positive and healthy interactions between the caregivers and the child, thereby resulting in a more secure parental/caregiver attachment and a more positive home environment. Intervention can be particularly useful to foster care and adoptive parents who may need a special skill set required to effectively parent the child in a way that will maximize their development.

According to the transactional model, the early caregiving environment—which includes parental perceptions of the infant, caregiving confidence, and the parent–infant relationship—is a critical intervention point for supporting the optimal development of a child (Meyer et al., 1994). Several interventions have been identified to support parent–infant interactions, including Watch, Wait, and Wonder (Muir, Lojkasek, & Cohen, 1999), Interactional Guidance (IG) therapeutic treatment (McDonough, 2005), and Individualized Family-Based Intervention (1994). In addition, Child–Parent Psychotherapy is another treatment model that has been found to be useful for infants, toddlers, and preschoolers who are experiencing mental health problems or parent–child relational problems due to parental factors (e.g., mental health), child constitutional factors that may influence the formation of a secure attachment, and/or discordant temperaments or styles between the parent and the child (Lieberman, 2005).

For children of school age, there are several recommendations for helping children who may be exhibiting symptoms related to prenatal substance exposure. Like all children, those who have been prenatally exposed to substances need structure, a simple and consistent routine, repetition for learning, and positive reinforcement to support healthy self-esteem. The following recommendations can be adapted for the child based on the unique symptoms and challenges within the home (National Organization of Fetal Alcohol Syndrome, 2004, p. 2).

Routine

- Keep the family's routine as much the same each day as possible.
- If the family's routine or schedule changes, remind the child about changes.

Behavior

- Learn how to tell when the child is getting frustrated, and help out early.
- Make sure the child understands the rules at home.
- Tell the child about what will happen if he or she has good behavior or bad behavior at home.

- Let the child know when he or she has good behavior.
- Teach self-talk to help the child develop self-control. Use specific, short phrases such as "stop and think."
- Repeat everything and give the child many chances to do what he/she is asked to do.
- Be patient.
- Give directions one step at a time. Wait for the child to do the first step in the directions before telling the second step.
- Tell the child before you touch him or her.
- Be sure the child understands the rules, and be firm and consistent with them.

It is also possible that parents of a child with FASD may also have been prenatally exposed to alcohol and have symptoms of FASD. When this is the case, it is essential that the practitioner also have the skills to engage both the child and the parent so that any individual challenges (on the part of the child and parent) are considered when implementing a family-based intervention. Likewise, it may benefit both the parent and the child if the parent is linked to the necessary case management or community services to optimize parental functioning.

Case of Donny

Donny is a 6-year-old Caucasian male who is a first grader at Crosby Elementary School in California. He was referred to the Child Guidance Center for a complete psychosocial assessment. He is the third child in a family of four children. Mary and John Kincaid, Donny's grandparents, have custody of the four children after Sarah Kincaid, Donny's mother, was incarcerated for drug possession. Donny's father, Alfred Collins, left the family after losing his job 3 years ago. Sarah and Alfred never married. Mary Kincaid describes her grandson as being very friendly and outgoing; however, he has had multiple problems since entering kindergarten last year. Donny has difficulty paying attention, staying in his chair, and requires constant reminders from his teacher in order to stay on task. While very friendly, he annoys other children with his "babyish" behaviors and appears to lack the social skills that many of his same-aged peers have. Mary Kincaid states that Donny is often teased and cries uncontrollably when other children call him names such as "smush face" or "four eyes." Donny has some characteristic facial features related to FASD such as small eye openings and narrow upper lip. Donny has quite pronounced vision problems and wears prescription glasses. The grandmother states that Donny and his younger sister have always seemed "different and strange" compared to the two older children.

During a short play session with Donny, the practitioner noted that Donny was highly distractible, immature, and had speech and language deficits. He seemed to have difficulty interacting with the practitioner and moved rapidly from one toy to the next. He often talked with almost a babbling quality and often used indiscernible language. After discussing her concerns with Donny's grandmother who confirmed that her daughter had a drinking problem, the practitioner referred Donny to a developmental pediatrician for a complete medical evaluation. The physician diagnosed Donny with FAS.

Following the evaluation, Donny's physician in collaboration with an interdisciplinary team developed a comprehensive intervention plan that encompassed parent training by a clinical social worker, referral for ongoing psychiatric evaluation, referral to a speech pathologist, and consultation with a school counselor with regard to an IEP and social skills training group. In addition, a social work case manager was assigned to coordinate services and provide support to the grandparents within the home.

SUMMARY

Despite the fact that alcohol, tobacco, and other drugs are known to lead to adverse pregnancy and child outcomes, many women continue to use one or more of these substances. The impact of these substances on children varies according to the woman's patterns of use, the environment, and the opportunity for children to receive early intervention. It is imperative that practitioners, teachers, and medical personnel are able to recognize the signs of ATOD exposure so that children can receive the assessment and intervention services that will maximize their functioning. It is also important to support the parent or caregiver of the child so that they will be able to provide a home environment that is warm and that accommodates the child's disabilities. Finally, a multi-systems and strength approach is useful when assessing or intervening with children prenatally exposed to ATOD and their families. While there are several interventions or approaches that have been developed to address the needs of children who have symptoms of FASD and ATOD, additional intervention development and research is necessary to better understand how to help these children.

REFERENCES

ACOG Committee on Ethics. (2004). At-risk drinking and illicit drug use: Ethical issues in obstetric and gynecological practice. *Obstetrics and Gynecology, 103,* 1021–1031.

Bertrand, J.; Interventions for Children with Fetal Alcohol Spectrum Disorders Research Consortium. (2009). Interventions for children with fetal alcohol spectrum disorders (FASDs): Overview of findings for five innovative research studies. *Research in Developmental Disabilities, 30,* 986–1006.

Bertrand, J., Floyd, R. L., & Weber, M. K. (2005, October 28). Guidelines for identifying and referring persons with fetal alcohol syndrome. *Morbidity and Mortatilty Weekly Report Centers for Disease Control and Prevention, 54*(RR11), 1–10.

Burd, L., Klug, M. G., Martsolf, J. T., & Kerbeshian, J. (2003). Fetal alcohol syndrome: Neuropsychiatric phenomics. *Neurotoxicology and Teratology, 25,* 697–705.

Centers for Disease Control and Prevention. (2004). Alcohol consumption among women who are pregnant or who might become pregnant—United States. *Morbidity Mortality Weekly Report, 53,* 1178–1181.

Centers for Disease Control and Prevention. (2007). *Preventing smoking and exposure to to secondhand smoke before, during, and after pregnancy.* Atlanta, GA: Author.

Centers for Disease Control and Prevention Task Force. (2008). *Fetal alcohol spectrum disorders: Competency based curriculum development guide for medical and allied health education and practice.* Atlanta, GA: Author.

Day, N. L., Richardson, G. A., Goldschimidt, L., Robles, N., Taylor, P. M., Stoffer, D. S., et al. (1994). Effect of prenatal marijuana exposure on the cognitive development of offspring at age three. *Neurotoxicology and Teratology, 16,* 169–175.

Delis, D. C., Kaplan, E., & Kramer, J. H. (2001). *Delis-Kaplan executive function system.* San Antonio, TX: The Psychological Corporation.

Delis, D. C., Kramer, J. H., Kaplan, E., & Ober, B. A. (1994). *California Verbal Learning Test—Children's version.* San Antonio, TX: The Psychological Corporation.

Delis, D. C., Kramer, J. H., Kaplan, E., & Ober, B. A. (2000). *California Verbal Learning Test* (2nd ed., CVLT-II). San Antonio, TX: Harcourt Assessment.

Floyd, R. L., Jack, B. W., Cefalo, R., Atrash, H., Mahoney, J., Herron, A., et al. (2008). The clinical content of preconception care: Alcohol, tobacco, and illicit drug exposures. *American Journal of Obstetrics and Gynecology, 199,* S333–S339.

Frank, D. A., Augustyn, M., Knight, W. G., Pell, T., & Zuckerman, B. (2001). Growth, development, and behavior in early childhood following prenatal cocaine exposure. *Journal of American Medical Association, 285,* 1613–1625.

Fried, P. A., Watkinson, B., & Gray, R. (2003). Differential effects on cognitive functioning in 13- to 16-year-olds prenatally exposed to cigarettes and marijuana. *Neurotoxicology and Teratology, 25,* 427–436.

Gold, D. R., Burge, H. A., Carey, V., Milton, D. K., Platts-Mills, T., & Weiss, S. T. (1999). Predictors of repeated wheeze in the first year of life: The relative roles of cockroach, birth weight, acute lower respiratory illness, and maternal smoking. *American Journal of Respiratory and Critical Care Medicine, 111,* 1176–1180.

Goldschmidt, L., Richardson, G. A., Willford, J., & Day, N. L. (2008). Prenatal marijuana exposure and intelligence test performance at age 6. *Journal of the American Academy of Child and Adolescent Psychiatry, 47*(3), 254–263.

Halstead, W. C. (1947). *Brain and intelligence.* Chicago: University of Chicago Press.

Heaton, R. K., Chelune, G. J., Talley, J. L., Kay, G. G., & Curtiss, G. (1993). *Wisconsin Card Sorting Test.* Lutz, FL: Psychological Assessment Resources.

Kable, J. A., Coles, C. D., & Taddeo, E. (2007). Socio-cognitive habilitation using the math interactive learning experience program for alcohol-affected children. *Alcoholism: Clinical and Experimental Research, 31*(8), 1425–1434.

Kesmodel, U., Wisbong, K., Olsen, S. F., Henriksen, T. B., & Secher, N. J. (2002). Moderate alcohol intake in pregnancy and the risk of spontaneous abortion. *Alcohol and Alcoholism, 37*(1), 87–92.

Korkman, M., Kirk, U., & Kemp, S. (2007). *NEPSY* (2nd ed.). San Antonio, TX: Harcourt Assessment.

Lewis, B. A., Kirchner H. L., Short, E. J., Minnes, S., Weishampel, P., Satayathum, S., et al. (2007). Prenatal cocaine and tobacco effects on children's language trajectories. *Pediatrics, 120*(1), 78–85.

Lieberman, A. F. (2005). Child-parent psychotherapy: A relationship-based approach to the treatment of mental health disorders in infancy and early childhood. In A. J. Sameroff, S. C. McDonough, & K. L. Rosenblum (Eds.), *Treating parent-infant relationship problems* (pp. 97–122). New York: Guilford Publications.

Lumeng, J. C., Cabral, H. J., Gannon, K., Heeren, T., & Frank, D. A. (2007). Prenatal exposures to cocaine and alcohol and physical growth patterns to age 8 years. *Neurotoxicology and Teratology, 29*(4), 446–457.

Lupton, C., Burd, L., & Harwood, R. (2004). Cost of fetal alcohol spectrum disorders. *American Journal of Medical Genetics, 127C*, 3–9.

May, P. A., & Gossage, J. P. (2001). Estimating the prevalence of fetal alcohol spectrum syndrome: A summary. *Alcohol Research Health, 25*, 159–167.

McDonough, S. C. (2005). Interaction guidance: Promoting and nurturing the caregiving relationship. In A. J. Sameroff, S. C. McDonough, & K. L. Rosenblum, (Eds.), *Treating parent-infant relationship problems* (pp. 79–96). New York: Guilford Press.

Meyer, E. C., Coll, C. T., Lester, B. M., Zachariah, B., McDonough, S. M., & Oh, W. (1994). Family-based intervention improves maternal psychological well-being and feeding interaction of preterm infants. *Pediatrics, 93*(2), 241–246.

Mokdad, A. H., Marks, J. S., Stroup, D. F., & Gerberding, J. L. (2004). Actual causes of death in the United States. *Journal of the American Medical Association, 291*, 1238–1245.

Muir, E., Lojkasek M., & Cohen N. (1999). *Watch, wait, & wonder: A manual describing a dyadic infant-led approach to problems in infancy and early childhood.* Toronto, ON: Hincks-Dellcrest Centre.

National Organization on Fetal Alcohol Syndrome. (2004). *Strategies for daily living: FAS/FASD throughout the lifespan.* Retrieved June 21, 2009, from http://www.nofas.org/living/strategy.aspx

O'Connor, M. J., Frankel, F., Paley, B., Schonfeld, A. M., Carpenter, E., Laugeson, E. A., et al. (2007). A controlled social skills training for children with fetal alcohol spectrum disorders. *Journal of Consulting and Clinical Psychology, 74*(4), 639–648.

Phibbs, C. S. (1991). The Economic implications of prenatal substance exposure. *The Future of Children: Drug Exposed Infants, 1*(1), 113–120. Retrieved from http://www.jstor.org/stable/1602621

Porath-Waller, A. J. (2009). Clearing the smoke on cannabis. *Canadian Centre on Substance Abuse.* Retrieved June 21, 2009, from http://www.ccsa.ca/2009%20CCSA%20Documents/ccsa0117832009_e.pdf

Project CHOICES Research Group. (2002). Alcohol-exposed pregnancy: Characteristics associated with risk. *American Journal of Preventative Medicine, 23,* 166–173.

Salihu, H. M., Aliyu, M. H., Pierre-Louis, B. J., & Alexander, G. R. (2003). Levels of excess infant deaths attributed to maternal smoking during pregnancy in the United States. *Maternal and Child Health Journal, 7,* 219–227.

Semel, E., Wiig, E. H., & Secord, W. A. (2003). *Clinical evaluation of language fundamentals* (4th ed.). San Antonio, TX: Harcourt Assessment.

Shiono, P. H., Kelbanoff, M. A., Nugent, R. P., Cotch, M. F., Wilkins, D. G., Rollins, D. E., et al. (1995). The impact of cocaine and marijuana use on low birth weight and preterm birth: A multicenter study. *American Journal of Obstetric Gynecology, 172,* 19–27.

Smith, A. M., Fried, P. A., Hogan, M. J., & Cameron, I. (2004). Effects of prenatal marijuana on response inhibition: An fMRI study in young adults. *Neurotoxicology and Teratology, 26,* 533–542.

Smith, A. M., Fried, P. A., Hogan, M. J., & Cameron, I. (2006). Effects of prenatal marijuana on response inhibition: An fMRI study in young adults. *Neurotoxicology and Teratology, 28,* 286–295.

Sokol, R. J., Delaney-Black, V., & Nordstrom, B. (2003). Fetal alcohol spectrum disorder. *Journal of the American Medical Association, 290,* 2996–2999.

Stratton, K., Howe, C., & Battaglia, F. (Eds.). (1996). *Fetal alcohol syndrome: Diagnosis, epidemiology, prevention and treatment.* Washington, DC: Institute of Medicine National Academy Press.

Streissguth, A. P., Bookstein, F. L., Barr, H. M., Press, S., & Sampson, P. D. (1998). A Fetal Alcohol Behavior Scale. *Alcoholism: Clinical and Experimental Research, 22*(2), 325–333.

Streissguth, A. P., Bookstein, F. L., Barr, H. M., Press, S., Sampson, P.D., O'Malley, K., et al. (2004). Risk factors for adverse life outcomes in fetal alcohol syndrome and fatal alcohol effects. *Developmental and Behavioral Pediatrics, 25,* 228–238.

Streissguth, A. P., & O'Malley, K. (2000). Neuropsychiatric implications and long-term consequences of fetal alcohol spectrum disorders. *Seminars in Clinical Neuropsychiatry, 5,* 177–190.

Substance Abuse and Mental Health Services Administration. (2001). *The NSDUH report: Pregnancy and illicit drug use.* Rockville, MD: Office of Applied Studies.

Substance Abuse and Mental Health Services Administration. (2002). *The DASIS report: Pregnant women in substance abuse treatment.* Rockville, MD: Office of Applied Studies.

Substance Abuse and Mental Health Services Administration. (2004). *The DASIS report: Pregnant women in substance abuse treatment: 2002.* Rockville, MD: Office of Applied Studies.

Substance Abuse and Mental Health Services Administration. (2007a). *Results from the 2006 national survey on drug use and health: National findings* (NSDUH series H-32, Department of Health and Human Services publication No. SMA 07-4923). Rockville, MD: Office of Applied Studies.

Substance Abuse and Mental Health Services Administration. (2007b). *The NSDUH report: Substance use treatment among women of childbearing age.* Rockville, MD: Office of Applied Studies.

Substance Abuse and Mental Health Services Administration. (2008a). *Results from the 2007 national survey on drug use and health: National findings* (NSDUH Series H-34, DHHS Publication No. SMA 08-4343). Rockville, MD: Office of Applied Studies.

Substance Abuse and Mental Health Services Administration. (2008b, September 11). *The NSDUH Report: Alcohol Use among Pregnant Women and Recent Mothers.* Rockville, MD: Office of Applied Studies.

Substance Abuse and Mental Health Services Administration. (2009, May 21). *The NSDUH Report: Substance use among women during pregnancy and following childbirth.* Rockville, MD: Office of Applied Studies.

U.S. Department of Health and Human Services. (2001). *Women and smoking: A report of the Surgeon General.* Washington, DC: U.S. Department of Health and Human Services, Public Health Service, Office of the Surgeon General.

U.S. Department of Health and Human Services, Centers for Disease Control and Prevention, National Center for Chronic Disease Prevention and Health Promotion, Office on Smoking and Health. (2004a). *The health consequences of smoking: A report of the Surgeon General* [Atlanta, GA]. Washington, DC: For sale by the Supt. of Docs., U.S. GPO.

U.S. Department of Health and Human Services. (2004b). *Fetal alcohol syndrome: Guidelines for referral and treatment.* Retrieved June 21, 2009, from http://www.cdc.gov/ncbddd/fas/documents/FAS_guidelines_accessible.pdf

U.S. Department of Health and Human Services, Center for Disease Control and Prevention, Coordinating Center for Health Promotion, National Center for Chronic Disease Prevention and Health Promotion, Office on Smoking and Health. (2006). *The health consequences of involuntary exposure to tobacco smoke: A report of the Surgeon General* [Atlanta, GA]: Washington, DC.

U.S. Department of Health and Human Services. (2009). *Rethinking drinking offers tools to assess and change risky drinking habits.* National Institute on Alcohol Abuse and Alcoholism (NIAAA). Doc: 301-443-3860.

Ventura, S. J., Hamilton, B. E., Matthews, T. J., & Chandra, A. (2003). Trends and variations in smoking during pregnancy and low birth weight: Evidence from the birth certificate. *Pediatrics, 111,* 1176–1180.

Warren, K. R., & Foudin, L. L. (2001). Alcohol related birth defects: The past, present and future. *Alcohol Research and Health, 25*(3), 153–158.

Wechsler, D. (1997). *Wechsler Adult Intelligence Scale* (3rd ed.). San Antonio, TX: The Psychological Corporation.

Wechsler, D. (2001). *Wechsler Individual Achievement Test* (2nd ed.). San Antonio, TX: The Psychological Corporation.

Wechsler, D. (2002). *Wechsler Preschool and Primary Scale of Intelligence* (3rd ed.). San Antonio, TX: The Psychological Corporation.

Wechsler, D. (2003). *Wechsler Intelligence Scale for Children* (4th ed.). San Antonio, TX: The Psychological Corporation.

Windham, G. C., Von Behren, J., Fenster, L., Schaefer, C., & Swan, S. H. (1997). Moderate maternal alcohol consumption and the risk of spontaneous abortion. *Epidemiology, 8,* 509–514.

RESOURCES

http://www.betterendings.org/FASFAE/
   parent.htm
http://www.psychiatry.emory.edu/
   PROGRAMS/GADrug/index.htm
http://www.guttmacher.org/statecenter/
   spib_SADP.pdf
http://www.nida.nih.gov/consequences/
   prenatal/
http://www.oig.hhs.gov/oei/reports/
   oei-03-90-02000.pdf

For Parents/Caregivers

http://www.archrespite.org/archfs49.htm
http://www.heretohelp.bc.ca

For Adoptive or Foster Parents

http://www.adoptivefamilies.com/articles
   .php?aid=741
http://drug-exposure.adoption.com/

5

Treatment Issues and Interventions with Young Children and Their Substance-Abusing Parents

Jeannette L. Johnson, Jan Gryczynski, and Jerry Moe

INTRODUCTION

Children of substance-abusing parents (COSAPs) are affected by the consequences of their parents' substance abuse, and some children are affected more than others. The risk factors that affect COSAPs include, but are not limited to, social support, opportunity structure, socio-economic status, education, and genetics. COSAPs appear to be especially vulnerable because they are exposed to multiple combinations of these factors. The single most potent risk factor, however, is their parent's substance-abusing behavior; this alone places them at biological, psychological, and environmental risk for a multitude of maladaptive behaviors (Johnson & Leff, 1999; Loukas, Zucker, Fitzgerald, & Krull, 2003; Peleg-Oren & Teichman, 2006; Stanger et al., 1999).

Between 2002 and 2007, an estimated 8.3 million children in the United States—over 1 in 10—lived with a parent who met criteria for substance abuse or dependence (Substance Abuse and Mental Health Services Administration [SAMHSA], 2009). Alcohol represents the most common substance of abuse: 7.3 million children lived with a parent who met criteria for past-year alcohol abuse or dependence. The 2001 National Household Survey on Drug Abuse (SAMHSA, 2009) estimated that almost 70 million children younger than 18 years of age lived with at least one parent who abused or was dependent upon alcohol or an illicit drug during the past year. While it is difficult to determine how many of these children fall into specific age categories, it has been estimated that COSAPs are over-represented in the youngest age groups (SAMHSA, 2009; see also SAMHSA, 1998). In the coming years as the youngest children mature, individuals with the life experiences and attendant vulnerabilities of growing up as a COSAP will constitute a growing proportion of adolescents and young adults.

The purpose of this chapter is to discuss the contribution of developmental processes to our understanding of COSAP experiences and to briefly present developmental psychopathology as a framework for the development of interventions for this group. We then review the intervention programs for young COSAPs that presently exist and argue for the strategy of promoting resilience as a unifying program component in the development of effective interventions.

EFFECTS OF LIVING WITH SUBSTANCE-ABUSING PARENTS

Since the turn of the twentieth century, many reports have described the lives of children of substance abusers (Elderton & Pearson, 1910; Pearson, 1910; Pearson & Elderton, 1910). As long ago as 1905, a physician in New York City who was studying the relationship between heredity and intelligence in over 55,000 school children noted how parental alcoholism affects children:

1. Alcohol at the threshold of life is a bar to success and a foe to health.
2. Alcohol, by destroying the integrity of nerve structures and lowering the standard of organic relations, launches hereditary influences which by continuous transmission gain momentum and potency and leave their impact upon gland and nerve until the mental faculties are demoralized, physical energies hopelessly impaired, and the moral nature becomes degenerate and dies.
3. If we are to make any material change in the ranks of mental deficients we must adopt methods of prevention as well as methods of cure.

    It is a momentous problem that confronts us. The spirit in which we meet it may be a possible aid or hindrance to its solution. (MacNicholl, 1905, p. 117)

Over 100 years have passed and the implications of these words are still with us. The life experiences of children living with substance-abusing parents are replete with stress, dislocation, or parental absence. In 1969, Margaret Cork described the life histories, feelings, and problems of children of alcoholics by conducting interviews with 115 boys and girls (aged 10 to 16) and gave us the first intimate look at the lives of children of alcoholics. The children described their lives as scary, without structure, and lonely. Later on, Kolar, Brown, Haertzen, and Michaelson (1994) interviewed 70 parents who were in methadone maintenance treatment about the life experiences of their children. Collectively, the parents reported on 188 children. Almost half of the parents reported that their children had repeated a grade in school, 19% of the children had been truant, and 30% had been suspended from school. A significant proportion of the COSAPs had been involved with the law or illicit substances. Many of the COSAPs had been in adoptive or foster care or a group home.

Early clinical observations recount the pain of childhood experiences among COSAPs (El-Guebaly & Offord, 1977, 1979; Jacob, Favorini, Meisal, & Anderson, 1978; Warner & Rosett, 1975). Later observations turned to scientific research that typically categorized studies into genetic, environmental, or psychosocial influences; family environment and disorders associated with a family history of substance abuse; biochemical and psychological factors; neuropsychological and neurophysiological functioning; and, drug-related factors (e.g., responsivity, sensitivity, exposure, and expectancies) (Hussong et al., 2008; Johnson & Leff, 1999; Sher, 1991). The reviews of the scientific literature consistently determined that COSAPs not only have different life experiences than children who are raised by non–substance abusers, but that these experiences affect the children differently and that there may even be familial subtypes (Johnson & Leff, 1999; Loukas et al., 2003; Puttler, Zucker, Fitzgerald, & Bingham, 1998). For example, Werner's (1986) longitudinal study comparing children of alcoholics without problems and children of alcoholics with problems (defined as serious delinquencies or mental health problems requiring treatment) revealed that the children of alcoholics with problems were primarily males who scored lower on verbal and quantitative cognitive measures. Cognitive deficits did not characterize the entire group of children of alcoholics; these deficits were only seen in a subgroup of male children. Werner (1986) subsequently proposed that the risks associated with parental alcoholism can be buffered by constitutional characteristics of the child. Additional research has argued that moderating variables or protective factors related to the intergenerational transmission of substance abuse can inhibit the expression of substance abuse in COSAPs (Luthar, 2003). The latest work in epigenetics suggests that this might be true; namely, that heritable alterations in gene expression may be caused by mechanisms other than changes in the DNA sequence, suggesting that resilience may prove to be a potent modifier of a genetic disease such as alcoholism or other drug abuse (Renthal & Nestler, 2008).

Parental substance abuse can disrupt family life significantly and especially raises stress within the family (Loukas et al., 2003). For example, Hussong et al. (2008) compared children of alcoholics and children of non-alcoholics on five classes of stressors that included physical health, general family stressors, family separation, financial difficulties, and peer relationships. Children of alcoholics reported more risk for general family stressors, family separation, and financial difficulty. Similarly, Bennett and her colleagues (Bennett & Wolin, 1986; Bennett, Wolin, Reiss, & Teitlebaum, 1987; Steinglass, Bennett, Wolin, & Reiss, 1987; Wolin, Bennett, & Noonan, 1979; Wolin, Bennett, Noonan, & Teitelbaum, 1980) showed that the degree of organization and disruption in the young child's alcoholic family can influence childhood outcome. Their research concluded that alcoholic families showing more stability, even when a parent drinks, produce fewer alcoholic adult children.

Clearly, young children who live with substance-abusing parents have different life experiences than children who live with parents who do not abuse substances (Sowder & Burt, 1980). Just how different these experiences are is what has been questioned and studied. Reports of violence, disruption, and neglect are common. For example, approximately 50–80% of all child abuse and neglect cases substantiated by child protective services involve some degree of substance abuse by the child's parents (U.S. Department of Health and Human Services [USDHHS], 1994). More recently, the National Council on Child Abuse and Family Violence (2010) reported that substance abuse exists in 40–80% of child-abusing families. Because circumstances vary from family to family, understanding the particular life experiences of COSAPs is essential if we are to develop effective interventions for them. In addition, it is essential to understand the impact of these experiences on normal childhood developmental processes.

DEVELOPMENTAL PROCESSES

Whether they grow up in alcohol- or drug-abusing homes or not, children face the challenges of each developmental stage with whatever psychological and biological resources they inherit, both those provided by their environment and those they intentionally or unintentionally develop themselves. What they inherit, what their environment provides, and what they create themselves interacts in every developmental stage and in every domain. Development may not be equal in all domains and, for example, biological development may be more advanced than social development. Nevertheless, it is a constantly interactive process across many different domains.

Across the life span, development is characterized by unique biological and psychosocial interactive changes in physical, cognitive, and psychological domains. Throughout development, physical appearance undergoes dramatic transformations, relationships with parents and others evolve in unique ways as the child moves from complete dependence to mutual independence, and biological and psychological functioning undergo rapid and sometimes dramatic fluctuation. In order to better understand the modifiers of behavior in young COSAPs, the issues facing each subsequent developmental period need to be addressed. Change, the primary activity of development manifested in the progression from earlier to later stages of maturation, is represented by constant flux. In infants, change, or developmental progression, may be apparent from day to day. In young children changes may appear from month to month, and as adulthood approaches, changes may only become apparent from year to year.

Developmental change is both a dynamic quantitative and qualitative process. Children do not simply learn more as they grow, they learn differently at different ages. When learning is quantitative, knowledge becomes additive; as children grow, they learn more. However, the qualitative process inherent in development is exemplified by *how* children learn; children learn about themselves and their environment in qualitatively distinct ways, depending upon their stage of development. Piaget's (1970, 1971) constructivist theory of equilibrium has described the nature of the developmental change process as one in which cognition is constantly being constructed through self-regulated activity (Kuhn, 1981). Self-regulated activity is characterized by adaption to the events, people, and objects in the environment in order to create balance, or equilibrium. Disruption of the normal developmental processes of childhood, such as those that occur in the families of substance abusers, has been posited to be a developmental pathway of risk (Zucker, Donovan, Masten, Mattson, & Moss, 2008). The background of this disruption is the child's attempt to create balance in a dysfunctional system. How can a child create balance, or equilibrium, in a home where the very nature of parental substance-abusing behavior constantly disrupts the balance of daily living? The child's self-regulated cognitive tasks (i.e., thinking, creating, remembering, etc.) are constantly in a state of disequilibrium.

DEVELOPMENTAL PSYCHOPATHOLOGY

Developmental psychopathology is an integrative perspective combining biological, psychobiological, and psychosocial paradigms from both normal developmental psychology and psychopathology in order to understand the continuities and discontinuities of behaviors over time (Rutter & Sroufe, 2000; Wenar & Kerig, 2006). For both the researcher and the clinician the dynamic process of development creates special problems, such as understanding the stability and instability of traits or the continuity and discontinuity of development. Developmental fluctuation is also complicated by the relationship between quantitative change (e.g., bone growth) and concurrent qualitative changes (e.g., increases in cognitive capacity), which vary as a function of individual developmental differences. The emergence of sex differences in cognition during early adolescence adds another layer of complexity to understanding the developmental process (Maccoby & Jacklin, 1974). These quantitative and qualitative processes underlie the unique experiences of the child living with substance-abusing parents.

Developmental Psychopathology as a Framework for Prevention and Intervention With Young COSAPs

In order to develop interventions for young COSAPs, it is necessary to unravel the nature of ontogenetic transactions and adopt an intervention model that takes into account the details of the child's developmental trajectory. Information gathered about the child should be sufficiently precise to identify the changes that have occurred and how these serve to preserve or modify more general bases of organization. The developmental perspective requires a comprehensive view of the individual child and the systems of which the child is a part. It is essential to take into account individual cognitive and emotional changes, and the family and social systems in which the children live. Assessment must focus on which problems tend to persist during development, and which do not; which early problems or combinations of problems predict later disorder; and which behaviors are normative and age-appropriate and which are not. Developmental psychopathology combines these multiple perspectives into one cohesive model (Rutter & Sroufe, 2000; Wenar & Kerig, 2006).

The framework of developmental psychopathology can be helpful in designing interventions for young COSAPs. If family disruption is a key consequence of parental drinking, young children from these families may not have the chance to progress through normal developmental stages. Instead, they often leap ahead and take on responsibilities for which they are not cognitively prepared. This disruption in the normal developmental progression has keen consequences for later behavior, as seen in the work of Jerry Moe (1993) and colleagues (Moe, Johnson, & Wade, 2007; 2008) who suggest that the main developmental tasks of COSAPs are disrupted by their chaotic family life and the compensatory role shifts they are required to take on. For example, young COSAPs are negatively affected when the main family caregiver (usually the mother) is heavily involved in alcohol or other drug abuse, when the child is still young, when the family becomes significantly involved in the abuse problem, when the family becomes socially isolated, and when there is a lack of an extended family to provide balance and encouragement to the child (Kumpfer, 1987; Kumpfer & DeMarsh, 1986b). Older children may have had to take care of the younger siblings by getting them ready for school in the morning if the parent was absent or not able to get up on time. Substance-abusing parents frequently do not provide the structure or discipline necessary for a family to function, but still expect their children to be competent at a wide variety of tasks (Kumpfer, 1987; Kumpfer & DeMarsh, 1986a). Interventions can be designed that help the older child understand that this caretaking role is not necessarily the norm for children.

Being the family caretaker is not the only consequence for children living in a home where the parents abuse substances. In some respects the parental behavior dictates the home environment for the child, and this behavior itself is dictated by what type of effects the drugs have on the parent. Methamphetamine has very different effects than heroin or alcohol, for example. It is in this environment that children must survive and they must act accordingly. Thus, caretaking is just one such role they take on prematurely. However, in the case of the child of a methamphetamine addict, the child is exposed to toxic chemicals, severely addicted adults wandering in the home, or the possibility of sexual abuse due to the nature of methamphetamine effects on adults which are known to increase sexuality. In this case, the child needs to focus on safety of self and would most likely find this safety outside of the home. The developmental task, then, would be to find the safe places in the environment where they could spend time (i.e., a friend's house, school clubs, church). Leaving the home is a premature developmental task and would require the child to learn advanced social skills.

Developmental psychopathology has been used to help design interventions for children of substance abusers. The developmental psychopathological model frequently forms the theoretical backdrop of the intervention and does not necessarily prescribe a particular intervention process or specific set of intervention activities. The model informs the intervention process. For example, family interventions have adopted developmental psychopathological models with great success (Alvarado & Kumpfer, 2000; Spoth, Redmond, Kahn, & Shin, 1997). In these family interventions, it is understood that child development occurs within the context of the family and that while the development of the child is adaptive within the family, outside of the family the same behavior would appear maladaptive. Successful family interventions using a developmental psychopathological foundation are based on the assumption that developmental change can be influenced by many different factors, and these interventions incorporate these factors into the environment. For example, they frequently educate parents not just about substance abuse, but about the basics of childhood development (to help parents understand what to expect from their child at different ages), the importance of dinnertime (to help parents understand the importance of appropriate social interaction in a family), or parenting skills (to help parents understand how to appropriately set limits, reward and discipline their children, for example). Thus, the developmental psychopathological model is inherent in many interventions for children of substance abusers because it does not decontextualize the intervention: It operates on many different levels in many different environments and assumes that the maladaptive behavior outside of the home can be adaptive inside of the home. In the next section, we will discuss the interventions designed specifically for COSAPs.

INTERVENTION PROGRAMS FOR COSAPs

Few programs for COSAPs can be considered truly evidence-based, rigorously evaluated, or specifically targeted for children of alcoholics or other substances abusers. Instead, most programs target the general youth population or children determined to be "at-risk" based on various criteria such as being a child of divorce, being homeless, or being a child living in a low socio-economic status neighborhood. Indeed, a review of prevention programs for children of problem drinkers expressed concern about the lack of demonstrated effectiveness for prevention interventions specifically targeting children of substance users (Cuijpers, 2005). There are numerous ethical and practical issues in designing, implementing, and evaluating programs for children of substance users. These issues have been previously discussed in great detail (Cuijpers, 2005; Emshoff & Anyan, 1991; Johnson & Leff, 1999; Kumpfer, 1999; Markowitz, 2004; Price & Emshoff, 1997; Williams, 1990). Different evaluation designs provide different levels of evidence, with the randomized experiment serving as the most rigorous design. Quasi-experimental designs utilizing non-randomized comparison groups (preferably matched on key characteristics) provide less conclusive evidence, although when properly formulated these can be a useful alternative when a randomized experiment is impractical or impossible. Evaluations that measure participants' change via a pre-/post-test without using another group as a basis of comparison represent the most basic design. While such designs certainly have a place in the literature, they are unable to provide definitive conclusions about program effectiveness.

Most programs for COSAPs have not been evaluated. While some programs show promising preliminary results, they are limited by small sample sizes (e.g., Clark, 1997; Horn & Kolbo, 2000; Izquierdo, 2001; Reinart, 1999). Some programs using sound theoretical and clinical frameworks were shown to be ineffective (see Gross & McCaul, 1992;

Scheer, 1996). The few published outcome studies in existence are generally dated, indicating a need for more evaluation research in this area. One exception is the Strengthening Families Program (SFP), which uses a holistic model to treat the whole family. The SFP is a family skills training program designed to increase resilience and reduce risk factors for behavioral, emotional, academic, and social problems in children 3–16 years old. It comprises three life-skills courses delivered in 14 weekly, 2-hour sessions to both parents and their children. It has shown exceptional success with multiple ethnic groups and in both rural and urban settings (DeMarsh & Kumpfer, 1986; Kumpfer, Alvarado, Smith, & Bellamy, 2002; Kumpfer, Alvarado, Tait, & Turner, 2002). Our search for evidence-based programs for young children of substance abusers identified only 17 programs. Appendix A lists 12 evidence-based intervention programs for COSAPs that were found in our search of the psychological, social work, and behavioral literature.

There is no common age range that is targeted in these programs, making it difficult to determine which programs are best for which ages. The age ranges of each of the programs vary considerably so that while some programs target the 6- to 12-year-old group, other programs target 8- to 13-year-olds, making it difficult to compare across programs or synthesize results. Despite this, most of the program findings show significant improvement in the measured outcomes (which also vary from program to program; there is no commonality among the programs in terms of outcome measurement). The third column of Appendix A lists the evaluation results for each intervention, as well as comments on the evaluation design (which is also variable). It is worth noting that the Student Assistance Program has consistently shown success across multiple studies, as has the Strengthening Families Program. Appendix B lists the remaining five programs found in our search that were evaluated without the application of a rigorous research design.

The successful programs for young children have as a common core a focus on the development of social skills and expression of feelings; this is exemplified by three programs: the Strengthening Families Program, Celebrating Families, and the Betty Ford Children's Program. While more program development and research is needed, such programs illustrate some of the strategies that have the potential to bolster resilience in the face of a challenging family environment. Two of the programs (Strengthening Families and Celebrating Families) are parent-skills training programs designed specifically for parents who have abused drugs but are in the early stages of recovery. Both parents and children receive education and experiential learning over multiple weeks with a focus on multiple themes such as goal setting, health, and communication. Many program components revolve around the development of social behaviors that increase communication, education about alcohol and drugs, and the experience of normative behaviors that exclude alcohol and drugs as a focal point of activity, such as having dinner together and talking about daily events. Family rituals, such as dinnertime, have been shown to protect against the adverse influences of parental substance abuse (Bennett et al., 1987). Conversely, the Betty Ford Children's Program is uniquely designed to work with children. In this program the children use art and games, along with storytelling and role plays, to help build social skills and increase their repository of resilience skills (see Moe, 1993; Moe et al., 2008 for more description).

SUMMARY

This chapter has discussed how a normal developmental trajectory in young children of substance abusers can be disrupted merely by being born to parents who abuse alcohol and/or other drugs. Successful programs for intervening in the lives of COSAPs typically focus on the development of resiliency in an effort to combat the deleterious effects of risk, which may not be possible to mitigate in many situations. This philosophy has met with great success with many children who experience stressful life situations (Radke-Yarrow & Sherman, 1990). Researchers and helping professionals have long identified a sub-group of children who grow up in homes with alcoholic parents and who seem to grow up relatively "invulnerable" to the detrimental effects of familial alcoholism. Early writing by Anthony and Cohler (1987) suggested that there may be sub-groups of children of substance abusers who, despite all odds, do, in fact, enjoy good health from birth, experience a positive environment at home, and develop rather normally into socialized, competent, and self-confident individuals. Certain children may be more competent in adapting to stressful living environments than others and are somehow able to compensate and cope with the various negative biological or environmental influences in their lives. Certain individuals may be able to manipulate their environment by choosing roles and goals that stabilize their developmental process and bring them the reinforcement they need to develop a positive self-image, and eventually a relatively healthy life. Other individuals may be able to master the processing of incoming data and to conceptualize these data in such a way as to choose positive behaviors in life which compensate for whatever problems are present. On the other hand, some children may not be able to do these things without the intervention of a caring adult (Werner & Johnson, 2004). This overview suggests these children can be taught skills in a relatively short period of time that will help them navigate an exceptionally difficult developmental terrain.

REFERENCES

Alvarado, R., & Kumpfer, K. L. (2000). Strengthening America's families. *Juvenile Justice, 7*(2), 8–18.

Anthony, E. J., & Cohler, B. J. (1987). *The invulnerable child.* New York: Guilford Press.

Apsler, R., Formica, S., Fraster, B., & McMahan, R. (2006). Promoting positive adolescent development for at-risk students with a student assistance program. *The Journal of Primary Prevention, 6,* 533–554.

Bennett, L. A., & Wolin, S. J. (1986). Daughters and sons of alcoholics: Developmental paths in transmission. *Alcoholism: Journal on Alcoholism and Related Addictions, 22*(1), 3–15.

Bennett, L. A., Wolin, S. J., Reiss, D., & Teitelbaum, M. A. (1987). Couples at risk for transmission of alcoholism: Protective influences. *Family Process, 26,* 111–129.

Clark, B. J. (1997). 'The fun kids club': Developing an effective school-based program for children at risk. *Journal of Psychohistory, 24*(4), 361–369.

Cork, M. R. (1969). *The forgotten children: A study of children with alcoholic parents.* Toronto, ON: General Publishing.

Cuijpers, P. (2005). Prevention programmes for children of problem drinkers: A review. *Drugs: Education, Prevention, and Policy, 12*(6), 465–475.

Davis, R. B., Wolfe, H., Orenstein, A., Bergamo, P., Buetens, K., Fraster, B., et al. (1994). Intervening with high risk youth: A program model. *Adolescence, 29*(116), 763–774.

DeMarsh, J., & Kumpfer, K. L. (1986). Family-oriented interventions for the prevention of chemical dependency in children and adolescents. *Journal of Children in Contemporary Society: Advances in Theory and Applied Research, 18*(122), 117–151.

DiCicco, L., Davis, R. B., Hogan, J., MacLean, A., & Orenstein, A. (1984). Group experiences for children of alcoholics. *Alcohol Health and Research World, 8,* 20–24.

Elderton, E. M., & Pearson, K. (1910). *A first study of the influence of parental alcoholism on the physique and intelligence of the offspring.* Eugenics Laboratory Memoir Series X (pp. 1–46). London: Cambridge University Press.

El-Guebaly, N., & Offord, D. R. (1977). The offspring of alcoholics: A critical review. *American Journal of Psychiatry, 134,* 357–365.

El-Guebaly, N., & Offord, D. R. (1979). On being the offspring of an alcoholic: An update. *Alcoholism: Clinical and Experimental Research, 3,* 148–157.

Emshoff, J. G. (1990). A preventive intervention with children of alcoholics. *Prevention in Human Services, 7*(1), 225–253.

Emshoff, J. G., & Anyan, L. L. (1991). From prevention to treatment: Issues for school-aged children of alcoholics. *Recent Developments in Alcoholism, 9,* 327–346.

Emshoff, J. G., & Price A. W. (1999). Prevention and intervention strategies with children of alcoholics. *Pediatrics, 103*(5, Pt. 2), 1112–1121.

Fertman, C. I., Fichter, C., Schlesinger, J., Tarasevich, S., Wald, H., & Zhang, X. (2001). Evaluating the effectiveness of student assistance programs in Pennsylvania. *Journal of Drug Education, 31*(4), 353–366.

Gross, J., & McCaul, M. E. (1992). An evaluation of a psychoeducational and substance abuse risk reduction intervention for children of substance abusers. *Journal of Community Psychology, Special Issue: Programs for Change: Office for Substance Abuse Prevention Demonstration Models,* 75–87.

Horn, K. A., & Kolbo, J. R. (2000). Using the cumulative strategies model for drug abuse prevention: A small group analysis of the choices program. *American Journal of Health Studies, 16*(1), 7–23.

Hussong, A. M., Bauer, D. J., Huang, W., Chassin, L., Sher, K. J., & Zucker, R. A. (2008). Characterizing the life stressors of children of alcoholic parents. *Journal of Family Psychology, 22*(6), 819–832.

Izquierdo, F. M. (2001). Un programa de prevencion con hijos de alcoholicos [A program of prevention with children of alcoholic parents]. *Anales de Psiquiatria, 17*(7), 313–318.

Jacob, T., Favorini, A., Meisel, S. S., & Anderson, C. M. (1978). The alcoholic's spouse, children and family interactions of the alcoholic: Substantive findings and methodological issues. *Journal of Studies on Alcohol, 39,* 1231–1251.

Johnson, J. L., & Leff, M. (1999). Children of substance abusers: Overview of research findings. *Pediatrics, 103*(5, Suppl.), 1085–1099.

Jrapko, A., Ward, D., Leakey, D., Hazelton, T., & Foster, T. (2003). *Family treatment drug court head start program.* Annual Report, October 1, 2002–September 20, 2003. Center for Applied Local Research.

Kolar, A. F., Brown, B. S., Haertzen, C. A., & Michaelson, B. S. (1994). Children of substance abusers: The life experiences of children of opiate addicts in methadone maintenance. *American Journal of Drug and Alcohol Abuse, 20*(2), 159–171.

Kuhn, D. (1981). The role of self-directed activity in cognitive development. In I. E. Sigel, D. M. Brodzinsky, & R. M. Golinkoff (Eds.), *New directions in Piagetian theory and practice* (pp. 353–358). Hillsdale, NJ: Lawrence Erlbaum Associates.

Kuhns, M. L. (1997). Treatment outcomes with adult children of alcoholics: Depression. *Advanced Practice Nursing Quarterly, 3*(2), 64–69.

Kumpfer, K. L. (1987). *Prevention services for children of substance-abusing parents.* National Institute on Drug Abuse Final Technical Report (R18-DA-02758-101/02 and DA-03888-01).

Kumpfer, K. L. (1999). Outcome measures of interventions in the study of children of substance-abusing parents. *Pediatrics, 103*(5, Suppl.), 1128–1144.

Kumpfer, K. L., Alvarado, R., Smith, P., & Bellamy, N. (2002). Cultural sensitivity and adaptation in family-based prevention interventions. *Prevention Science, 3*(3), 241–246.

Kumpfer, K. L., Alvarado, R., Tait, C., & Turner, C. (2002). Effectiveness of school-based family and children's skills training for substance abuse prevention among 6-8-year-old rural children. *Psychology of Addictive Behaviors, 16*(Suppl. 4), S65–S71.

Kumpfer, K. L., & DeMarsh, J. (1986a). Family-oriented interventions for the prevention of chemical dependency in children and adolescents. In S. G. Ezekoye, K. L. Kumpfer, & W. J. Bukoski (Eds.), *Childhood and chemical abuse: Prevention and intervention* (pp. 219–233). New York: Haworth Press.

Kumpfer, K. L., & DeMarsh, J. (1986b). *Prevention strategies for children of drug-abusing parents.* Proceedings of the 34th Annual International Congress on Alcoholism and Drug Dependence, Calgary, Alberta.

Kumpfer, K. L., Molgaard, V., & Spoth, R. (1996). The Strengthening Families Program for the prevention of delinquency and drug use. In R. D. Peters &

R. J. McMahon (Eds.), *Preventing childhood disorders, substance abuse, and delinquency* (pp. 241–267). Thousand Oaks, CA: Sage.

Loukas, A., Zucker, R. A., Fitzgerald, H. E., & Krull, J. L. (2003). Developmental trajectories of disruptive behavior problems among sons of alcoholics: Effects of parent psychopathology, family conflict, and child undercontrol. *Journal of Abnormal Psychology, 112*(1), 119–131.

Luthar, S. S. (2003). Maternal drug abuse versus other psychological disturbances: Risk and resilience among children. In S. S. Luthar (Ed.), *Resilience and vulnerability: Adaptation in the context of childhood adversities* (pp. 104–129). New York: Cambridge University Press.

Maccoby, E. E., & Jacklin, C. N. (1974). *The psychology of sex differences.* Stanford, CA: Stanford University Press.

MacNicholl, T. A. (1905). A study of the effects of alcohol on school children. *The Quarterly Journal of Inebriety, 27,* 113–117.

Maguin, E., Zucker, R. A., & Fitzgerald, H. E. (1994). The path to alcohol through Conduct problems: A family-based approach to very early intervention with risk. *Journal of Research on Adolescence, 4*(2), 249–269.

Markowitz, R. (2004). Dynamics and treatment issues with children of drug and alcohol abusers, In S. Straussner & L. Ashenberg (Eds.), *Clinical work with substance-abusing clients* (2nd ed., pp. 284–302). New York: Guilford Press.

Moe, J. (1993). *Discovery: Finding the buried treasure.* Dallas, TX: ImaginWorks.

Moe, J., Johnson, J. L., & Wade, W. (2007). Resilience in children of substance users: In their own words. *Substance Use & Misuse, 42*(2), 381–398.

Moe, J., Johnson, J. L., & Wade, W. (2008). Evaluation of the Betty Ford Children's Program. *Journal of Social Work Practice in the Addictions, 8*(4), 464–489.

Morehouse, E., & Tobler, N. S. (2000). Preventing and reducing substance use among institutionalized adolescents. *Adolescence, 35*(137), 1–28.

National Abandoned Infants Assistance Resource Center. (2005). Celebrating families: an innovative approach to working with substance abusing families. *The Source Newsletter, 14*(1), 6–10.

National Council on Child Abuse and Family Violence. (2010, January 24). *Parental substance abuse: A major factor in child abuse and neglect.* Retrieved from http://www.nccafv.org/parentalsubstanceabuse.htm

Pearson, K. (1910). *Supplement to the memoir entitled: The influence of parental alcoholism on the physique and ability of the offspring: A reply to the Cambridge economists. Questions of the day and of the fray, No. I*(1–3). London: Cambridge University Press.

Pearson, K., & Elderton, E. M. (1910). *A second study of the influence of parental alcoholism on the physique and intelligence of the offspring. Eugenics Laboratory Memoir Series XIII, 1–35.* London: Cambridge University Press.

Peleg-Oren, N. (2002). Drugs—Not here!—Model of group intervention as preventive therapeutic tool for children of drug addicts. *Journal of Drug Education, 32*(3), 245–259.

Peleg-Oren, N., & Teichman, M. (2006). Young children of parents with substance use disorders (SUD): A review of the literature and implications for social work practice. In S. L. A. Straussner & C. H. Fewell (Eds.), *Impact of substance abuse on children and families: Research and practice implications* (pp. 49–62). New York: Haworth.

Piaget, J. (1970). *Genetic epistemology.* New York: Norton and Company.

Piaget, J. (1971). *Biology and knowledge: An essay on the relations between organic regulations and cognitive processes.* Chicago: University of Chicago Press.

Price, A. W., & Emshoff, J. G. (1997). Breaking the cycle of addiction: Prevention and intervention with children of alcoholics. *Alcohol Health and Research World, 21*(3), 241–247.

Puttler, L. I., Zucker, R. A., Fitzgerald, H. E., & Bingham, C. R. (1998). Behavioral outcomes among children of alcoholics during the early and middle childhood years: Familial subtype variations. *Alcoholism: Clinical and Experimental Research, 22*(9), 1962–1972.

Quittan, G. A. (2004). *An evaluation of the impact of Celebrating Families program and Family Drug Treatment Court (FDTC) on parents receiving family reunification services.* Retrieved from www.preventionpartnership.us/pdf/recent_evaluation2.pdf

Radke-Yarrow, M., & Sherman, T. (1990). Hard growing: children who survive. In J. Rolf, A.S. Masten, D. Cicchetti, K. H. Nüechterlein, & S. Weintraub (Eds.), *Risk and protective factors in the development of psychopathology* (pp. 97–119). New York: Cambridge University Press.

Reinart, D. F. (1999). Group intervention for children of recovering alcoholic parents. *Alcoholism Treatment Quarterly, 17*(4), 15–27.

Renthal, W., & Nestler, E. J. (2008). Epigenetic mechanisms in drug addiction. *Trends in Molecular Medicine, 14*(8), 341–350.

Rutter, M., & Sroufe, L. A. (2000). Reflecting on the past and planning for the future of developmental psychopathology. *Development and Psychopathology, 12*(3), 265–296.

Scheer, D. A. (1996). *Group therapy for children of alcoholics: An outcome study of a group curriculum for children of alcoholic parents.* Unpublished doctoral dissertation, University of Louisville.

Sher, K. J. (1991). *Children of alcoholics: A critical appraisal of theory and research.* Chicago: University of Chicago Press.

Short, J. L., Roosa, M. W., Sandler, I. N., Ayers, T. S., Gensheimer, L. K., Braver, S. L., et al. (1995). Evaluation of a preventive intervention for a self-selected subpopulation of children. *American Journal of Community Psychology, 23*(2), 223–248.

Sowder, B. J., & Burt, M. (1980). *Children of heroin addicts: An assessment of health, learning, behavioral, and adjustment problems.* New York: Praeger.

Spoth, R. L., Redmond, C., Kahn, J. H., & Shin, C. (1997). A prospective validation study of inclination, belief, and context predictors of family-focused prevention involvement. *Family-Process, 36*(4), 403–429.

Springer, J. F., Phillips, J. L., Phillips, L., & Cannady, L. P. (1992). CODA: A creative therapy program for children in families affected by abuse of alcohol or other drugs. *Journal of Community Psychology. Special Issue: Programs for change: Office for Substance Abuse Prevention Demonstration Models,* 55–74.

Stanger, C., Higgins, S. T., Bickel, W. K., Elk, R., Grabowski, J., Schmitz, J., et al. (1999). Behavioral and emotional problems among children of cocaine- and opiate-dependent parents. *Journal of the American Academy of Child Psychiatry, 38*(4), 421–428.

Steinglass, P., Bennett, L. A., Wolin, S. J., & Reiss, D. (1987). *The alcoholic family.* New York: Basic Books.

Substance Abuse and Mental Health Services Administration, Office of Applied Studies. (1998). *Analyses of substance abuse and treatment need issues, OAS Analytical Series #A-7*. Publication No. SMA 98-3227. Rockville, MD: Department of Health and Human Services.

Substance Abuse and Mental Health Services Administration. (2006). *Model programs Web site*. Retrieved February 12, 2006, from www.modelprograms. samhsa.gov

Substance Abuse and Mental Health Services Administration, Office of Applied Studies. (2009, April 16). *The NSDUH Report: Children living with substance-dependent or substance-abusing parents: 2002 to 2007*. Rockville, MD: U.S. Department of Health and Human Services.

U.S. Department of Health and Human Services. (1994). *Protecting children in substance abusing families*. Washington, DC: National Center on Child Abuse and Neglect.

Warner, R. H., & Rosett, H. L. (1975). The effects of drinking on offspring. *Journal of Studies on Alcohol, 36*(11), 1395–1420.

Wenar, C., & Kerig, P. (2006). *Developmental psychopathology: From infancy through adolescence* (5th ed.). Boston: McGraw-Hill.

Werner, E. E. (1986). Resilient offspring of alcoholics: A longitudinal study from birth to age 18. *Journal of Studies on Alcohol, 47*, 34–40.

Werner, E. E., & Johnson, J. L. (2004). The role of caring adults in the lives of children of alcoholics. *Substance Use and Misuse, 39*(5), 699–720.

Williams, C. N. (1990). Prevention and treatment approaches for children of alcoholics. In M. Windle, & J. S. Searles (Eds.), *Children of alcoholics: Critical perspectives* (pp. 187–216). New York: Guilford.

Wolin, S. J., Bennett, L. A., & Noonan, D. L. (1979). Family rituals and the recurrence of alcoholism over generations. *American Journal of Psychiatry, 136*(4B), 589–593.

Wolin, S. J., Bennett, L. A., Noonan, D. L., & Teitelbaum, M. A. (1980). Disrupted family rituals: A factor in the intergenerational transmission of alcoholism. *Journal of Studies on Alcohol, 41*(3), 199–214.

Zucker, R. A., Donovan, J. E., Masten, A. S., Mattson, M. E., & Moss, H. B. (2008). Early developmental processes and the continuity of risk for underage drinking and problem drinking. *Pediatrics, 121*, S252–S272.

Appendix A

Evidence-Based Programs
for COSAPs

Program	Format and Content Overview	Evaluation Results	Client Profile	Source
Strengthening Families Program (SFP)	**Format:** Intervention includes entire family, 14–18 2–3 hour sessions in the community. **Content:** *Parents:* AOD education, communication skills, and techniques to guide children's behavior. *Family:* Practice skills through role playing.	Randomized controlled trial—Program reduced risk factors such as delinquency, increased resilience, decreased AOD use among children of AOD abusers. Note: Program has been modified for various ethnocultural groups. Minor cultural revisions were more effective than major revisions. 15 replications have had favorable results. Originally developed for families with parents in AOD treatment, but has been used with various populations.	Originally for at-risk families with 6–12-year-old children. Adaptations have included younger children and teenagers as well.	Kumpfer, Molgaard, & Spoth (1996); Review in Price & Emshoff (1997); Emshoff & Price (1999)
CASASTART	**Format:** Comprehensive services, with intensive case management. **Content:** social support, family services, educational services, activities, mentoring, juvenile justice intervention, incentives.	Randomized quasi-experimental evaluation in multiple sites. Results: higher positive peer influences, less association with deviant peers, reduced AOD use. SAMHSA Model Program.	8–13-year-old children at-risk. Family substance abuse is one of four risk areas necessary for eligibility.	SAMHSA (2006)
Celebrating Families! (CF!)	**Format:** Program implemented through drug courts; 15 weekly, 90-minute sessions, followed by 30-minute structured family activity. **Content:** various components aiming at fostering resilience, social support, activities, parenting classes, anger management, refusal skills, AOD education, providing recovery resources for parents, etc.	Early evaluation results (purposive sample, 78 parents: study demonstrated that Celebrating Families had 72% reunification rates, where standard services had 37% reunification rates) (Quittan, 2004). Another evaluation (Jrapko, Ward, Leakey, Hazelton, & Foster, 2003) showed increases in knowledge about AOD and its impact on the family, healthy living skills, and parental reports of improvements in their children's coping skills, decision making, and ability to positively express feelings.	Families affected by parental substance abuse through CJ involvement, separate age-appropriate groups (adolescent, pre-adolescent, children, parents).	Quittan (2004); Jrapko et al. (2003); Review in NAIARC (2005)

Stress Management and Alcohol Awareness Program (SMAPP)	**Format:** 8-week, school-based competency-building group intervention. **Content:** building self-esteem, alcohol education, coping skills. Later, a "personal trainer" component was added, where someone met with children once weekly to reinforce skills learned in program.	Used randomized delayed-treatment control group. 9–11-year-old COAs more likely than nonparticipant COAs to display increased knowledge, social support, and emotion-focused coping behavior. Increased problem-solving and social competence reported by teachers. No difference in outcome for groups who received personal trainer component vs. those who did not. Unintended effect: significantly more participants believed alcohol can reduce tension.	Elementary school COAs.	Short et al. (1995); Review in Price & Emshoff (1997); Emshoff & Price (1999)
Students Together and Resourceful (STAR)	**Format:** Group school-based intervention. **Content:** Alcohol education and effects on family, increase social competence skills (problem-solving, decision making, stress management, and alcohol refusal).	Randomized wait-list control design comparing participants with nonparticipant COAs over time. Results: participants established stronger social relationships, sense of control, improved self-concept, increases in number of friends and perceived social support. Decreased loneliness and depression.	Children 11–14 with substance abuse in family.	Emshoff (1990); Review in Price & Emshoff (1997); Emshoff & Price (1999)
Cambridge and Sommerville Program for Alcoholism Rehabilitation	**Format:** As part of comprehensive treatment program, COA service sessions provided by staff in school and community settings and by peer leaders in after-school sessions. **Content:** Basic family and alcohol education and coping skills. COA-specific groups and basic open group.	Comparison of COAs in COA-specific group with COAs and non-COAs in basic open groups. COA-specific groups resulted in more COAs being willing to discuss problems and feelings than COAs and non-COAs in basic groups. More COAs in basic group drank less compared with COAs in COA-specific group or non-COAs in basic group.	High school students; Open to all children, but COA-specific groups also used.	DiCicco, Davis, Hogan, MacLean, & Orenstein (1984); Davis et al. (1994); Review in Price & Emshoff (1997); Emshoff & Price (1999)

(Continued)

119

Program	Format and Content Overview	Evaluation Results	Client Profile	Source
Dando Fuerza a La Familia	**Format:** Culturally-appropriate adaptation of Strengthening Families Program. 14-week intervention, once per week for 2 hours. **Content:** Monthly focus groups with parents, 16 educational/recreational activities per year for families, monthly 2-hour psycho-educational groups. Children were taught prosocial skills.	Experimental design with pre-/post-test. Increased educational aspirations, school performance, attendance, and knowledge of ATOD consequences between pre-/post-test for experimental group. Children in the experimental group also showed improved interaction with peers and reduction of violent behavior between pre- and post-test. Parents showed increase in bonding with children and effective control techniques between pre-/post-tests. (Precise differences between experimental and control group are not shown in source document.)	Mexican-American COSAPs ages 6–8 whose parents had been in treatment in the last year.	SAMHSA (2006)
Strengthening the Bonds of Chicano Youth and Families	**Format:** Community-based program for at-risk rural Chicano youth using interventions for youth and families. COSAP status is one of the risk factors for admission. Youth involved for an average of 1.6 years. **Content:** Four domains: Barrio life (community), School, Family, and Individual/Peer. Also uses camps, informal talks, peer support, and workshops. Also includes a homework center and a theater project.	Experimental design with control groups, but used pre-post only. Significant differences in pre-/post-test scores in family relations domain for intervention group, but not control. Significant decrease in AOD use from pre-post test for treatment group, no difference in control.	At-risk Chicano youth. Recruitment of siblings of SAs, COSAPs, juvenile delinquents, at-risk of teen parenthood, school failure risk, and youth living in public housing.	SAMHSA (2006)

Program	Description	Sample	Citation
Michigan State University Multiple Risk Child Outreach Program	**Format:** 10-month intervention with 28 sessions based on Oregon Social Learning Center's Parent-training protocol. **Content:** Two phases—*Phase 1:* child management skills through weekly sessions with families and telephone contacts 3 times a week. *Phase 2:* 12 bi-weekly face-to-face sessions with at least weekly phone contacts.	Families of fathers in sample were assigned to one of three groups—both parents, mothers only, or control. Intervention showed significant effects on negative, prosocial, and affectionate behavior at post-test. However, only prosocial behavior remained significant after 6-month follow-up. Intervention was specifically to prevent the development of conduct problems.	Families, but focus on the parents. Sample of 104 alcoholic fathers convicted of drunk driving (final $N = 81$ families). Children's mean age at time of contact was 4.4 yrs.	Maguin, Zucker, & Fitzgerald (1994)
Name not available	**Format:** Group format, either self-help or psychotherapy. **Content:** Alcohol prevention information and social support.	Randomized clinical trial with quasi-experimental design comparing psychotherapy, self-help, and control—both psychotherapy and self-help were effective in decreasing depression compared to control.	College-aged children of alcoholics.	Kuhns, 1997
Children of Drug Abusers and Alcoholics	**Format:** Two 12-week components, one each for families and children. **Content:** Small group activities including art and play therapy. Family interaction group once a week with parent.	Results showed increased competence and improved behavior measured by Child Behavior Checklist. However, this was only a pre-post design with no control group.	4-10-year-old at-risk children living with parent/guardian who abuses substances.	Springer, et al. (1992); Review in Emshoff & Price (1999).

(Continued)

Program	Format and Content Overview	Evaluation Results	Client Profile	Source
Student Assistance Programs (RSAP)	**Format:** Comprehensive program providing a range of prevention and early intervention services for high-risk adolescents institutionalized in residential facilities. Individual and small group services. **Content:** Includes assessment, small group role playing, prevention and education, group counseling, referral, facilitation of 12-step involvement, all integrated into the residential facility, specialized group, and individual services for COAs/ COSAPs.	Outcome evaluation with cross-sectional internal and external comparison groups of youth who were institutionalized but did not participate in program. Participants showed marked reductions in alcohol, marijuana, and tobacco use from pre-post compared with comparison groups. Program was effective in preventing and reducing substance use, with greater impact related to higher intervention dosage.	High-risk adolescents (14–17 years old) living in residential facilities. (Parental AOD abuse a typical risk factor in intervention population).	Apsler, Formica, Fraster, & McMahan (2006); Fertman et al. (2001); Morehouse & Tobler (2000)
Betty Ford Children's Program	**Format:** Four full days of program activities that include caretaker involvement on the last 2 days. **Content:** Playtime, AOD knowledge, problem solving, social skills, talking about family experiences.	Pre-post test using comprehensive psychological battery. COSAPs showed positive changes in social skills, decreases in loneliness, and the ability to recognize that they cannot control their parent's substance use behavior.	160 male and female children aged 7–12.	Moe et al. (2008)

Appendix B

Nonevaluated Programs
for COSAPs

Program	Format and Content Overview	Evaluation Results	Client Profile	Source
"The Fun Kids Club"	**Format:** Small group, school-based program. **Content:** Eight group sessions targeting various risk factors including hyper-activity, low self-esteem, poor impulse control, etc.	Two pilot groups of 6 or 7 children, total *N* = 13. All participants showed improvement in grades and reduction in hyperactivity or withdrawal behavior.	6–7-year-old 1st and 2nd graders from families with history of alcohol abuse who were at-risk of school failure.	Clark (1997)
Name not given, group intervention for children of parents in treatment for alcoholism	**Format:** Weekly 1-hr meetings for COAs whose parents were in treatment, led by a family thera-pist. **Content:** Various experiential activities and games.	Pre-/post-test only. *N* = 9 in treatment group, comparison group matched on age and sex. However, comparison group was drawn from a private school (non-COAs, whose parents were not in treat-ment), with higher mean family income for children in the comparison group. Evaluation based on parent and teacher reports, COA screening test, Behavior Assessment System for Children, and re-searcher scoring of various drawings by children. Results showed improvements in self-reliance and fewer signs of depres-sion. No improvements in self-esteem or social skills, but COA subjects within nor-mal range at baseline.	Mean age 9.4 years, children of parents in treatment for alcoholism.	Reinart (1999)

CHOICES Program	**Format:** 11 sessions, 1 hour a week. School-based, using a "cumulative strategies model" utilizing a synthesis of different approaches to prevention. **Content:** Three components: Structured support groups, Healthy Lifestyle Peer Mentors, and Academic Channels to Ensure Success. Program led by school counselor.	Random assignment to various combinations of program components and a delayed intervention group ($n = 3$). Total N = 16. Repeated Measures Baseline design. Results: Children who did two components as opposed to one or none had improvements in self-esteem, social skills, and attachment to school.	8–11-year-old 3rd and 4th grade COAs (COA status judged by self-report and subsequent counselor assessment).	Horn & Kolbo (2000)
Constructivist Program of Prevention (Spanish Study)	**Format:** Autobiographic group based on constructive activities and the life story. Eight sections applied in two sessions. **Content:** Positive and negative experiences, family, AOD, critics, decision making and problem solving.	Pre-/post-test. All group members increased their self-concept, locus of control, and self-esteem.	9 teenage COAs, 14–16 yrs old, 2 females and 7 males in Spain.	Izquierdo (2001)

6

Treatment Issues and Interventions With Adolescents From Substance-Abusing Families

Judy Fenster

INTRODUCTION

Parents who abuse substances place their children at environmental, biological, and psychological risk of developing dysfunctional or maladaptive behaviors. The adolescent, neither a child nor an adult, and more prone to impulsive actions and risky behaviors than either the child or the adult, may be especially vulnerable to the consequences of parental substance abuse. By the same token, adolescents may be endowed with strengths and competencies that uniquely equip them to endure the stresses and demands of living with a substance-involved parent.

In the decade between ages 10 and 20, children face distinct developmental challenges. The tasks of adolescence, including going through puberty and discovering and constructing one's social and sexual identities, can be daunting. Ego psychologist Erik Erikson (1982) posited that adolescents in this stage of psychosocial development are struggling to form their own identity, and that those who fail to do so transition into adulthood ill-prepared to handle the social-emotional demands of that era. On the other hand, the adolescent has newly acquired cognitive and psychological tools with which to confront life, as noted by theorist Jean Piaget, who viewed adolescents entering this "stage of formal operations" as capable of abstraction and rational thinking (Inhelder & Piaget, 1958).

Adolescent children of substance-abusing parents are likely to confront a constellation of stress factors within the family and larger ecosystem. Depending upon individual characteristics, such as temperament, intellectual abilities, and personality, as well as a host of environmental factors, some teens may have the resiliency to bounce back and even learn from adverse experiences related to their parents' substance use. Most will not face long-term negative consequences. However, those who falter under the burden of parental substance use and its correlates may need help getting back on track developmentally.

This chapter outlines the demographic patterns and the risk and protective factors faced by adolescents with a substance-abusing parent. Assessment and treatment issues are discussed, and strategies for working with adolescents in various stages of development are presented.

THE IMPACT OF PARENTAL SUBSTANCE ABUSE ON THE ADOLESCENT

It has been estimated that upwards of 10% of adolescent children live with a mother or father who actively abuses alcohol or illicit drugs (Substance Abuse and Mental Health Services Administration [SAMHSA], 2008). Moreover, about 23% of children are raised by a parent who has abused alcohol at some point in his or her life (Eigen & Rowden, 2000). Although less susceptible than younger children to physical harm by a parent abusing alcohol or other drugs, adolescents with substance-involved parents are at high risk for suffering other negative consequences affecting their physical, emotional, and behavioral health. In fact, it has been argued that, compared with younger children, teenage children of substance abusers are at greater risk, since, on average, they have had more prolonged exposure to their parents' substance use and its consequences (Moss, Clark, & Kirisci, 1997). The section below summarizes the research on social-emotional, behavioral, and substance use outcomes of adolescent children with substance-involved parents.

Health, Mental Health, and Behavioral Consequences of Parental Substance Abuse

Children of alcoholics are two-to-four times more likely than peers with nonalcoholic parents to develop a psychiatric disorder by the time they reach age 15 (Lynskey & Fergusson, 1994) and are also more apt to have health problems (Woodside, Coughey, & Cohen, 1993). Impulsivity and sensation-seeking—personality traits often found in younger children of alcoholics—are also prevalent among adolescents from alcoholic homes (Sher, 1997). Emotional problems reported in this group include depression, anxiety, and feelings of isolation (Chassin, Pitts, DeLucia, & Todd, 1999). Additionally, female adolescents from alcoholic families are at increased risk for eating disorders and teen pregnancy (Mylant, Ide, Cuevas, & Meehan, 2002).

Adolescent children of illicit drug-users have been reported to have similar outcomes as those from alcoholic homes. Teenagers raised by drug-addicted parents have been found to have higher rates of depression and anxiety, to exhibit a more negative self-image, and to feel more fearful or lonely, compared with other teenagers (Bauman & Dougherty, 1983; Fisher & Harrison, 2000; Perez-Bouchard, Johnson, & Ahrens, 1993). They are also more likely than other teens to experience behavioral problems such as conduct disorder, school problems such as truancy and lower academic functioning, and run-ins with the law (McGrath, Watson, & Chassin, 1999).

Positive Outcomes in Teens With Substance-Abusing Parents

A small number of studies have reported positive outcomes such as greater resiliency among teens exposed to parental substance abuse. For example, Gavriel-Fried and Teichman (2007) found mid-adolescent-aged children of alcoholics to possess a greater sense of ego identity and genuineness than a comparison group of peers with nonaddicted parents. It has been hypothesized that experiencing unpleasant effects of a parent's addiction may motivate some adolescents to eschew using alcohol or other drugs while aiding them in developing coping strategies, skills, and values that protect them from experiencing negative effects and engaging in destructive behaviors, including substance abuse (Wolin & Wolin, 1993). However, to date, this link has not been established.

Parental Drug Use Patterns and the Effect on the Adolescent

Several studies have focused on specific characteristics of parental substance use and the subsequent impact on the social, emotional, and behavioral well being of their progeny. The parent's stage of recovery from addiction has been examined, with contradictory results. A longitudinal study of drug-using parents with HIV found that parental relapse increased substance use, peer conflict, and emotional distress in their adolescent children, though parental recovery, even when transient, had a positive effect on their teenagers' social-emotional behaviors (Lester et al., 2009). However, focusing only on alcohol use behaviors, an earlier research team found problematic drinking among middle adolescents to be unrelated to whether their alcoholic fathers were currently drinking or in recovery (Chassin et al., 1999). Chassin and her colleagues concluded that, while parental modeling of alcohol use may have an effect on preadolescent alcohol misuse, teenage drinking may be influenced and maintained through a different set of factors. It is also possible that gender mediates the impact of parental substance use, as there is some evidence that adolescent youth are more affected by maternal than paternal drug abuse (Ohannessian et al., 2004; Peiponen, Laukkanen, Korhonen, Hintikka, & Lehtonen, 2006).

Severity of substance use and drug use preferences have also been examined for their impact on the adolescent. Parents with more entrenched substance use problems have progeny who suffer more negative consequences than parents who are less severely addicted (Gance-Cleveland, Mays, & Steffen, 2008). Regarding drug of choice, though cannabis is the most commonly used illicit drug, it is least likely to result in a parent being unable to fulfill their filial duties (Marmorstein, Iacono, & McGue, 2009; SAMHSA, 2007). On the other extreme, methamphetamine users can develop dependence quickly, often causing parents to neglect or abuse their children (Swetlow, 2003). Those who produce methamphetamine in their homes may further expose their children to harm via hazardous chemicals released in the process of manufacturing the drug.

Research suggests that children learn drug use habits from their parents differentially based on gender. Adolescent girls have been found to mimic their mothers' pill-taking habits (most commonly tranquilizers and painkillers), while sons share their fathers' preferences for cigarettes and alcohol (Annis, 1974). Since parenting a teenager can be challenging in the best of circumstances, the effect of the teen's behavior on the parent's substance use has also been examined. Studies have found deviant behavior in adolescents to raise stress levels in their substance-involved parents, thereby increasing the likelihood of more severe substance misuse among the latter (Lang, Pelham, Atkeson, & Murphy, 1999).

RISK AND PROTECTIVE FACTORS FOR ADOLESCENTS WITH SUBSTANCE-ABUSING PARENTS

During the past two decades, a number of studies have investigated factors that increase or decrease risk of negative consequences to the adolescent with a substance-abusing parent. These variables can be categorized as related to the individual adolescent, his or her family, and the broader environment.

Individual Characteristics

Children of substance abusers who affiliate with peers with deviant behaviors are more likely to abuse substances and engage in other deviant behaviors themselves. Additionally, teenagers with impulsive or sensation-seeking traits are more apt to engage in risky behaviors of all kinds. Poor school performance or attendance has also been identified as a risk factor in this group (National Institute on Drug Abuse [NIDA], 2002).

Factors that protect adolescent children of addicted parents have not been as thoroughly researched as risk factors. The focus has been mostly on identifying and analyzing "competence" among children of alcoholics. Other potential sources of resilience among adolescent offspring of substance users include average or above-average cognitive functioning, good coping skills, ability to follow rules, low tolerance for risk taking, optimistic outlook, moderate self-esteem, and self-awareness (Roosa, Beals, Sandler, & Pillow, 1990).

Familial Factors

Individuals who are more severely addicted and those with comorbid disorders (chemical dependency and mental illness) are least able to function adequately as parents, and thus place their children at greater risk for a range of adverse consequences (Bailey Hill, Oesterle, & Hawkins, 2006; Peiponen et al., 2006). The co-occurrence of antisocial personality and substance abuse in the parent is especially linked with poor outcomes for children and adolescents (Barnow, Ulrich, Grabe, Freyberger, & Spitzer, 2007). Among alcoholic parents, meting out overly harsh punishment and exposing their teenage children to more severe consequences of parental addiction are both related to alcohol abuse in the latter (Hill, Nord, & Blow, 1992). On the other hand, youth living with parents who, despite their addiction, are able to avoid divorce or separations, maintain family routines, enforce expectations for behavior, and meet their children's emotional needs fare better socially, emotionally, and behaviorally than youth with parents whose substance abuse results in a disruption of family ties and rituals (Bowser & Word, 1993; Brook, Brook, Whiteman, Gordon, & Cohen, 1990; Perez-Bouchard et al., 1993; Stewart & Brown, 1993).

Environmental and Cultural Factors

Environmental factors include school and community characteristics. Adolescents who perceive their school teachers as supportive are less likely to associate with deviant peers and, subsequently, less drawn to risky behaviors such as substance use (Suldo, Mihalas, Powell, & French, 2008). Having greater involvement in religious groups can also protect teens from negative effects of parental substance use (Szewczyk & Weinmuller, 2006; Wallace & Forman, 1998). Conversely, disorganized neighborhoods and those in which there is more violence and drug dealing are thought to increase risk to the child (Hawkins, Catalano, & Miller, 1992).

Cultural influences can sometimes mediate risk and protective factors. Puerto Rican teens who have drug-abusing fathers and who identify strongly with their culture—defined as having a high degree of Hispanic awareness, preferring the Spanish to the English language, and identifying with Puerto Rican friends—are less likely to use drugs than peers with weaker cultural ties (Brook, Whiteman, Balka, Win, & Gursen, 1998). Similarly, while black youth are more likely than white youth to say they have seen someone selling drugs in their neighborhood (USDHHS, 1995), living in such surroundings does not appear to increase rates of illicit drug use among black adolescents. It is hypothesized that this greater exposure serves a protective function in this group, in that black youth are forced to confront the negative consequences of drug use and learn a lesson from it (Wallace, 1999).

The Relationship Between Parental and Adolescent Substance Abuse

It has yet to be established whether children of illicit drug users inherit a tendency toward illicit drug use, since initial findings supporting this notion have failed to be replicated (Johnson & Leff, 1999). However, substantial research has proven children of alcoholics vulnerable to developing alcohol dependence (Chalder, Elgar, & Bennet, 2006; Ehringer, Rhee, Young, Corley, & Hewitt, 2006; Young et al., 2006). Alcohol is the drug of choice for adolescents in general as well as for teenage children of alcoholics. Once a teen with an alcoholic parent initiates alcohol use, they are at greater risk for developing alcohol problems earlier, escalating use more quickly, and developing more serious dependency than a child of non-addicted parents. Besides being correlated with interpersonal violence and a number of risky behaviors, alcohol and other drug use in adolescents is linked to accidental injuries, which is the primary cause of death among children in this age group (United States Department of Health and Human Services [USDHHS], 2007).

Adolescents are less sensitive than adults to negative effects of alcohol such as sedation and motor impairment (Spear & Varlinskaya, 2005; White et al., 2002). Thus, when they drink, they are physically able and more apt to consume more alcohol than the average adult and to engage in activities—such as drunk driving, fighting, or unprotected sex—that increase the risk of harm to self or others. Adolescents are also less prone to experience other negative effects of drinking such as intoxication and hangovers. This relative insensitivity to negative consequences—coupled with an increased sensitivity to positive effects of alcohol, such as stress reduction—may encourage greater alcohol consumption. Teenage children of alcoholics may be at even greater risk, since, when these teens drink, they experience greater stress reduction than teens of nonaddicted parents who drink (Finn, Zeitouni, & Pihl, 1990). Such a greater positive effect may lead children of alcoholics to drink more in order to ward off negative affects or otherwise decrease their stress levels.

PATHWAYS TO ADOLESCENT SUBSTANCE USE

Since adolescent substance abuse is the problem most frequently associated with having a substance-abusing parent, understanding mechanisms leading to adolescent substance use can help the clinician predict which teenagers are most at risk for encountering this type of trouble. The following are the three models that have been proposed to explain the onset of substance abuse in adolescents (Rice, Dandreaux, Handley, & Chassin, 2006):

- *Deviance Proneness.* Poor parenting and an unstable family environment lead to temperamental problems and cognitive dysfunction in the child, which in turn leads to poor academic performance and association with other children at risk for school failure, which raises the odds for initiation of substance use.
- *Stress and Negative Affect.* Offspring of substance-involved parents are exposed to stressful life events (such as numerous geographical relocations, financial crises, parental separation, legal problems, etc.) that may lead to chronic emotional distress in the adolescent and, subsequently, to substance use.
- *Substance Use Effects.* Teens who experience more positive and fewer negative side effects of using alcohol or other drugs may increase their intake, thus raising their risk of developing dependency.

Unfortunately, most of the research on pathways to substance initiation combined samples of children who have and those who have not endured parental substance abuse, making it difficult to separate out results by subgroup (see Ohannessian & Hesselbrock, 2008). In an effort to differentiate pathways for children of alcoholics and children of nonalcoholics, Molina, Chassin, and Curran (1994) utilized a control group. They discovered that low parental monitoring and negative affect increase the likelihood of teens associating with a peer group that supports the use of substances, thus leading to a higher risk of substance use disorders in young adolescent children of alcoholics. However, since they found the same mechanism to predict substance misuse among children of nonalcoholics, it remains to be seen whether teenage children of alcoholics who drink or use drugs are unique in the process through which they initiate substance use.

Long-Term Impact of Parental Substance Abuse on the Adolescent

A lack of longitudinal research has left open the question of whether problems occurring during adolescence are truly deficits, or just developmental "road bumps" that recede as the teen matures into adulthood. The few existing longitudinal studies of children of alcoholics suggest that the majority do *not* develop serious long-term social-emotional problems (Velleman & Orford, 1999; Werner & Smith, 1992). However, some lasting negative effects have been documented. Adults who as youths endured more adverse consequences of their parents' alcohol or drug addiction are more likely to experience depression and substance abuse as grown-ups, compared with those who suffered less adversity related to parental substance abuse (Anda et al., 2002). Adult children of alcoholics are also less likely to marry than those not raised in alcoholic homes. Those who do wed are more likely to marry into a family in which alcohol abuse is prevalent (Schoenborn, 1991) and to divorce (Call, 1998).

ASSESSMENT

Assessment of the adolescent with a substance-involved parent should be comprehensive and should focus on the previously identified psychological, behavioral, cognitive, and social-emotional spheres, as well as possible dysfunction in the family and greater environment. Protective processes, strengths, and resources should also be delineated.

Screening to Identify Adolescents
With a Substance-Involved Parent

It has been recommended that, since familial substance abuse can be insidious and family members secretive about it, health care providers screen *all* adolescents for substance use problems within their families, asking them simple questions such as "Have you ever felt that someone in your family or household should cut down on their drinking or drug taking?"

(Werner, Joffc, & Graham, 1999). Alternatively, standardized instruments can be used. Two screening tools appropriate for use with adolescent children of alcoholics are the Children of Alcoholics Screening Test (CAST), and the Family Drinking Survey. The CAST is a 30-item self-report measure that gauges the experiences and feelings of adolescents regarding their parents' drinking behaviors (Jones, 1982). The Family Drinking Survey, which assesses the effect of a parent's drinking on an adolescent's physical, emotional, and social health, can help clarify the impact on the teen of the parent's substance use (Whitfield, 1991). Both screening tools have been found to have the sensitivity and specificity to discern parental alcohol abuse and consequences to the adolescent (Sheridan, 1995).

Despite the existence of easy-to-use screening instruments, the stigma attached to having a substance-involved parent and fear of consequences to the family unit can make some adolescents reluctant to discuss problems of this sort with a professional. Thus, the clinician should possess good engagement skills and the ability to tune-in to indirect and nonverbal signs of possible dysfunction. Moreover, the issue of confidentiality can create barriers to collaboration unless it is clearly addressed at the beginning of the treatment process. Concern that their parents will be notified about information they share with their doctors is the number one reason adolescents cite for skipping health care appointments (Miller, Tebb, Williams, Neuhaus, & Shafer, 2007; Reddy, Fleming, & Swain, 2002). This result can be extrapolated to suggest the importance of informing adolescent clients early on of their right, as well as any limits, to confidentiality within the clinical setting, and dealing with any concerns adolescents may have about discussing their own and their parents' problems.

Assessment Issues

As is true with younger children, adolescent children of substance abusers may feel ashamed about their parent's drug use or the family disruption that often accompanies it, may have the added stress of trying to hide it from peers and adults, or may feel responsible to ameliorate its impact on the family system. Additionally, if a teen's parent uses illicit drugs, there may be feelings related to knowing that the parent is involved in illegal behaviors, or teen is being coerced into criminal activity to obtain, hold, or sell drugs for the parent (Dore, Kaufman, Nelson-Zlupko, & Granfort, 1996).

Some adolescents may have witnessed or been the victims of physical, sexual or emotional abuse in the home related to substance use (Brookoff, O'Brien, Cook, Thompson, & Williams, 1997). Others may have been forced to prematurely assume parenting duties, such as caring for younger siblings, managing the household, or supporting the family financially, which may have sharply limited their spending time with peers and engaging in other age-appropriate activities. These stresses, sacrifices, and additional responsibilities may burden them or tax them beyond their developmental capacities. Consequently, they may feel overwhelmed and may experience resentment, anxiety, depression, social inhibition, lack of trust, and low or labile self-esteem (Lynskey & Fergusson, 1994; Perez-Bouchard et al., 1993).

Adolescents with addicted parents may have a decreased learning capacity or may underperform academically (McGrath et al., 1999). They may experience problems in executive functioning such as planning, regulating emotion, and controlling impulses. Rather than signaling intellectual impairment, such cognitive dysfunction typically stems from worry or other negative feelings about the parent's substance use or its effect on the family. Irregular school attendance may also occur and may contribute to poor grades.

On a social-emotional level, adolescents from a substance-abusing family may feel alienated from their peers or family, may expect perfection from their every endeavor, may be excessively self-conscious, or may exhibit phobias. The younger adolescent may be afraid or averse to going to school, while the older adolescent may complain of feeling isolated, lonely, or emotionally numb. Even when performing adequately in school, they may underrate their academic ability and exhibit anxiety around educational assignments and exams. Teens reared in chaotic households may come to believe that they have no power to change or improve their lives. They may adapt an *external locus of control*, in which they believe that outside forces, rather than they themselves, control their destiny (Robinson & Rhoden, 1997). This can lead to a lack of initiative and motivation to learn how to navigate life's challenges and work toward personal goals.

The clinician should ask the adolescent about his or her parent's drug use patterns and its effect on the family. Is the substance misuse limited to one parent, or are both parents affected? How severe and how chronic is the parent's substance problem? To what degree has the adolescent been exposed to the parent's substance use and associated negative consequences? In what stage of recovery is the parent—are they currently using, relapsing, or abstaining?

How the family functions as a dynamic system should also be explored for strengths and vulnerabilities. Does the family eat dinner together most nights or participate in other family rituals? Do the parents maintain appropriate boundaries? To what extent do the parents monitor their adolescent children? What is the quality of the relationship among the adolescent, his or her siblings, and the parent(s)? Does conflict among family members occur, and if so, what is the nature and severity of it? Is the emotional atmosphere in the home one of warmth or coldness? Stability or unpredictability? Closeness, enmeshment, or disengagement? Is there any history of mental illness in the family? The extent of extrafamilial support from teachers, clergy, and other potential role models should also be explored, and data on the adolescent's physical and emotional health, coping strategies, peer relationships, and school performance obtained.

Since adolescents with an addicted parent are at increased risk for developing a substance use disorder, an assessment of substance use should be conducted. Although marijuana and alcohol problems are those most prevalent among general population teenagers admitted to substance abuse treatment, the clinician should also ask about stimulants, opiates, and prescribed medications, since misuse of these types of drugs is not uncommon among adolescents presenting for treatment (SAMHSA, 2007). The adolescent's substance use patterns, that is, whether the substance use is experimental, occasional, binge-related or chronic, should also be explored, as each pattern suggests different risks.

Professionals are advised to use caution when diagnosing adolescent substance abuse or dependence using standard criteria from the *Diagnostic and Statistical Manual of Mental Disorders (DSM-IV)*. Due to age, unique usage patterns, and decreased sensitivity to the effects of alcohol and other drugs, substance-involved adolescents may experience few of the negative symptoms described in the *DSM-IV*. Clinicians should instead look for disturbances in behavior, cognition, or mood, such as those described in the paragraphs above, that often accompany drug abuse (Segal & Stewart, 1996). Standardized instruments designed specifically for adolescents can also help determine the existence, extent, and impact of teenage substance misuse. One such instrument, the CRAFFT, which consists of six age-appropriate questions related to substance use, has been found to have good reliability and validity (Knight, Sherrit, Shrier, Harris, & Chang, 2002).

The teen's attitudes toward substance use and misuse should also be ascertained. Clarifying what the individual believes the alcohol or drug use will do for them can help uncover underlying personal and interpersonal dynamics that reinforce drug use. Outcome expectancies have been found to be an important predictor of drinking behaviors among adolescents and young adults. Teens who believe that drinking will help decrease stress, ease boredom, lift depression, or absolve them from responsibility for engaging in risky behaviors are likely to drink more and more often than those with less favorable attitudes toward alcohol (National Center on Addiction and Substance Abuse, 2003).

INTERVENTIONS

Treatment Strategies

To date, there have been few major studies evaluating the effectiveness of clinical interventions specifically for adolescents with substance-involved parents. One important investigation by Leichtling, Gabriel, Lewis, and Vander Ley (2006) utilized a sample of 221 adolescents in substance abuse treatment to compare treatment experiences and outcomes of offspring of substance abusers to those from non–substance-involved families. The authors found that adolescent children of substance abusers were more likely to have participated in both family and individual counseling sessions, in combination with group treatment. Although outcome data collected 1-year posttreatment demonstrated gains for both cohorts, children of substance abusers showed an even greater degree of change than their counterparts, manifested as greater decreases in substance use and externalizing behaviors. Type of treatment influenced outcome, in that teens with substance-involved parents were most likely to show psychosocial improvement if they participated in individual counseling, either in lieu of or in combination with group and/or family counseling.

Interestingly, at the 6-month data-collection point, involvement in family counseling was linked with an *increase* in substance use among adolescents from substance-involved families, an effect that was not observed among teens living with non–substance-abusing parents. The results of this study indicate that adolescents with substance-involved parents can benefit from treatment. Furthermore, though the study would need to be replicated before definitive principles for treatment could be inferred, results suggest that, for parents or teens in earlier stages of recovery, individual and group treatment for adolescents may be more effective than family treatment.

Despite the scarcity of published outcome studies on this population, the existing literature does provide principles and guidelines for professionals working with adolescents from substance-involved families. Below are suggestions for best practice drawn from research literature on interventions for adolescents in general and, where available, adolescent children of substance-abusing parents as well as clinical experiences of seasoned practitioners. Prior to discussing the specific intervention, it is important to be aware of the different needs of adolescents at different stages of development.

Intervention at Early, Middle, and Late Stages of Adolescence

Adolescents at various stages of development have diverse needs and experiences, and are involved differentially in social systems. Although best practice guidelines for working with adolescents from substance-involved families based on substage of development have yet to be established, substantial research has delineated psychological aspects of early, middle, and late adolescence. Issues that the clinician should be aware of when working with teenagers from specific age groups are discussed below.

Early adolescents (ages 10–14) are still somewhat attached to the family unit and more influenced by and dependent upon their parents. They need and expect more structure from parents and other adults. Toward the end of this first substage, puberty often begins, bringing with it physical and emotional changes that can be confusing and disorienting.

Typically, it is at this age that teens begin their journey toward discovering and choosing their social and sexual identities. Rebellion in the form of minor rule-breaking is not uncommon. This is also the age at which many children begin using alcohol and experimenting with other drugs. For these reasons, and toward the goal of early intervention, school-based and other preventive services providing psycho-education and support are often targeted to children in this cohort (Emshoff & Price, 1999).

In the middle stage of adolescence (ages 15–17), peers become more influential. This is the age at which many teens learn to drive, thus achieving a greater degree of physical independence from their parents. The middle-stage teen may also be expected to take on additional responsibility for household and caregiving duties. Concerns about dating, sexuality, and socializing are common. An adolescent entering this stage of development may resist efforts to "put the family back together" precisely at the point at which they are struggling to separate physically and emotionally from their parents and family. Thus, they may be less enthusiastic about entering family treatment or engaging in family activities prescribed by treatment providers (White & Savage, 2005). Helping youth in this age range strengthen their resolve and ability to resist peer influences to use drugs or engage in other risky behaviors can protect them from harmful consequences. Concurrently, their parents can be coached to support their striving for autonomy by providing them with age-appropriate responsibilities and granting them age-appropriate liberties, though continuing to monitor their activities and set limits as needed. Additionally, encouraging the entire family's participation in activities and traditions can promote or enhance bonds between parent and child.

Those in late adolescence (ages 18–20) are seen in the American culture as transitioning to adulthood. Older adolescents desire and expect more independence and less monitoring, and will need less structure from their parents and other adults. Some are at college, and others may be living on their own elsewhere. Vocational goals become a focus for most. Older adolescents will need to hone their skills in negotiating the larger world beyond their family and peer groups. Some may need help dealing with low self-esteem or other behavioral or mental health problems that arise as the environment demands more from them cognitively, socially, and emotionally. At this stage of development, it may be more feasible to treat the young adult separate from the family unit. Strategies that support autonomous functioning and build self-efficacy while providing guidance as needed around decision making and problem solving can be productive.

Individual-Level Intervention Strategies for Adolescents

Individual treatment of the adolescent should focus on issues identified during assessment, and should include educational, developmental, and psychosocial aspects of intervention. Regardless of the approach utilized, the overarching goal of treatment is to enhance adolescents' abilities to care for themselves emotionally, physically, and socially. Mitigating risk factors and strengthening resilience are additional objectives transcending treatment orientation.

The clinician working from a *psychodynamic* perspective will encourage the adolescent to access and express feelings—such as guilt, shame, or resentment—related to parental substance abuse and its effect on them. Helping teens "tell their story," the clinician guides them in reflecting on current and past events, and encourages them to ventilate feelings, sometimes referred to as "abreaction" or "catharsis." This process allows the release of emotional tensions and brings forth issues that can then be discussed and, optimally, ameliorated. Helping adolescents realize that they can acknowledge and express losses and disappointments related to their parents' substance use without becoming emotionally overwhelmed can aid them in learning to tolerate and accept negative feelings, rather than shutting down or acting out. Additionally, teenagers can be helped to develop coping strategies to deal with negative affects that may arise when feelings are identified and expressed. It may also be productive to ask teenage clients to reflect on what, if anything, they have gained or learned from their experiences. A search of the literature revealed no studies evaluating the use of psychodynamic techniques with adolescent offspring of substance abusers. However, psychodynamic therapies for adults have been tested and found effective for those with a variety of mental health problems (Leichsenring & Leibing, 2007), and psychodynamic techniques have been successfully applied to work with general population children and adolescents (Kazdin & Weisz, 2003).

Cognitive therapy and cognitive-behavioral therapy can help teens with impulsive or sensation-seeking traits develop awareness of their own thinking processes and build skills in problem-solving, interpersonal communication, conflict resolution, and negotiation. Whereas psychodynamic techniques emphasize how past experiences shape present perspectives and behaviors, cognitive techniques focus on developing healthy thinking patterns and solving current problems, while behavioral techniques focus on developing healthy behavior. Adolescents participating in cognitive or cognitive-behavioral therapy may be encouraged to examine their thoughts and beliefs and how they influence their choices, to identify and challenge distorted beliefs, to reflect on the risks and benefits of their choices, to choose positive roles and role models, and to build relationships with supportive peers who help them feel good about themselves. Teaching relaxation techniques and other strategies for distracting oneself from upsetting events or worries can help mitigate anxiety or other negative mood states in adolescents from substance-involved families. Helping teens set and follow through with educational and vocational goals may also be useful, since adolescents with clear goals are less likely to use drugs and to become parents during their teenage years (Fletcher, Harden, Brunton, Oakley, & Bonell, 2008). Cognitive and cognitive-behavioral therapies have been proven to help adolescents exhibiting depression, anxiety, and disruptive behaviors (David-Ferdon & Kaslow, 2008; Eyberg, Nelson, & Boggs, 2008; Silverman, Pina, & Viswesvaran, 2008).

If an assessment reveals a substance use problem for the adolescent, this will need to be addressed as well. Depending on the severity of this problem, a decision should be made whether to refer the teen to substance abuse treatment or integrate harm reduction strategies into the current treatment. In a systematic review of 56 alcohol prevention interventions for teenagers, those that incorporated skills training were found to have the most positive outcomes for prevention and early intervention with adolescents at risk for substance abuse and related problem behaviors (Foxcroft, Ireland, Lowe, & Breen, 2002).

Regardless of the treatment orientation utilized, clinical experience suggests that helping youth develop a relationship with a caring adult who can model healthy behaviors can be beneficial. Community supports (teachers, extended family, religious institutions) can also provide positive role models and growth experiences. In addition, making teens aware of their increased risk to inherit a substance use problem, and helping them come to terms with that risk, are essential parts of treatment planning.

Intervention Strategies for Families

A substance-abusing parent who provides inconsistent or overly punitive discipline and less emotional support to the child increases the risk of substance use and conduct disorder in that child when he or she reaches adolescence (Brody et al., 2001). Thus, parents should be helped to establish reasonable and effective expectations, and discipline for the adolescent appropriate for their stage of development. If needed, a referral for substance abuse treatment for the parent should be made.

Family treatment should be strengths based, culturally competent, and integrated into other treatments and services provided. The family may need information on the effects of parental substance abuse on the child, or help in connecting or reconnecting with each other. Regardless of the status of their substance use, parents can learn to listen to, empathize with, show interest in, hug, and spend time with their adolescent children, and to keep familial conflict to a minimum. Families should be encouraged to reinstitute and follow through with family routines and rituals such as church attendance, holiday celebrations, family meals, and school events, as these can help strengthen bonds and restore a sense of normalcy to the family.

Adolescents can be expected to test the limits of parental control. Rather than viewing this as a deliberate challenge of parental authority, such behaviors can be reframed as a normal, albeit awkward, struggle for autonomy in a child transitioning to adulthood. Parents can be trained to respond to such behaviors decisively without overreacting. They can be encouraged to monitor their teenage children appropriately. They may also receive education on how to respond to rule-breaking by their teenager by providing corrective consequences without resorting to threats or violence.

There have been few rigorous studies assessing interventions for substance-involved families with adolescent children. A notable exception is the *Strengthening Families Program* (SFP). Originally designed by Karol Kumpfer and colleagues for drug-abusing families with younger children (Kumpfer, DeMarsh, & Child, 1989), SFP was later adapted for use with other populations, including adolescents and their substance-involved parents. This highly structured intervention teaches parents and teenagers skills in problem-solving, interpersonal communication, and conflict resolution. Each week begins with a family group dinner, followed by separate group meetings for parents and youth, and ending with a family session. SFP has been evaluated and found to improve social skills and decrease delinquency and substance use in adolescents, to enhance parenting skills, and to strengthen bonds within families (Foxcroft et al., 2002). Over a dozen other studies evaluating the program in diverse settings and with diverse populations have reported similar positive results (Foxcroft, Ireland, Lister-Sharp, Lowe, & Breen, 2003).

Another program evidencing success in treating drug-addicted parents and their adolescent children is *Celebrating Families!*, which was originally developed for parents involved in drug court proceedings and later adapted for use with substance-involved families receiving residential and outpatient treatment services (Lutra Group, 2006). However, to date, this program has not been as widely replicated as the SFP.

Although the programs described provide primary prevention services, a number of family interventions have been developed to help teens already identified as having substance use and other problem behaviors. Several of these family treatments have been tested and deemed effective or promising. *Brief Strategic Family Therapy* was developed to treat drug use and related behaviors in adolescents. Treatment consists of 12–24 sessions and utilizes a family systems approach in which anything that happens to one member of the family is assumed to affect all other members (Szapocznik, Hervis, & Schwartz, 2003). *Family Support Network* provides case management, parent education groups, and in-home therapy sessions for the adolescent and family (Hamilton, Brantley, Tims, Angelovich, & McDougall, 2001). *Multidimensional Family Therapy* consists of 14–16 sessions, utilizing a combination of individual and family modalities and focusing on the family system as well as school, peer, and other systems in which the teen is involved (Liddle, 2002). Lastly, *Multisystemic Therapy* engages the family and community in mitigating adolescent antisocial behaviors (Henggeler, Schoenwald, Borduin, Rowand, & Cunningham, 1998).

Group Interventions

Group treatment is the most commonly utilized format for intervention with adolescent children of substance abusers (Price & Emshoff, 1997). Treatment is typically short term, although some groups are longer term or ongoing.

Groups have several advantages for this population. They can provide information and support, instill hope, and empower the teen to seek and receive help and to consider their own needs. In the group, adolescents learn that they are not alone in dealing with the consequences of having a substance-involved parent, which can reduce feelings of guilt and shame. Group members can share reactions to and strategies for living with an addicted parent, and can also practice social skills. Group modalities may be especially appropriate in cases where adolescents are hesitant to hurt their parents by confronting them in a family session, feel anger or hatred toward a parent that they are unwilling or unable to productively express, or fear how their parents will react if they reveal their own drug use attitudes or behaviors. Since teens who associate with peers with deviant behaviors are more likely to abuse substances and engage in other deviant behaviors themselves, groups can also provide opportunities to interact with peers engaged in more prosocial behaviors.

Group dynamics, when properly utilized, can play an important role in helping teens experiencing anger and low self-esteem related to parental substance abuse. Accordingly, the group leader should possess knowledge of group stages, themes, and processes, and skill in facilitating self-disclosure and encouraging mutual aid among group members.

As an adjunct to treatment, the clinician may also consider a referral to *Alateen* (http://www.alateen.org), a community-based mutual-aid support group for teens who have a significant other with a substance use problem. Alateen is based on tenets of the 12-step program of Alcoholics Anonymous and operates similarly to the Al-Anon program for adults concerned about a loved one with a substance abuse problem. Another resource is a Web-based discussion board run by the National Association for Children of Alcoholics (www.nacoa.org), where teens can go online to discuss their experiences of living with alcoholic parents.

Treating Adolescents: A Caveat

It is worth noting that, regardless of the treatment modality provided, and even when satisfied with the services they have received, adolescents may end treatment abruptly. In one clinical study, psychotherapists reported that, in contrast to their work with adults, termination with their teenage clients was almost always unplanned and unannounced (Mirabito, 2006). The clinicians saw developmental issues as contributing to this phenomenon, in that teens struggling with separation–individuation may have difficulty attaching and detaching from a therapeutic relationship, and may not want to face the pain of saying goodbye. This may be especially true for an adolescent who has previously suffered interpersonal losses or disappointments related to parental substance abuse.

CASE EXAMPLE

The following case vignette illustrates the presenting problems and concerns of an adolescent from a substance-involved family, and how these issues were addressed in treatment.

> G is a 16-year-old male living with his mother. His father, a poly-drug user, left when G was 5 years old. His mother, formerly a heroin addict, has been on methadone maintenance for the past 2 years, and continues to use marijuana occasionally. G and his mother survive on social security checks, supplemented by intermittent gifts of food and cash provided by what G calls "my mother's boyfriend-of-the-month."
>
> G was referred to the mental health clinic by the school counselor, after he began skipping classes and was caught smoking marijuana on school

property. An above-average student in elementary school, G's grades started to slip in middle school, and continued to decline after he transferred to a high school with a larger student body where he had fewer connections to teachers or school administrators. G started hanging out with a peer group known to experiment with drugs, and began isolating in his room after school.

Initially reticent to talk in treatment, G gradually opened up about his feelings of sadness over his father's abandonment of the family, his growing awareness of his mother's addiction, his fears related to her struggles to stay clean, and his belief that he was doomed to follow in his parents' footsteps.

After some individual sessions, the social worker referred G to a nearby support group for adolescents with substance-abusing parents. There G met other teens with similar experiences and feelings who provided him with a new, more positive peer group, and helped instill in him a sense of hope. The social worker also conducted some family sessions with G and his mother, in which G was encouraged to share his concerns about his mother's battles with addiction. Realizing the impact on her son, she made more efforts to curb her marijuana use. At the same time, she set some ground rules around his drug use, and insisted that he attend school and work to raise his grades. As she said to him, "I don't want you to have the life I've had—I expect better for you and I expect more from you."

CONCLUSION

In assessing and intervening with adolescent offspring of substance-abusing parents, it is important to note that each individual adolescent is unique. The clinician must carefully attend to the teen's strengths, vulnerabilities, attitudes, and aspirations. Regardless of modality or orientation, establishing a treatment alliance with the teenager is crucial, and engendering a sense of realistic optimism is vital.

As do younger children, adolescents often feel guilt and shame about their parents' chemical addiction. Professionals working with such youth can help them develop coping strategies and learn to manage their own lives. These treatment goals are encapsulated in advice offered by the National Association for Children of Alcoholics (2009, p. 25), which recommends teaching children and adolescents affected by parental substance abuse the "seven Cs":

I didn't **Cause** it
I can't **Cure** it
I can't **Control** it
But I can take better **Care** of myself
By **Communicating** my feelings
Making healthy **Choices**, and
Celebrating me.

REFERENCES

Anda, R. F., Whitfield, C. L., Felitti, V. J., Chapman, D., Edward, V. J., Dube, S. R., et al. (2002). Adverse childhood experiences, alcoholic parents, and later risk of alcoholism and depression. *Psychiatric Services, 53*(8), 1001–1009.

Annis, H. M. (1974). Patterns of intra-familial drug use. *British Journal of Addiction, 69*, 361–369.

Bailey, J. A., Hill, K. G., Oesterle, S., & Hawkins, J. D. (2006). Linking substance use and problem behavior across three generations. *Journal of Abnormal Child Psychology, 34*(3), 273–292.

Barnow, S., Ulrich, I., Grabe, H., Freyberger, H. J., & Spitzer, C. (2007). The influence of parental drinking behavior and antisocial personality disorder of adolescent behavioural problems: Results of the greifwalder family study. *Alcohol & Alcoholism, 42*(6), 623–628.

Bauman, P. S., & Dougherty, F. E. (1983). Drug-addicted mothers' parenting and their children's development. *International Journal of the Addictions, 18*(3), 291–302.

Bowser, B. P., & Word, C. O. (1993). Comparison of African-American adolescent crack cocaine users and nonusers: Background factors in drug use and HIV sexual risk behaviors. *Psychology of Addictive Behaviors, 7*(3), 155–161.

Brody, G. H., Ge, X., Conger, R., Gibbons, F., Murry, V. M., Gerrard, M., et al. (2001). The influence of neighborhood disadvantage, collective socialization, and parenting on African American children's affiliation with deviant peers. *Child Development, 72*(4), 1231–1246.

Brook, J. S., Brook, D. W., Whiteman, M., Gordon, A. S., & Cohen, P. (1990). The psychosocial etiology of adolescent drug use: A family interactional approach. *Social & General Psychology Monographs, 116*(2), 112–267.

Brook, J. S., Whiteman, M., Balka, E. B., Win, P T., & Gursen, M. D. (1998). Drug use among Puerto Ricans: Ethnic identity as a protective factor. *Hispanic Journal of Behavioral Sciences, 20*, 241–254.

Brookoff, D., O'Brien, K. K., Cook, C. S., Thompson, T. D., & Williams, C. (1997). Characteristics of participants in domestic violence. *Journal of the American Medical Association, 277*, 1369–1373.

Call, J. (1998, November 15). Alcoholics' kids face marital woes. *Deseret News,* Provo, UT.

Chalder, M., Elgar, F. J., & Bennet, P. (2006). Drinking and motivations to drink among adolescent children of parents with alcohol problems. *Alcohol & Alcoholism, 41*(1), 107–113.

Chassin, L., Pitts, S. C., DeLucia, C., & Todd, M. (1999). A longitudinal study of children of alcoholics: Predicting young adult substance use disorders, anxiety and depression. *Journal of Abnormal Psychology, 108*(1), 106–119.

David-Ferdon C., & Kaslow N. (2008). Evidence-based psychosocial treatments for child and adolescent depression. *Journal of Clinical Child and Adolescent Psychology, 37*(1), 62–104.

Dore, M. M., Kaufman, E., Nelson-Zlupko, L., & Granfort, E. (1996). Psychosocial functioning and treatment needs of latency-age children from drug-involved families. *Families in Society, 77*(10), 595–604.

Ehringer, M., Rhee, S. H., Young, S. E., Corley, R. P., & Hewitt, J. K. (2006). Genetic and environmental contributions to common psychopathologies of childhood and adolescence: A study of twins and their siblings. *Journal of Abnormal Child Psychology, 34*(1), 1–17.

Eigen, L., & Rowden, D. (2000). A methodology and current estimate of the number of children of alcoholics in the United States. In S. Abbott (Ed.), *Children of alcoholics: Selected readings* (Vol. 2). Rockville, MD: National Association for Children of Alcoholics.

Emshoff, J. G., & Price, A. W. (1999). Prevention and intervention strategies with children of alcoholics. *Pedriatrics 103*, (S 1112–1111).

Erikson, E. (1982). *The life cycle completed.* New York: Norton.

Eyberg, S. M., Nelson, M. M., & Boggs, S. R. (2008). Evidence-based psychosocial treatments for children and adolescents with disruptive behavior. *Journal of Clinical Child and Adolescent Psychology, 37*(1), 215–237.

Finn, P. R., Zeitouni, N., & Pihl, R. O. (1990). The effects of alcohol on psychophysiological hyper-reactivity to non-aversive and aversive stimuli in men at high-risk for alcoholism. *Journal of Abnormal Psychology, 99*, 79–85.

Fisher, G. L., & Harrison, T. C. (2000). *Substance abuse: Information for school counselors, social workers, therapists, and counselors* (2nd ed.). Boston: Allyn & Bacon.

Fletcher, A, Harden, A., Brunton, G., Oakley, A., & Bonell, C. (2008). Interventions addressing the social determinants of teenage pregnancy. *Health Education, 108*, 29–39.

Foxcroft, D. R., Ireland, D., Lister-Sharp, D. J., Lowe, G., & Breen, R. (2003). Longer-term primary prevention for alcohol misuse in young people: A systematic review. *Addiction, 98*, 397–411.

Foxcroft, D. R., Ireland, D., Lowe, G., & Breen, R. (2002). Primary prevention for alcohol misuse in young people. *Cochrane Database of Systematic Reviews,* Issue 3 (Article no: CD003024).

Gance-Cleveland, B., Mays, M. Z., & Steffen, A. (2008). Association of adolescent physical and emotional health with perceived severity of parental substance abuse. *Journal for Specialists in Pediatric Nursing, 13*(1), 15–25.

Gavriel-Fried, B., & Teichman, M. (2007). Ego identity of adolescent children of alcoholics. *Journal of Drug Education, 37*(1), 83–95.

Hamilton, N. I., Brantley, L. S., Tims, F. M., Angelovish, N., & McDougall, B. (2001). *Family support network for adolescent cannabis users, cannabis youth treatment (CYT) series* (DHHS Publication Number 01-3488, Vol. 3). Rockville, MD: Center for Substance Abuse Treatment, Substance Abuse and Mental Health Services Administration.

Hawkins, J. D., Catalano, R. F., & Miller, J. Y. (1992). Risk and protective factors for alcohol and other drug problems in adolescence and early adulthood: Implication for substance abuse prevention. *Psychological Bulletin, 112*(1), 64–105.

Henggeler, S. W., Schoenwald, S. K., Borduin, C. M., Rowand, M. D., & Cunningham, P. B. (1998). *Multisystemic treatment of antisocial behavior in children and adolescents.* New York: Guilford Press.

Hill, E. M., Nord, J. L., & Blow, F. C. (1992). Young-adult children of alcoholic parents: Protective effects of positive family functioning. *British Journal of Addiction, 87*, 1677–1690.

Inhelder, B., & Piaget, J. (1958). *The growth of logical thinking from childhood to adolescence.* New York: Basic Books.

Johnson, J. L., & Leff, M. (1999). Children of substance abusers: Overview of research findings. *Pediatrics, 103,* 1085–1099.

Jones, J. (1982) *Preliminary test manual: The children of alcoholics screening test.* Chicago, IL: Family Recovery Press.

Kazdin, A. E., & Weisz, J. R. (Eds.). (2003). *Evidence-based psychotherapies for children and adolescents.* New York: Guilford Press.

Knight, J. R., Sherrit, L., Shrier, L. A., Harris, S. K., & Chang, G. (2002). Validity of the CRAFFT substance abuse screening test among adolescent clinic patients. *Archives of Pediatrics and Adolescent Medicine, 156*(6), 607–614.

Kumpfer, K. L., DeMarsh, J. P., & Child, W. (1989). *Strengthening families program: Children's skills training curriculum manual, Parent training manual, children's skill training manual, and family skills training manual (Prevention services to children of substance-abusing parents).* Social Research Institute, Graduate School of Social Work, University of Utah.

Lang, A., Pelham, W. E., Atkeson, B. M., & Murphy, D. A. (1999). Effects of alcohol intoxication on parenting behavior in interactions with child confederates exhibiting normal or deviant behaviors. *Journal of Abnormal Child Psychology, 27,* 177–189.

Leichsenring, F., & Leibing, E. (2007). Psychodynamic psychotherapy: A systematic review of techniques, indications and empirical evidence. *Psychology and Psychotherapy, 80*(2), 217–228.

Leichtling, G., Gabriel, R. M., Lewis, C. K., & Vander Ley, K. J. (2006) *Adolescents in treatment: Effects of parental substance abuse on treatment entry characteristics and outcomes. Journal of Social Work Practice in the Addictions, 6*(1), 155–174.

Lester, P. E., Weiss, R. E., Rice, E., Comulada, W. S., Lord, L., Alber, S., et al. (2009). The longitudinal impact of HIV+ parents' drug use on their adolescent children. *American Journal of Orthopsychiatry, 79*(1), 51–59.

Liddle, H. A. (2002). *Multidimentional family therapy for adolescent cannabis users, cannabis youth treatment series* (DHHS Publication Number 02-3660, Vol. 5). Rockville, MD: Center for Substance Abuse Treatment, Substance Abuse and Mental Health Services Administration.

Lutra Group. (2006). *Year one (FY 05-06) evaluation report for the celebrating families! Grant.* Unpublished report, Salt Lake City, UT: Author.

Lynskey, M. T., & Fergusson, D. M. (1994). The effect of parental alcohol problems on rates of adolescent psychiatric disorders. *Addiction, 89*(10), 1277–1286.

Marmorstein, N. R., Iacono, W. G., & McGue, M. (2009). Alcohol and illicit drug dependence among parents: Associations with offspring externalizing disorders. *Psychological Medicine, 39,* 149–155.

McGrath, C. E., Watson, A. L., & Chassin, L. (1999). Academic achievement in adolescent children of alcoholics. *Journal of Studies on Alcohol and Drugs, 60*(1), 18–26.

Miller, C. A., Tebb, K. P., Williams, J. K., Neuhaus, J. M., & Shafer, M. A. (2007). Chlamydial screening in urgent care visits: Adolescent-reported acceptability associated with adolescent perception of clinician communication. *Archives of Pediatrics and Adolescent Medicine, 161*(8), 777–782.

Mirabito, D. (2006). Revisiting unplanned termination: Clinician perceptions of termination from adolescent mental health treatment. *Families in Society, 87*(2), 171–180.

Molina, B. S., Chassin, L., & Curran, P. (1994). A comparison of mechanisms underlying substance use for early adolescent children of alcoholics and controls. *Journal of Studies on Alcoholism, 55,* 269–275.

Moss, H. B., Clark, D. B., & Kirisci, L. (1997). Timing of paternal substance use disorder cessation and effects on problem behavior in sons. *American Journal of Addictions, 6,* 30–37.

Mylant, J., Ide, B., Cuevas, E., & Meehan, M. (2002). Adolescent children of alcoholics: Vulnerable or resilient? *Journal of the American Psychiatric Nurses Association, 8*(2), 57–64.

National Association for Children of Alcoholics. (2009). *Children of alcoholics: A kit for educators.* Retrieved May 30, 2009, from http://www.nacoa.org/pdfs/EDkit_web_06.pdf

National Center on Addiction and Substance Abuse. (2003, February). *The formative years: Pathways to substance abuse among girls and young women ages 8–22.* Retrieved October 5, 2010, from http://www.casacolumbia.org/templates/Publications_Reports.aspx#r29

National Institute on Drug Abuse. (2002, February). U.S. Department of Health and Human Services. *NIDA Notes, 16*(6), 5.

Ohannessian, C. M., & Hesselbrock, V. M. (2008). A comparison of three vulnerability models for the onset of substance use in a high-risk sample. *Journal of Studies on Alcohol & Drugs, 69*(1), 75–84.

Ohannessian, C. M., Hesselbrock, V. M., Kramer, J., Bucholz, K. K., Schuckit, M. A., Kuperman, S., et al. (2004). Parental substance use consequences and adolescent psychopathology. *Journal of Studies on Alcoholism, 65*(6), 725–730.

Peiponen, S., Laukkanen, E., Korhonen, V., Hintikka, U., & Lehtonen, J. (2006). The association of parental alcohol abuse and depression with severe emotional and behavioral problems in adolescents: A clinical study. *International Journal of Social Psychiatry, 52*(5), 395–407.

Perez-Bouchard, L., Johnson, J. L., & Ahrens, A. H. (1993). Attributional style in children of substance abusers. *American Journal of Drug and Alcohol Abuse, 19*(4), 475–489.

Price, A. W., & Emshoff, J. G. (1997). Prevention and intervention with children of alcoholics. *Alcohol Health and Research World, 21*(3), 241–246.

Reddy, D. M., Fleming, R., & Swain, C., (2002). Effect of mandatory parental notification on adolescent girls' use of sexual health care services. *Journal of the American Medical Association (JAMA), 288*(6), 710–714.

Rice, C. E., Dandreaux, M. S., Handley, E. D., & Chassin, L. (2006). Children of alcoholics: Risk and resilience. *The Prevention Researcher, 13*(4), 3–6.

Robinson, B. E., & Rhoden, J. L. (1997). Psychological adjustment of children of alcoholics. In B. E. Robinson & J. L. Rhoden (Eds.), *Working with children of alcoholics: The practitioner's handbook* (2nd ed.). Thousand Oaks, CA: SAGE Publications.

Roosa, M., Beals, J., Sandler, I., & Pillow, D. (1990). The role of risk and protective factors in predicting symptomology in adolescent self-identified children of alcoholics. *American Journal of Community Psychology, 18,* 725–741.

Schoenborn, C. A. (1991). Exposure to alcoholism in the family: United States, 1988. *Advance Data, 205,* 1–13.

Segal, B. M., & Stewart, J. C. (1996). Substance use and abuse in adolescence: An overview. *Child Psychiatry Human Development, 26*(4), 193.

Sher, K. (1997). Psychological characteristics of children of alcoholics. *Alcohol Health and Research World, 21,* 247–254.

Sheridan, M. (1995). A psychometric assessment of the Children of Alcoholics Screening Test (CAST), *Journal of Studies on Alcoholism, 56,* 156–160.

Silverman, W. K., Pina, A. A., & Viswesvaran, C. (2008). Evidence-based psychosocial treatments for phobic and anxiety disorders in children and adolescents. *Journal of Clinical Child and Adolescent Psychology, 37*(1), 105–130.

Spear, L. P., & Varlinskaya, E. I. (2005). Adolescence: Alcohol sensitivity, tolerance and intake. *Recent Developments in Alcoholism, 17,* 143–159.

Stewart, M. A., & Brown, S. A. (1993). Family functioning following adolescent substance abuse treatment. *Journal of Substance Abuse, 5,* 327–339.

Substance Abuse and Mental Health Services Administration, Office of Applied Studies. (2007). *Results from the 2006 national survey on drug use and health: National findings.* Rockville, MD: Author.

Substance Abuse and Mental Health Services Administration, Office of Applied Studies. (2007, May 24). *The DASIS report: Adolescent treatment admissions by gender: 2005.* Rockville, MD. Retrieved from http://www.oas.samhsa .gov/2k7/youthTX/youthTX.htm

Substance Abuse and Mental Health Services Administration, Office of Applied Studies. (2008, April 16). *The NSDUH report: Children living with substance-dependent or substance-abusing parents: 2002 to 2007.* Rockville, MD: Author.

Suldo, S. M., Mihalas, S., Powell, H., & French, R. (2008). Ecological predictors of substance use in middle school students. *School Psychology Quarterly, 23*(3), 373–388.

Swetlow, K. (2003). *Children at clandestine methamphetamine labs: Helping meths's youngest victims. OVC Bulletin.* Retrieved April 11, 2009, from the Web site of the Office for Victims of Crime, U.S. Department of Justice: www.ojp.usdoj .gov/ovc/publications/bulletins/children/197590.pdf

Szapocznik, J., Hervis, O., & Schwartz, S. (2003). *Brief strategic family therapy for adolescent drug use* (NIH Publication Number 03-4751). Washington, DC: National Institute on Drug Abuse.

Szewczyk, L. S., & Weinmuller, E. B. (2006). Religious aspects of coping with stress among adolescents from families with alcohol problems. *Mental Health, Religion and Culture, 9*(4), 389–400.

U.S. Department of Health and Human Services. (1995). *Drug use among racial/ ethnic minorities.* Washington, DC: U.S. Government Printing Office.

U.S. Department of Health and Human Services. (2007). *The surgeon general's call to action to prevent and reduce underage drinking.* U.S. Department of Health and Human Services: Office of the Surgeon General.

Velleman, R., & Orford, J. (1999). *Risk and resilience: Adults who were children of problem drinkers.* Amsterdam: Harwood Academic.

Wallace, J. M., Jr. (1999). Explaining race differences in adolescent and young adult drug use: The role of racialized social systems. *Drugs & Society, 13*(1–2), 21–36.

Wallace, J. M., & Forman, T. A. (1998). Religion's role in promoting health and reducing risk among American youth. *Health Education & Behavior: Special Issue: Public Health and Health Education in Faith Communities, 25*(6), 721–741.

Werner, E. E., & Smith, R. (1992). *Overcoming the odds: High risk children from birth to adulthood.* Ithaca, NY: Cornell University Press.

Werner, M. J., Joffe, A., & Graham, A. V. (1999). Screening, early identification and office-based intervention with children and youth living in substance-abusing families. *Pediatrics, 103*(5), 1099–1112.

White, A. M., Truesdale, M. C., Bae, J. G., Ahmad, S., Wilson, W. A., Best, P. J., et al. (2002). Differential effects of ethanol on motor coordination in adolescent and adult rats. *Pharmacology, Biochemistry and Behavior, 73*(3), 673–677.

White, W., & Savage, B. (2005). All in the family: Alcohol and other drug problems, recovery, advocacy. *Alcoholism Treatment Quarterly, 23*(4), 3–37.

Whitfield, C. (1991). *Co-dependence: Healing the human condition.* Deerfield Beach, FL: Health Communications, Inc.

Wolin, S. J., & Wolin, S. (1993). *The resilient self: How survivors of troubled families rise above adversity.* New York: Villard Books.

Woodside, M., Coughey, K., & Cohen, R. (1993). Medical costs of children of alcoholics—pay now or pay later. *Journal of Substance Abuse, 5,* 281–287.

Young, S. E., Rhee, S. H., Stallings, M. C., Corley, R. P., Crowley, T. J., & Hewitt, J. K. (2006). Genetic and environmental vulnerabilities underlying adolescent substance use and problem use: General or specific? *Behavior Genetics, 36*(4), 603–615.

7

Treatment Issues and Psychodrama Interventions With Adults Who Grew Up With Substance-Abusing Parents

Tian Dayton

INTRODUCTION

Over the past decade, research in neurobiology has validated what many in the addiction-treatment field have long understood from our own clinical experience. Namely, the adult children of alcoholics (ACA) syndrome is, in fact, a posttraumatic stress reaction in which unresolved childhood wounds that lay dormant for decades resurface in adulthood as a delayed reaction to childhood trauma. In 1980 when the term "adult child of an alcoholic" or ACA was coined, ACAs literally self-identified with a host of "ACA characteristics" described by Sharon Wegscheider-Cruse (1980), Claudia Black (1981), Janet Woititz (1983), and Tim Cermack (1985). They testified to the pain that the child within them seemed still to be hanging onto long after they had left their alcoholic homes. They reported feeling at times like "children walking around in the bodies of grownups," and stuffed animals held onto by adults who felt small and vulnerable began popping up in treatment centers as they finally shared their childhood anxieties, confusion, and hurt.

When these children of alcoholics reached adulthood and found the ACA movement, they talked about having parts of themselves—the wounded, angry, and disillusioned aspects of their inner world—that had gone unidentified and unexpressed for years. These "hidden parts," not surprisingly, were becoming triggered when, as adults, they began choosing partners and having children of their own. The very closeness, vulnerability, and dependence that are part of any intimate relationship triggered all of their unresolved childhood pain. As John, a 42-year-old married man, shared:

> I feel like a soldier who hits the dirt when he hears a car backfire because he thinks it's gunfire. Only I "hit the dirt" emotionally when my wife yells at me. All I can see is my drunk mother. No, that's not it. I can't stand to remember my drunk mother, it feels too weird 'cause sometimes my Mom was so great. I feel like I'm being disloyal to the part of her I loved. So I put all that pain on my wife, even though she doesn't even drink. I can't tell when she's just mad at something little that might go away; everything feels big. Nothing ever went away in my house. Criticism was just the tip of the iceberg. It could mean days of nobody cooking any meals, or being yelled at if I went to a friend's for dinner or brought a friend home, which I learned fast not to do. Sometimes when my wife and I are having a fight I get these creepy images of my mom walking through the house in her bathrobe, drunk and looking out of it, I just freeze inside. Then I look at my wife and say all the stuff I wanted to say to my mom but couldn't. Somehow it's easier to yell it out at my wife, I guess 'cause I'm bigger now. When I was just a little kid if I'd said it to my mom, she'd have made my life miserable. She'd anywhere have told me to get out of the house. I was just a kid and didn't have anywhere to go.

John is typical of the clients who, at about 35–40 years of age, wander into therapists' offices confused and worried because they can't seem to get comfortable with closeness. Their old ghosts keep reemerging and scaring them, making them feel they have made a bad choice in partners, or that they just don't know why they feel so reactive inside. They get the sorts of flashbacks that John described, fragments of barely visible but disturbing memories that they want to bat away and remove from their minds. These fragments, if not identified for what they are, can become mixed up with relationship dynamics of the present and make them seem fraught with the potential for hurt. Through projection and transference, unconscious and unprocessed pain from the past gets layered onto their relationships in the present, making them confusing and difficult to deal with. This chapter will discuss the personality characteristics that may develop as a result of the trauma of living with an addicted parent and will look at how specific techniques, such as psychodrama, can be used to help these adults to heal.

HOW TRAUMA AFFECTS CHILD DEVELOPMENT

Children make meaning out of situations with the psychological and emotional equipment available to them at their particular stage of development. For the small child, the parent is all-powerful and of vital importance for his or her survival. Because children need to stay connected to their parents to meet their most basic needs, they can be severely challenged when their intoxicated parent loses control. Because children don't really have a well-developed sense of their own identity as separate from their parents, they may have trouble recognizing that their parent's behavior is not caused by them. "If only I were smarter or behaved better, Daddy wouldn't shout at me and Mommy wouldn't feel so depressed and need to drink all the time . . . they would stop fighting and saying such horrible things to each other." Left to make sense out of a painful situation without the aid of an intelligent and caring adult, they extract the meaning that any age-appropriate child would make and conclude, "I must be the problem." To complicate matters even further, this may be exactly what their parents, in the heat of their own pain and anger, are telling them as well.

A child's particular level of brain development literally defines his ability to process emotional information. The amygdala, which is the brain center for the fight/flight/freeze response, is fully functional at birth. This means that a baby is capable of a full-blown trauma response. However, the hippocampus, which is where we comprehend our surrounding context and assess stimuli to determine whether or not it is threatening, is not fully functional until the age of 4 or 5 (Cozolino, 2006). This means that children can be deeply frightened and have absolutely no idea what is frightening them or how frightened they need to be. They are totally dependent upon the adults around them to decode the surrounding world and explain it to them. The prefrontal cortex, where we do our critical reasoning and planning, is not fully mature until around age 11 or older. Its function is to allow the child to translate feeling states into words so that the child can think about what he or she is feeling, and use this ability to think in abstractions to get some emotional perspective on a situation. Until this capacity develops at 11 or 12 years of age, the child is left to either make his or her own immature meaning of the situation, or to depend upon the adults surrounding him or her to explain what is going on. Because of this immature level of brain development, childhood experiences may not get elevated to a conscious level and processed by thinking about them. Instead, they are either repressed or defended against in some other manner, or stored away with the original childlike meaning attached to them.

When these memories get triggered by an adult child of a substance-abusing parent (COSAP) during adulthood, they can be very confusing to decode. One reason for this is that the prefrontal cortex, which is where we do much of our critical thinking and meaning making, where we *think* about what we're *feeling* and make sense of it, shuts down when we are in a state of terror or high stress. When people perceive impending trauma, they are prone to an extreme startle or "deer in the headlights" reaction. Following that is the attempt to *fight* or *flee*. If escape is possible, the experience of the near-trauma will be temporarily stressful, but the person is unlikely to develop full-blown posttraumatic stress disorder (PTSD). If the intention to flee is thwarted, however, the result is a "freeze" response (van der Kolk, 2003). The freeze response creates an inability to process what is happening and increases the PTSD symptoms. For children who grew up in homes with addicted adults, there may have been nowhere to run or any debriefing of what they had been exposed to. After a traumatic event, the fear-laden memories may have remained unconscious and unprocessed because the adults to whom they would normally go to for comfort and closure were unavailable. To make matters worse, it may have been the adults themselves causing the fear and stress.

When the ability to think is temporarily frozen or "out of order," we need to make sense of frightening or traumatic moments after the fact. Feelings about what happened and the sensorial impressions and responses need to be elevated to a conscious level and thought about *after the threat is over and we feel safe again*. When this does not happen, the memories and the feelings that surround them can remain locked in the unconscious, limbic, or body memory waiting to be triggered (van der Kolk, 1994). However, when these feelings do surface, they often get projected onto the situation that triggered them with little or no awareness of their deeper origins. This can cause adult intimacy to feel very confusing and unmanageable since the present may become difficult to distinguish from the past. The result is that the problems become bigger and more complicated than necessary.

HOW DO COSAPs RE-CREATE DYSFUNCTIONAL FAMILY DYNAMICS?

When COSAPs attempt to form and sustain relationships in adulthood, they may overreact to the difficulties that inevitably arise. Intimacy and parenthood may trigger feelings of dependency and vulnerability in which they expect chaos, out-of-control behavior, and abuse to be inevitable since this was their early childhood experience. They may unconsciously be so convinced that distress is at hand that they may experience mistrust and suspicion if problems are solved too smoothly. They may even push a situation in a convoluted attempt at self-protection until, through their relentless efforts to avoid it, they actually create it. Thus, the pattern of strong feeling leading to chaos, rage, and tears is once again reinforced and passed along (Dayton, 2007). As pointed out by Bessel van de Kolk (1994), people with PTSD often organize their lives after a trauma by either being dominated by intrusive experiences in the form of flashbacks, nightmares, or anxiety, or the opposite: They may avoid involvement in many aspects of life in order to avoid feelings that might trigger the dangerous feelings related to the original trauma. When the trauma experienced is about intimate family relationships, people with PTSD may alternate between overcloseness and undercloseness, or between enmeshment and avoidance.

When COSAPs enter treatment, they may present a wide variety of clinical syndromes, such as anxiety disorders, reactive and endogenous depression, psychosomatic symptoms, psychotic episodes, eating disorders, and substance abuse. If the clinician can get a clear picture of whether or not having an addicted, pain-inducing parent has been a major influence in their lives, an appropriate treatment plan can more clearly emerge.

CHARACTERISTICS FREQUENTLY SEEN IN TRAUMATIZED COSAPs

The following is a list of symptoms and dynamics that emerge most frequently in COSAPs with a history of traumatic early life. These symptoms and dynamics are drawn from both research and clinical observations and serve as the focus of treatment using psychodrama, which is described later in this chapter.

Rigid Psychological Defenses

People who are consistently being wounded emotionally and are not able to address or process what's hurting them openly and honestly may develop rigid psychological defenses to manage or ward off pain. Dissociation (remaining physically present but inwardly absent), denial (rewriting reality to be more palatable), splitting (seeing life and people as alternately all good or all bad), repression (pushing feelings down out of consciousness), minimization (minimizing the impact of situations or behavior), intellectualization (using thinking to rationalize and analyze in order to avoid feeling), and projection (disowning one's own pain by projecting it outwardly) are some examples of these defenses (Dayton, 2007).

Problems With Self-Regulation

The limbic system can become deregulated through emotional trauma. Deregulation of the limbic system can translate into a lack of ability to regulate feeling states, appetite, sleep, or sex drive as well as broad swings between states of emotional intensity and numbing. COSAPs who have become used to living in emotional extremes can find themselves uncomfortable living in a more regulated, middle range of thinking, feeling, and behavior.

Hypervigilance/Anxiety/Hyperreactivity

When one is hypervigilant, one tends to scan the environment and relationships for signs of potential danger or repeated relationship insults and ruptures (van der Kolk, 1987). The individual is constantly trying to read the faces of those in the environment in order to protect the self against perceived pain or humiliation—a constant state of "waiting for the other shoe to drop." Unfortunately, this hair-trigger reactivity can lead to perceptions of problems that do not exist and inadvertently to their development, or to an exaggeration of problems that might have been easily managed if the individual was not projecting pain from the past onto situations and relationships in the present.

Cultivation of a False Self

COSAPs often learn not to tell the truth about what they see going on around them. For the family that is in denial about the progressive addiction in its midst, telling the truth can be dangerous. Family members can quickly turn against the one who tries to make the growing problems resulting from addiction evident, and ostracize this individual. "Looking good" becomes a critical survival strategy. Because of the need to "look good," the COSAP may take refuge in creating a persona that is acceptable within the family at the expense of his/her authentic self. Although it may feel easier to adopt a false self, which feels like a clever solution to a pressing identity problem, in the long run such a solution can cost a great deal in terms of one's self-honesty and genuineness. Though we all, to some extent, cultivate a false self for protection (Horney, 1950), the COSAP may *become* the false self and lose touch with who he or she really is.

Emotional Constriction

Children raised in trauma-inducing families that do not encourage the expression of genuine emotion, or that make the child want to hide or shut down what is being experienced, may develop a limited or restricted range of emotions that they are comfortable feeling and sharing (Dube et al., 2003).

Unresolved Grief

Children who have experienced parental loss through divorce, parental incarceration, or being removed from the home and put into foster care are likely to suffer a profound sense of grief. Others may have experienced childhood losses of family members to addiction and the disruption of family rhythms and rituals. They all may need to mourn not only those various childhood loses, but also what they never had an opportunity to experience (Rando, 1993).

Learned Helplessness

When an individual feels that nothing can be done to affect or change a situation for the better, he or she may develop what has been termed "learned helplessness" (Peterson, Maier, & Seligman, 1995). Subsequently, they may lose their ability to take actions to change or influence a situation, or give up easily, and adopt a permanent position of victimhood.

Somatic Disturbances

Because the body is neurologically wired to process emotions, strong feelings can make one feel impelled to take an action. For example, one gets scared, then runs or freezes in place; one feels loved, then reaches out and touches or hugs (van der Kolk, 1987).When the person is unable to experience or act on powerful emotions, those emotions may then be experienced somatically as back pain, chronic headaches, muscle tightness or stiffness, stomach problems, heart pounding, or headaches.

High-Risk Behaviors

Trauma can engender a flattened, emotional world. High-risk behaviors can be seen as an attempt to jump start a numbed inner world by overstimulating the nervous system and body through excitation. Adrenaline is highly addictive to the brain and may act as a powerful mood enhancer. Speeding, sexual acting out, spending, fighting, drugging, working compulsively, or other behaviors done in a way that puts one at risk for emotional, relationship, and other problems are some examples of high-risk behaviors that may be encountered when working with COSAPs.

Survivor's Guilt

The COSAP who "gets out" of an unhealthy family system while others remain mired within it may experience what is referred to as "survivor's guilt" (Dayton, 2000; Lifton, 1986). Survivor's guilt can lead to self-sabotage or becoming overly preoccupied with fixing one's family. Adult COSAPs may seesaw between wanting to cut off their family because being close makes them feel that they are sliding "backwards," and wishing to reconnect with their family so that they do not have to tolerate their painful feelings of separateness and guilt. Over time, the adult COSAP needs to learn what children who grew up in healthy families tend to learn—how to be in the presence of another person while still hanging onto their own, autonomous sense of self and trusting what they themselves feel and see.

Shame

For the person growing up in an addicted environment, shame becomes not so much a feeling that is experienced in relation to an incident or situation, as is the case with guilt, but rather a basic attitude toward and about the self. "I am bad" as opposed to "I did something bad." Shame can be experienced as a lack of energy for life, an inability to accept love and caring on a consistent basis, or a hesitancy to move into self-affirming roles. It may play out as impulsive decision making or an inability to make decisions at all (Bradshaw, 1988).

Distorted Reasoning

Watching a parent slowly become emotionally or mentally unstable or dysfunctional due to prolonged use of substances can shake us to the core. It can be deeply disrupting, humiliating, and frightening. Family members may twist or distort their own reasoning in order to make this destabilizing experience easier to manage, or less "real." Also, as children, one makes sense of situations with the developmental equipment one possesses at any given age; when one is young, one either borrows the reasoning of surrounding adults or makes one's own child-like meaning. This "child think" may be saturated with interpretations that are laced with immature or even fantastical conclusions, which may also be influenced by the natural egocentricity of the child who feels that the world circulates around and because of them. This immature and distorted reasoning can be carried into and played out in adult relationships.

Tendency to Isolate

People who have felt traumatized may isolate and avoid emotionally connecting with others, reasoning that by avoiding connection they will avoid further feelings of being hurt. Isolation is also a feature of depression. Unfortunately, social connectedness, though natural to our species, still needs to be learned and practiced. The more one isolates, the more out of practice one becomes at making connections with other people, which further increases one's isolation and loneliness (van der Kolk, McFarlane, & Weisauth, 1996).

Loss of Ability to Accept Caring and Support From Others

Even if one does not isolate completely from others, the numbing response, fear, and mistrust, along with the emotional constriction that is a natural part of a trauma response, may influence one's ability to accept caring and support from others (van der Kolk, 1987). Consequently, one's willingness to allow love and support to feel good may be lessened due to a fear of potentially experiencing more loss or pain.

Loss of Trust and Faith

When one's personal world and the relationships within it become very unpredictable or unreliable, one may experience a loss of trust and faith in relationships, as well as in life's ability to repair and renew itself. This is why the restoration of hope is so important when working with COSAPs. In addition, having a spiritual belief system can play an important role in personal healing by providing both hope and a sense of security despite any ongoing familial and intrapsychic chaos (Dayton, 2007).

Traumatic Bonding

Because it is so deeply disruptive to one's sense of normalcy, early traumatic relationships can impel people not only to withdraw from close connection, but also to seek it desperately. This results in unhealthy bonding styles, particularly among children experiencing a high degree of fear at home. Children who are feeling lost and frightened may "rescue" each other, or carry a sense of "surviving together," which can create a belief that loyalty should be maintained at all costs, even if "close" bonds become problematic or dysfunctional (Carnes, 1997). Traumatized adult COSAPs may repeat this type of bonding style in relationships throughout their lives, often without their conscious awareness.

Cycles of Reenactment/Repetition Compulsion

Repetition compulsion is a psychological phenomenon in which one repeats the emotional, psychological, or behavioral aspects of a traumatic event over and over again (Freud, 1922). This can take the form of repeated recreating or reenacting the painful, warded off, or feared contents of the traumatic dynamic or putting oneself in situations where the dysfunctional dynamics or similar events are likely to happen again. This "reliving of the trauma" can also emerge in flashbacks or dreams in which fragments of memory and feelings of what happened are reexperienced in the dream state. In this way, COSAPs may find themselves repeating painful and dysfunctional relationships from childhood well into adulthood.

Desire to Self-Medicate

All of the characteristics discussed previously can create emotional, psychological, and somatic disturbance and disequilibrium. Self-medication can then seem to be a solution, a way to calm an inner storm and restore "balance." Although the use of various forms of medications can make pain, anxiety, and body symptoms temporarily abate, in the long run, it creates many more problems than it solves. Teenage and adult children of substance-abusing parents all too often become addicts themselves, engaged in a compulsive relationship with alcohol, drugs, food, sex, work, or money as a form of mood and pain management. Part of getting and staying sober for these people will be facing childhood pain so that it does not remain unresolved and trigger future relapses.

Co-Occurring Disorders

In addition to the risk of developing a substance use disorder, adult COSAPs often develop other mental disorders, such as depression or anxiety (Anda et al., 2006). In a review of studies of co-occurring disorders, Sacks and colleagues found that 50–75% of clients in substance abuse treatment programs were reported to have a co-occurring disorder (S. Sacks, J. Sacks, De Leon, Bernhardt, & Staines, 1997). These disorders may be undiagnosed and untreated even if the individual receives help for family issues or for his or her own addiction. When addicts remove the substance that they have been using to manage or self-medicate their depression, for example, they will then need to be treated for that depression. It can be very discouraging for both adult COSAPs and their family members to go through all that treatment for addiction demands only to be faced with a new form of mental illness.

RESILIENCE IN ADULT COSAPs

Though, as indicated, there are numerous pathological problems that can stem from growing up with the trauma of addiction, it is clear that not everyone develops these problems. Many who have experienced such problems develop significant strength from facing and overcoming childhood challenges—what has been termed as resilience (Werner, 1996).

Early researchers (e.g., Werner, 1996; Werner & Smith, 1992; Wolin & Wolin, 1993) observed that resilience seems to develop out of the *challenge to maintain self-esteem*. Troubled families often make their children feel powerless and bad about themselves. But resilient children find ways to feel good about themselves and their lives in spite of the negative influence of their parents and their environment. A more recent exploratory study of resiliency in families affected by parental alcohol abuse suggested that there is a continuum of family functioning that allows some families to function well despite parental alcohol abuse and that such positive family functioning serves as a protective mechanism (Coyle et al., 2006).

According to S. J. Wolin and S. Wolin (1993), resilient people often move their lives forward by *establishing goals* for themselves, reaching them, and moving beyond them; they *tend not to let adversity define them*. Rather they continually marshal their strengths and propel themselves out of their present circumstances. Additionally, they *see their problems as temporary* rather than as a permanent state of affairs. They tend not to globalize their problems and find reasons and ways, whether they be religious, creative, or just good common sense, to place a temporary framework and perspective around the problems in their lives. Resilient individuals often report having an inborn feeling that life will work out. Although they may struggle, they keep going, stay engaged with life, and continue to function. Resilience is not the ability to escape unharmed. It is the ability to thrive in spite of the odds. Nonetheless, even some resilient people have emotional and psychological scars due to their early life experience. They can, for example, have stormy relationships, health problems, or be somewhat aloof. Consequently, even some resilient adult COSAPs may need professional help to address some of the issues of growing up with an alcohol or drug-addicted parent.

INTERVENTIONS WITH ADULT COSAPs

Because the types of trauma that occur in homes of COSAPs often constitute ruptures in relationships at the hands of primary caretakers upon whom a child depends for nurturance and survival, treatment becomes complicated. That is, the very vehicle that will lead them eventually back to health, that is, connection with others, are those situations that have become fraught with pain and anxiety. Entering into an intimate relationship with a helping professional or a group therapy setting can seem like a "really bad idea" to the adult COSAP who has learned that people cannot necessarily be trusted. Also, fears of disloyalty to the family or being ostracized for "telling the truth" can keep adult COSAPs not only telling a lie to the outside world but living a lie within themselves well into adulthood. Treatment threatens to expose that lie. Twelve-step programs, such as Al-Anon and ACA (Adult Children of Alcoholics), can be wonderful adjuncts or even initial initiation to therapy since they provide a safe and constantly available container in which adult COSAPs can slowly identify with the stories of others and feel both held and less alone in their pain (Spiegel & Fewell, 2004). There are also a variety of other 12-step programs that address common issues faced by some adult COSAPs, such as those designed for eating problems (Overeaters Anonymous), spending (Debtors Anonymous), or sexual problems (Sex and Love Addicts Anonymous).

Another helpful approach to treatment of adult COSAPs is via the use of psychodrama, which is described below.

The Use of Psychodrama With Adult COSAPs

Psychodrama is a role-playing method of therapy developed by J. L. Moreno in Vienna at the turn of the twentieth century. Moreno is considered to be the father of group psychotherapy and his work represents the first attempts to treat people in groups rather than exclusively in a one-to-one setting (Moreno, 1953; 1964). Psychodrama allows conflicts and unresolved issues to be concretized by casting group members to play roles from the life of the protagonist or client whose "story" is being examined. It allows the protagonist to have a physical "encounter" with the self; to see and experience what is carried within the mind and body so that it can be made explicit, concrete, and can be dealt with in the here and now.

The purpose of psychodramatic role plays is to bring about insight through action rather than talk alone and, thus, to resolve conflicts (Dayton, 2005). Through role play, thinking, feeling, and behavior emerge simultaneously to allow a fuller picture to come into view of what is being carried in the psyche. Group members can be allowed to double when they identify with the protagonist in order to shed light on what might be going on in their inner world. The "double" puts into words the protagonist's interior thought, sensations, and emotions that may be locked within the limbic system in a wordless, actionless state.

Psychodrama, which allows body as well as emotional memory to emerge through action and role play, is an ideal form of therapy for trauma resolution and is therefore a helpful treatment tool for helping adult COSAPs. Repressed limbic memory can rise naturally to the surface in a "safe enough" container so that the cortex, rather than shutting down when reexperiencing fear, can remain alert enough to "self-observe" and make sense of the emotion that is emerging. According to van der Kolk (1994), the clinician's task is to ensure that the client does not shut down physiologically so that he or she will be able to process the trauma rather than relive it. The goal is to get the client to become curious about what he or she is feeling and engaged in what is going on inside and consequently process those emotions. Less is more. The goal is engagement rather than any specific agenda or expectation of intense emotions. Although they may emerge in time, they should not be forced.

As mentioned previously, fear is at the base of the trauma response. Fear is what signals the fight/flight/freeze survival defenses to engage. Being overwhelmed by fear leads to helplessness and terror at being confronted with circumstances that feel out of control and this desperation activates the trauma response. Consequently, we need to remember that once a fear is triggered, there is the additional fear of being frozen or unable to respond. During a psychodrama, clients may freeze when confronted with even a surrogate of someone who has frightened them in the past. This response needs to be recognized as the way they may have coped early in their lives when something frightened them. As they "thaw out," they begin to realize that feeling will lead them to actions and words. They are able to say what they wanted to say, do what they wanted to do, or even think what they wanted to think but didn't dare. Their thwarted intentions, whether in thought, word, feeling, or action can be experienced in a safe and supportive space. They can then make many choices as to how to proceed in their drama. In this way, adult COSAPs can learn to reeducate this fear response and regulate their emotions.

Moreno (1964), the father of psychodrama, understood that "the body remembers what the mind forgets," recognizing far before his time that there is such a thing as somatic memory and that the body as well as the mind need to participate in therapy in order for healing to occur. Because the cortex was not fully involved in the storage of traumatic memories, those experiences may not have been thought about and put into a logical context and sequence. Consequently, they can be difficult to access through reflective talking alone. Though this may be interpreted by some therapists as resistance, it is more likely to be related to a loss of access not only to repressed feeling, but to any cognitive understanding of what actually may have occurred. When asked to tell their story, therapists may well be faced by a client who is drawing a complete blank (van der Kolk, 2003).

Psychodrama Is Relational

Another key component of the unusual healing potential of psychodrama is its ability to allow for a contained reexperiencing of split-off emotion while in the presence of others. As clients experience the full range of affect including anger and rage, shed the tears, and feel the fear that may have been banished from their consciousness, several things occur simultaneously. They can reintegrate the split-off emotion into the self-system, at the same time that they take in support and caring from others and rebuild their affiliative bonds. Clients are also witnessing themselves and others in action so that they can reflect upon their own behavior in its concrete form. This process includes using all of the senses to rework a situation that was, of course, experienced with all senses to begin with. This multilayered approach may, in part at least, account for the deep and profound feeling of healing and release that clients report having after successful psychodramatic work.

And most importantly, clients are able to access and experience deeply held limbic memory and sensation and translate both into words so that feelings and sensorial imprints (such as touch, smell, sights, and sounds) can be elevated to a conscious level where they can be thought about, made sense of, and placed into an overall framework within the self. They thus can become part of an integrated and multisensory trauma narrative. Clients who have been traumatized have likely experienced some dysregulation of their limbic system, which governs mood, appetite, sleep cycles, emotional coloring, and intensity. In this way psychodrama, sociometry, and group psychotherapy allow clients to slowly create new neural imprints, to repattern their limbic system.

When protagonists experience their bodies during a psychodrama, whether it be through shutting down, a queasy stomach, feeling of tightness in the chest, or unsteady legs, the therapist can slowly explore what is going on. "What is going on inside of you right now? What's getting triggered? What's happening in your body?" Taking the time to ask these questions, whether in group treatment or individual psychodrama, can help the client to learn to integrate the material being triggered rather than getting stuck in a defensive position to get away from it. The group also may become triggered as the process moves ahead. As the director/therapist checks in with the protagonist as to what's going on in the body, the group members learn to check in with themselves in a similar fashion. They become educated as to how to process their own trauma as they witness what is happening with the protagonist. It is important that plenty of time be reserved for sharing so that all members of the group can process what is going on for them. The knowledge that they are and will continue to be in a group healing process helps group members to stay with what's happening inside of them and use the protagonist's drama to better understand their own inner world. As they witness and identify, their minds make a thousand small connections as their inner world moves through cycles of fuzziness and clarity while the veils of illusion lift and truth emerges.

It is important to remember that the material that is getting triggered is largely unconscious, stuck in the body, as it were. Even asking trauma survivors to answer questions like, "What's going on with you?" can baffle them. They go into a sort of "speed think" and try to come up with the answer they think the therapist wants to hear. It is much more useful to say, "What's going on in your body? Where is it going on, can you put your hand there? If that part of your body had a voice, what would it say?" Once the body starts talking through the mouth, the head, the intellect, can quiet down. Once the client knows that it's okay for the body to open up and tell its story, the cortex can take a break and work at normal speed, where it can make sense of what's being said. What we want to do is to help traumatized persons to calm down enough so that they can tune in to what's going inside of them and begin to become curious about it, to want to know more, and to articulate it. In this way, adult COSAPs can heal themselves and come to understand both what is happening to them and the process of healing, so that when they get triggered outside of therapy, they can avoid becoming retraumatized. They become capable of integrating fragments of memory and modulating the intensity of the whole response system, namely the thinking, feeling, and behavior that get triggered, and thus are able to continue healing.

The other question that is useful to ask clients is, "What does your body want to do?" When these states are triggered the body often wants to do something—to take some action related to the suppressed emotion or suppressed actions associated with the painful or traumatic dynamics or events. Often, this may include yelling, kicking, screaming, hitting, or running and hiding. Psychodrama allows those actions to be undertaken while in a safe clinical setting. If done mindfully, if the need to act is understood by the client and is seen in its therapeutic context, it can produce a deep sense of relief and help to unblock emotions long stored in the body. As these feelings come forward, the thinking that was frozen in place starts to come forward, too. The body moves and the mind and heart follow. Oftentimes, this takes the form of the kind of reasoning one sees in confused children trying to make sense of what to them made no sense. Sentences such as "Am I bad?" "Stop yelling at me!" "I hate you!" "Why can't you see how much I love you," and so on, sputter out as they gain their footing on the new soil that is rapidly accumulating beneath their feet. This is psychodrama in slow motion (Dayton, 2005).

Having the therapist follow the lead of the protagonist very slowly and carefully helps adult COSAP trauma survivors feel that they are at the locus of control in their psychodrama; that they will not be pushed beyond capacity and coerced into areas that they are not ready or willing to explore (Dayton, 2005). The trauma survivor initially may come forward tentatively, frightened of retaliation for even thinking angry thoughts. Contrary to what many people think, the material in psychodrama does not necessarily come pouring forth; it is slow and painstaking work. It requires much time with protagonists in order to help them to tune in on their bodies and slowly move from there. The Chinese have a saying: "The deepest pain has no words." To work with adult COSAPs with a history of trauma means working with this sort of pain, which comes out of hiding like a disembodied spirit that has not seen the light of day, a spirit coming back from the world of the dead.

Sensory, Emotional, and Psychological Integration

Psychodrama allows for a level of sensory, intellectual, emotional, and behavioral integration that is the foundation of its unusual therapeutic efficacy and healing power. It incorporates all of the senses along with language, thought, emotion, and concrete behavior. Psychodrama provides a framework in which clients can experience themselves not simply as victims of circumstance, but as courageous victors willing to revisit painful material in service of healing, to view the early landscape through the eyes of today with the help and support of therapeutic allies, or to take a plunge into dreams, fantasies, and hopes for the future. Clients are allowed a full range of expression. The unique combination of talking, movement, natural behavior, whether it be tears or laughter, yelling or whispers, physical closeness or distance, allows for a full engagement with the material. If direct involvement is too intense or confusing for an adult COSAP, a stand-in can be enrolled to portray the self of the protagonist, providing the effect of viewing one's life in a mirror, in a more distanced manner.

In addition to diving into past conflicts, psychodrama can also address the present, illuminating and concretizing current life choices, examining and infusing them with new emotional intelligence and awareness. Psychodrama can also allow an adult COSAP client to peer into and practice future life scenarios, playing out the dreams, fears, and possible choices that can become the tomorrows, consciously and with the support and attention of others. It is a virtual laboratory where the client is his or her own self-chosen study. It is life imitating life—a second chance at living.

CONCLUSION

Psychodrama, a role-playing method that involves surrogates representing roles from the protagonist's world, can re-create the relational context in which the family pain of many ACAs first occurred. Visiting what is referred to in psychodrama as the *status nascendi,* or that place from which a complex grew, can allow adult COSAPs to identify, revisit, and hopefully gain insight into what might be driving their own dysfunctional patterns of relating. Because of its ability to reach back into the psyche and the early internalized object relationships, psychodrama can be an ideal vehicle for affect regulation as it helps to mirror the level of both internal and relational intensity that adult COSAPs "understand" and often re-create and reenact throughout their adulthood. When this emotional, psychological, and behavioral "intensity" is reenacted through role play, it is effectively being brought from an unconscious to a conscious state. This allows clients to see themselves in action so that they can recognize the need to modulate their behavior.

The use of psychodrama allows old behaviors to be brought forward and new behaviors to be practiced. It helps the adult COSAP to use the *thinking mind* to reregulate the *limbic mind* so that a new narrative can be formed and new meanings can be made, and a recovery process can begin and continue.

REFERENCES

Anda, R., Felitti, V., Bremner, J., Walker, J. D., Whitfield, C., Perry, B. D., et al. (2006). The enduring effects of abuse and related adverse experiences in childhood. *European Archives of Psychiatry and Clinical Neuroscience, 256*(3), 174–186.
Black, C. (1981). *It will never happen to me.* Denver, CO: Ballentine Books.
Black, C. (1982). *Double duty: Help for the adult child.* Deerfield Beach, FL: Health Communications.
Bradshaw, J. (1988). *Healing the shame that binds you.* Deerfield Beach, FL: Health Communications.
Carnes, P. (1997). *The betrayal bond: Breaking free of exploitive relationships.* Deerfield Beach, FL: Health Communications.
Cermack, T. L. (1985). *A primer on adult children of alcoholics.* Pompano Beach, FL: Health Communications.
Coyle, J. P., Nochajski, T., Maguin, E., Safyer, A., DeWit, D., & Macdonald, S. (2006). An exploratory study of the nature of family resilience in families affected by parental alcohol abuse. *Journal of Family Issues, 10*(12), 1606–1623.
Cozolino, L. (2006). *The neuroscience of human relationships.* New York: W.W. Norton.
Dayton, T. (2000). *Trauma and addiction.* Deerfield Beach, FL: Health Communications.
Dayton, T. (2005). *The living stage: A step by step guide to psychodrama, sociometry and experiential group therapy.* Deerfield Beach, FL: Health Communications.

Dayton, T. (2007). *Emotional sobriety: From relationship trauma to resilience and balance*. Deerfield Beach, FL: Health Communications.

Dube, S. R., Miller, J. W., Brown, D. W., Giles, W. H., Felitti, V. J., Dong, M., et al. (2006). Adverse childhood experiences and the association with ever using alcohol and initiating alcohol use during adolescence. *The Journal of Adolescent Health, 38*(4), 444.e1–444.e10.

Freud, S. (1922). *Beyond the pleasure principle*. London: International Psycho-Analytical Press.

Horney, K. (1950). *Neurosis and human growth*. New York: W.W. Norton.

Lifton, R. J. (1968). *Death in life: Survivors of Hiroshima*. New York: Random House.

Moreno, J. L. (1953). *Who shall survive: Foundations of sociometry, group psychotherapy and psychodrama*. Beacon, NY: Beacon House.

Moreno, J. L. (1964). *Psychodrama: Foundations of psychotherapy*. Beacon, NY: Beacon House.

Peterson, C., Maier, S. F., & Seligman, M. E. P. (1995). *Learned helplessness: A theory for the age of personal control*. New York: Oxford University Press.

Rando, T. A. (1993). *Treatment of complicated mourning*. Chicago: Research Press.

Sacks, S., Sacks, J., De Leon, G., Bernhardt, A. I., & Staines, G. L. (1997). Modified therapeutic community for mentally ill chemical "abusers": Background; influences; program description; preliminary findings. *Substance Use and Misuse, 32*(9), 1217–1259.

Spiegel, B. R., & Fewell, C. H. (2004). 12-Step programs as a treatment modality. In S. Straussner (Ed.), *Clinical work with substance-abusing clients* (2nd ed., pp. 125–145). New York: Guilford Press.

van der Kolk, B. A. (1987). *Psychological trauma*. Washington, DC: American Psychiatric Press.

van der Kolk, B. A. (1994). The body keeps the score: Memory and the evolving psychobiology of post-traumatic stress. *Harvard Review of Psychiatry, 1*(5), 253–265.

van der Kolk, B. A. (2003). Posttraumatic stress disorder and the nature of trauma. In M. F. Solomon & D. J. Siegel (Eds.), *Healing trauma: Attachment, mind, body, and brain* (pp. 168–195). New York: W.W. Norton.

van der Kolk, B. A., McFarlane, A., & Weisauth, L. (Eds.). (1996). *Traumatic stress: The effects of overwhelming experience on mind, body, and society*. New York: The Guilford Press.

Wegscheider-Cruse, S. (1980). *Another chance: Hope and health for the alcoholic family*. Deerfield Beach, FL: Health Communications.

Werner, E. E. (1996). How children become resilient: Observations and cautions. *Resiliency in Action, 1*(1), 18–28.

Werner, E. E., & Smith, R. S. (1992). *Overcoming the odds: High risk children from birth to adulthood*. New York: Cornell University Press.

Woititz, J. G. (1983). *Adult children of alcoholics*. Deerfield Beach, FL: Health Communications.

Wolin, S. J., & Wolin, S. (1993). *The resilient self: How survivors of troubled families rise above adversity*. New York: Villard Books.

8

Prevention and Intervention Programs for Pregnant Women Who Abuse Substances

Iris E. Smith

INTRODUCTION

Fetal Alcohol Syndrome (FAS) was first identified in the United States in the early 1970s by Jones, Smith, Ulleland, and Streissguth (1973). Although much of the early research focused on FAS as a categorical diagnosis resulting from a mother's use of alcohol during pregnancy, subsequent research revealed a continuum of developmental outcomes ranging from subtle neurobehavioral effects to mental retardation and other significant medical problems. This continuum of developmental outcomes has become known as Fetal Alcohol Spectrum Disorder or FASD. With an estimated incidence of 2–6 cases per 1,000 live births, FASD is now recognized as one of the leading causes of mental retardation and birth defects (Centers for Disease Control and Prevention [CDC], 2009). Research on FASD has also led to questions about the developmental impact of other drugs used during pregnancy such as cocaine and more recently methamphetamine as well as effective strategies for intervening with women who use these substances. Though heavy alcohol consumption during pregnancy appears to create the greatest threat to an unborn child, any drug use (including tobacco) during pregnancy increases the risk of medical problems and developmental disabilities (Schempf, 2007).

In the 36 years since FAS was first identified, we have increased our understanding of the underlying mechanisms and developmental impact of prenatal alcohol and other drug exposures, but have made little progress in our efforts to prevent it. The 2005 National Survey on Drug Use and Health indicated no significant change in illicit drug use among women between 15 and 44 from 1999 to 2005 (SAMHSA, 2005). According to the results of the 2005 survey, 3.9% of pregnant women and 9.9% of nonpregnant women between the ages of 15 and 44 used illicit drugs, with marijuana being the drug most frequently used, indicating little change in the prevalence of drug use in the past 30 years (SAMHSA, 1997). Similarly, data from the CDC indicates that the prevalence of alcohol use and binge drinking among pregnant and nonpregnant women of childbearing age remained unchanged from 1991 to 2005, despite widespread prevention and intervention efforts (CDC, 2009).

Although the most recent results from the Pregnancy Risk Assessment Monitoring System (PRAMS) in 31 states did report a significant decrease in the prevalence of smoking during pregnancy (from 15.2% in 2000 to 13.8% in 2005; $p \leq 0.01$), the prepregnancy rates essentially remained unchanged, ranging from 21% to 22% for this period (CDC, 2009). Rates of smoking appeared to be highest for women 20–24 years of age.

Rising rates of alcohol and drug use among nonpregnant younger women is a reason for concern and certainly merits our attention. A 2009 study examining trends in alcohol binge drinking among youth and young adults from 1979 to 2006 ($n = 500,000+$) found that although the overall prevalence of binge drinking among youth under the age of 20 had declined, binge drinking rates among young women between the ages of 12 and 20 has been rising. This study, which examined data from the National Household Survey on Drug Abuse and the National Survey on Drug Use and Health, also found that the risk of binge drinking was increasing fastest among minority females in this age group (Grucza, Norberg, & Bierut, 2009). Another important finding from this study was that while the drinking rates among nonstudents had declined, drinking among male college students remained unchanged and binge drinking among female college students (21–23 years of age) was increasing. The fact that these women are just entering the peak reproductive years highlights the need for targeted intervention to nonpregnant young women on college campuses.

It is evident from these data that efforts to raise public awareness of the risks associated with alcohol and other drug use during pregnancy have not been sufficient to deter women from using these substances. The considerable social and economic costs associated with prenatal alcohol and drug exposure highlight the need for effective, evidence-based intervention strategies to motivate and support women in discontinuing the use of harmful substances even before they become pregnant. Studies of adolescents and young adult women suggest that many younger women may be more tolerant toward alcohol and at higher risk for combining alcohol use and sexual activity, increasing the risk of an unplanned, alcohol-exposed pregnancy (Walker, Fisher, Sherman, Wybrecht, & Kyndely, 2005). This chapter will review evidence-based prevention and early intervention programs for women at risk of alcohol- or drug-exposed pregnancies.

SCREENING WOMEN FOR RISK OF ALCOHOL- OR DRUG-EXPOSED PREGNANCY

Valid and reliable screening and assessment tools are essential in identifying and intervening with substance-using women. There are a number of well-validated, brief, self-report questionnaires that have been used to screen women for alcohol use including the Michigan Alcoholism Screening Test (MAST), the T-ACE, TWEAK, and the CAGE. All of these measures have performed reasonably well in identifying heavy drinkers in a variety of populations, with the T-ACE and the TWEAK being more sensitive and specific for assessing periconceptional drinking (Bradley, Boyd-Wickizer, Powell, & Burman, 1998; Russell et al., 1994). Scores on the Maternal Substance Abuse Checklist (MSAC), a cumulative index developed by Coles, Krable, Drews-Botsch, and Falek (2000) have been found to correlate with developmental delays observed in children prenatally exposed to alcohol. The most effective screening tools incorporate multiple measures of drinking and drug use and the associated problems.

Self-report measures have been the most commonly used method for identifying alcohol or other drug exposure. However, self-report instruments may not always yield accurate information on use. Many women may be reluctant to admit to using alcohol or drugs during pregnancy because of perceived social stigma, fear of legal sanctions such as loss of child custody, guilt, poor recall, or other factors (CDC, 2009; Koren, Hutson, & Gareri, 2008; Smith & Coles, 1991). While many biological measures such as toxicology screens of blood or urine have limited utility due to the rapid metabolism and clearance of many drugs from the maternal and/or infant system, recently developed techniques for assessing biomarkers show considerable promise, especially for identifying drug exposed infants not detected through maternal self-report measures. Biomarkers present in maternal and infant hair have been used to detect cocaine, methamphetamine, opioids, marijuana, and other drugs commonly abused, and can be useful in identifying more long-term use of these substances. Fatty acid ethyl esters in meconium and maternal hair have also been used to assess prenatal alcohol exposure (Koren, Hutson, & Gareri, 2008).

In addition to screening for alcohol and drug use, a comprehensive assessment of other associated risk factors is highly recommended. Women with a history of heavy prepregnancy drinking and/or drug use are also more likely to have multiple risk factors for negative pregnancy outcomes in addition to those associated with alcohol or drug use during pregnancy. Lifestyle factors such as poor nutrition, lack of health care, and exposure to violence and sexual abuse place female drug users at risk for a number of reproductive and gynecologic problems including sexually transmitted diseases, amenorrhea, infertility, premature delivery, stillbirth, and spontaneous abortions (Smith & Coles, 1991).

PREVENTION STRATEGIES

It has been difficult to establish a clear risk threshold for alcohol and other recreational drugs. For that reason, the best advice for women who are either pregnant or planning to become pregnant is abstinence. Studies of FASD, for example, have consistently raised questions about whether there is a "safe" level of alcohol exposure during pregnancy (Coles, Smith, Fernhoff, & Falek, 1984; Landesman-Dwyer, Keller, & Streissguth, 1978; Mattson & Riley, 1998). In addition to the patterning and levels of alcohol exposure, factors such as maternal ability to metabolize alcohol (which may in part be genetically determined) may also influence outcomes. Peak blood alcohol levels during pregnancy and binge drinking (consuming four or more alcoholic drinks per occasion) are associated with an increased risk of negative developmental outcomes (Barr et al., 2006; Eckardt et al., 1998; Jacobson, Jacobson, Sokol, & Ager, 1998; Sampson, Streissguth, Barr, & Bookstein, 1989). High peak blood alcohol levels have also been found to increase fetal risk in animal studies (Ramadoss et al., 2006).

The timing of alcohol exposure during pregnancy is also an important consideration. Studies that have examined the effects of discontinuing alcohol use during pregnancy have found that both the amount of alcohol consumed and the length of prenatal exposure affect the range and severity of deficits observed (May et al., 2008). Thus, even if a woman has been drinking heavily during early pregnancy, discontinuing alcohol or drug use at any point during the pregnancy can be beneficial for both mother and child.

Although the more severe manifestations of FASD are generally associated with heavier drinking during pregnancy, not all heavy-drinking women give birth to an FAS child and the milder manifestations of

FASD may occur at drinking levels within most cultural norms. The fact that some mother–child dyads appear to be more vulnerable than others to alcohol's effects suggests that there may be biological and/or environmental factors which mediate alcohol's effects. Empirical support for genetic influences in the etiology of FAS is limited. Case studies of identical and nonidentical twins suggest that genetic predisposition may play a role (Christoffel & Salafsky, 1975). Epidemiologic studies suggest that the incidence of FAS and FAE is higher among certain ethnic groups most notably Native Americans and African Americans and populations residing on the Western Cape of South Africa (May, Hymbaugh, & Aase, 1983; National Institute on Alcohol Abuse and Alcoholism [NIAAA], 1997). More recent research to identify polymorphisms that might contribute to FASD has identified several potential genetic mediators of risk, but thus far only one of the genes for the alcohol dehydrogenase enzyme has been linked to FASD (Warren & Li, 2005).

Preventing FASD and other prenatal drug effects requires a multi-pronged approach ranging from patient education to alcohol and drug treatment for substance-dependent women. The Institute of Medicine (IOM) defines three levels of prevention based on the intended target population and anticipated outcomes, which provide a useful conceptual framework for reviewing strategies for the prevention of prenatal alcohol and other drug effects. The IOM definitions are as follows (Gordon, 1983):

Universal: These interventions are directed toward the general public or a subgroup of the general public who show no signs of risk factors, but for whom these strategies could reduce the likelihood that they will develop risk behaviors.

Selected: These interventions focus on subgroups whose risk of problems is believed to be higher than the general population, due to certain characteristics.

Indicated: These interventions focus on families and individuals who are already exhibiting specific risk factors, but have not progressed to the behavior being targeted.

Universal Prevention Strategies

Public education has been the most widely used strategy for the prevention of prenatal alcohol and other drug effects. Beginning in 1989, federal law required alcoholic beverage containers to carry a warning label that read: "GOVERNMENT WARNING: (1) According to the Surgeon General, women should not drink alcoholic beverages during pregnancy because of the risk of birth defects. (2) Consumption of alcoholic beverages impairs your ability to drive a car or operate machinery, and may cause health problems" (PL 100-690, 1988). During the 1980s many states passed laws that required signage with similar warnings in establishments that served alcoholic beverages.

Research on the effectiveness of the warning labels and signs in changing attitudes and behavior has not been encouraging. Although population surveys have indicated that people are reading the labels, research has consistently failed to demonstrate that the labels have affected beliefs or behaviors over time (Craig, 1995; MacKinnon, Nohre, Pentz, & Stacy, 2000). The ineffectiveness of warning labels may be due to several factors. Foremost among these is the fact that the populations at highest risk are those who may have the least amount of control over their drinking or drug using behavior. In addition, the phenomenon of "cognitive dissonance" may cause some individuals to disregard the warning or even to increase their drinking in defiance of it (Abel, 1998).

Although public education strategies, such as community-wide health promotion and warning labels, are the most common universal approaches to the prevention of prenatal alcohol and other drug effects, legal strategies such as prohibition also fall into this category. Bowerman (1997) reports on such a strategy in Barrow, Alaska, where in 1994 a law was passed prohibiting the possession of alcohol. A pre- and post-legislation comparison of self-reported alcohol use by pregnant women in the six affected villages found that alcohol use dropped from 42% to 9% during the first 5 months of the ban. The most significant decrease was for alcohol use in the first trimester. Although use in the third trimester also decreased, it did not achieve significance. Changes in the use of tobacco, cocaine, amphetamines, and marijuana were not significant, supporting the hypothesis that the alcohol specific legislation was responsible for the change observed. The results of this study are certainly intriguing, although it is possible that the legal sanctions attached to alcohol use may have compromised the validity of the self-reported data.

Selected Prevention Strategies

Health promotion and public education are likely to be effective for non–substance-dependent women whose alcohol or drug use falls within socially acceptable boundaries. For these women, concern about the possibility of developmental problems in their children is a sufficient motivation for them to either reduce substance use or postpone pregnancy.

Provider perceptions and attitudes can also influence the success of intervention programs as well as the perceived accessibility to prenatal care (Sculpholme, Robertson, & Kamons, 1991). A study of mandatory reporting of perinatal substance abuse in Pinellas County, Florida, found that although rates of drug use were comparable among African American and Caucasian women in this region, African American women were 10 times as likely to be reported to the local health department for substance use during pregnancy (Chasnoff, Landress, & Barrett, 1990). This observed bias in reporting was consistent with the widely held belief that prenatal cocaine abuse was a problem of poor minority women. Moreover, many women may have avoided prenatal clinics for fear of being reported and losing custody of their children.

Teagle and Brindis (1998) found that provider perceptions of the prevalence of drug use and the characteristics of drug users often differed significantly from the reality. These researchers found higher use of alcohol, cigarettes, and marijuana among Caucasian adolescents compared to African American girls. However, African American adolescents were more likely to discontinue or reduce their use of drugs during pregnancy. Service providers surveyed and believed that the prevalence of drug use to be lower than what was reported, although they correctly identified Caucasian girls as being more likely to use drugs.

One of the most promising intervention approaches for drug using women is the Brief Motivational Intervention (BMI). During the past decade, there has been a proliferation of studies demonstrating the effectiveness of this approach in changing a number of health related behaviors including alcohol and drug use (Burke, Arkowitz, & Menchola, 2003). BMIs are based on the Transtheoretical Model of Change and are designed to facilitate behavior change through a combination of information, supportive counseling, concrete assistance, and service brokering (Prochaska, DiClemente, & Norcross, 1992).

Brief Interventions in the Prenatal Clinic

Most of the early intervention models were developed for alcohol-using women who were already pregnant. Many of the most successful interventions were implemented in prenatal clinics and integrated into routine prenatal care. Outcome studies of these programs indicated that the developmental impact of alcohol use may be reduced if women discontinue alcohol use during pregnancy (Coles et al., 1991; Corse & Smith, 1998; Rossett & Weiner, 1985; Smith, Lancaster, Moss-Wells, & Falek, 1987; Weiner & Morse, 1988). One of the most important findings from these studies was the value of targeted intervention even as late as the second trimester of pregnancy.

The success of prenatal clinic based interventions such as those cited above depend upon the provider's ability to engage and retain pregnant alcohol and other drug users in prenatal care. However, heavy alcohol and drug-using women may be less likely to initiate and comply with prenatal care (Friedman, Heneghan, & Rosenthal, 2009; Melnikow, Alemangno, Rottman, & Zyzanski, 1991; Sculpholme et al., 1991; Sunil, Spears, Hook, Castillo, & Torres, 2008).

Brief Interventions in Other Health Care Settings

While pregnant women are the most critical audience for alcohol and drug interventions, the most effective prevention efforts are those that reach women before they become pregnant. Ideally screening and intervention should occur during routine primary care, in the emergency department, and in other health care settings where women receive care.

BMIs have been found effective in a variety of settings, including emergency departments. Anderson (1986) reported the results of an intervention program implemented in a hospital emergency department utilizing a personalized nursing model that found program participants ($n = 72$) reported lower rates of drug use and less perceived stress and emotional distress than a comparison group ($n = 83$) of women who were not involved in the program. All women in this study had refused referrals to alcohol or drug treatment programs and had been identified primarily through emergency department admissions. The intervention involved home visits by project nurses with the goal of assisting participants with client-identified needs. This model may hold promise for working with women who are resistant to seeking drug treatment or who have received inadequate prenatal care.

The Healthy Moms study, a clinical trial ($n = 235$) examining the efficacy of a brief alcohol intervention for postpartum women receiving care at 34 obstetrical practice clinics in Wisconsin, focused on women who had already given birth (Fleming, Lund, Wilson, Landry, & Scheets, 2008). The goal of the intervention was to reduce the risk of a subsequent alcohol exposed pregnancy and reduce other risks associated with alcohol use. This program employed a brief alcohol intervention delivered in four sessions to women receiving routine postpartum care from a primary healthcare provider. The evaluation of the program found statistically significant reductions in alcohol and drug use among participants at 6-month followup. The results of this study provide further evidence of the efficacy of BMIs in encouraging changes in alcohol use.

In addition to venues where parents receive care, pediatric practice settings provide another opportunity for identifying alcohol or drug users. A study by Wilson et al. (2008) that explored the feasibility of screening for parental alcohol use in pediatric practices found that 12% ($n = 879$) of the parents receiving care at one of the three pediatric primary care clinic sites screened positive on either the TWEAK or the AUDIT for alcohol problems.

The majority (89%) of parents who participated in this study also indicated that they would be willing to be screened by a pediatrician for alcohol use and would likely provide honest responses (Wilson et al., 2008).

More widespread implementation of alcohol and drug screening and brief interventions would not only help to identify risky alcohol and drug users prior to conception, but would also open the door to early intervention with substance-abusing families. Women who have already given birth after an alcohol-exposed pregnancy are at high risk for another. Previous alcohol exposed pregnancies may also be identified during routine pediatric visits, creating an opportunity for early assessment and intervention with FASD children. Nonexposed siblings of FASD children are also at higher risk of abuse, neglect, psychological and other health problems, and early mortality compared to children of non–substance-using parents (Burd, Klug, & Martsolf, 2004). In general, children of alcoholics and other substance-dependent parents are at higher risk of social and developmental problems (Harter & Taylor, 2000; Silverman & Schonberg, 2001; Whitaker, Orzoi, & Kahn, 2006).

Indicated Prevention Strategies

The population at highest risk for FAS and other prenatal drug effects are women within the child bearing age range who are heavy users of drugs and alcohol. Women who have developed a dependency on alcohol or other drugs will require more intensive interventions than women who are light or social drinkers or drug users. The results of selective strategies such as those employed at Boston City Hospital and elsewhere suggest that even heavy drinkers in the prenatal clinic setting may respond to education and supportive counseling (Rossett & Weiner, 1985). However, women enrolled in prenatal care may not be representative of the population at risk. Many drug addicted women may seek prenatal care late in pregnancy, if at all (Abma & Mott, 1991; Chan, Wingert, Wachsman, Schuetz, & Rogers, 1986; Petitti, Coleman, Binsacca, & Allen, 1990). Effective intervention programs are needed in venues that heavy drinking and drug using women tend to frequent.

The compulsive nature of substance dependency may make it difficult for addicted women to discontinue their use without intensive, focused interventions including drug treatment. At least two studies have found that women who discontinue or reduce their alcohol or drug use during pregnancy may differ from those who do not on a number of characteristics, most notably the length and severity of their addiction (Corse & Smith, 1998; Smith et al., 1987).

In 1997, CDC funded a study to examine the effectiveness of a selective intervention for preconceptional women at high risk for an alcohol exposed pregnancy. This program known as Project CHOICES provided women with a brief intervention focused on both the reduction of alcohol use and the use of contraception to postpone pregnancy. In this study, Project CHOICES was implemented in a variety of community settings where the prevalence of heavy alcohol use was likely to be higher than in the general population such as correctional facilities, alcohol and drug treatment centers, and county health departments (Floyd, Ebrahim, & Boyle, 1999; Floyd et al., 2007). The study was conducted in collaboration with Nova Southeastern University, the University of Texas Health Sciences Center at Houston, and Virginia Commonwealth University at Richmond. The results of the multisite randomized control trial found that targeting both risky drinking and contraception use was effective in reducing the risk of an alcohol exposed pregnancy even in dependent or risky drinkers. The intervention consisted of four sessions focused on increasing a woman's commitment to change and helping her to work through the pros and cons of either changing alcohol use or postponing pregnancy. Women who elected to postpone pregnancy were scheduled for an additional appointment for contraceptive counseling. Project CHOICES is one of the few selected interventions that have been tested in large scale randomized controlled trials ($n = 4,626$ women). A detailed description of the program can be found at www.cdc.gov/ncbddd/fas.

Barriers to Treatment for Substance-Dependent Women

Despite the increased attention to the prevention of FASD and other drug related birth defects, even women who desire addiction treatment may face significant challenges in obtaining it. According to Substance Abuse Mental Health Services Administration (2007), of the 6.3 million women between the ages of 18 and 49 who needed substance abuse treatment in 2006 only 10.4% received it through a specialty substance use treatment facility. According to this study, poor women (family incomes less than $20,000) were more likely to receive treatment than those with higher incomes. The study also found that 84.2% of those who were classified as needing substance abuse treatment did not believe that they needed it. Among women who desired treatment but did not receive it, barriers included not being able to stop using alcohol or illicit drugs (36%), lack of health insurance coverage (34%), and social stigma (30%).

Another significant barrier to treatment for substance-dependent women is the fact that they are more likely than men to be the primary caretakers of their children. The lack of child care provisions in most traditional treatment programs is often a deterrent to seeking help. Outcome studies of participants in therapeutic community programs have found that retention rates for women tend to improve when they are allowed to have their children with them (DeLeon & Jainchill, 1991).

Recovery for women is often compromised by the fact that they tend to return to environments that are not supportive of continued abstinence. Several studies have found that addicted women tend to have a number of other family members who are alcohol and drug users (Lex, Teoh, Lagomasino, Mello, & Mendelson, 1990; Wallace, 1991). Thus, many recovering women must return to an environment that is, at best, not supportive of their recovery. Women are also more likely to be single at the time that they enter treatment, a fact which adds to feelings of loneliness and isolation, which in turn can be triggers for relapse.

Many researchers point out that the treatment needs of women, particularly women who are pregnant or parenting, are different from those of men (Kosten, Gawin, Kosten, & Rounsaville, 1993). Most traditional treatment models have been designed for males and thus give little attention to gender-specific treatment components. A 2007 review of the literature on treatment entry, retention and outcome in women found that while women may be slightly less likely to enter treatment compared to men, gender is not a significant predictor of treatment retention, completion, or outcome (Greenfield et al., 2007). However, effective treatment models that incorporate components specific to the psychosocial development and experiences of women are more effective in promoting long-term changes in drug use (Greenfield et al., 2007; Greenfield, Trucco, McHugh, Lincoln, & Gallop, 2007).

Unlike men, women tend to view themselves in the context of their social roles and interpersonal relationships (Stenius, Veysey, Hamilton, & Anderson, 2005). Disruptions in important intimate relationships can contribute both to the development of drug dependency and to relapse following treatment. Use of alcohol and drugs often exacerbates feelings of loneliness and alienation, leading to a vicious cycle (Finkelstein, 1996). Perceived inadequacy in her role as caregiver may seriously impact a woman's self-esteem. Limited psychological resources and social supports coupled with deficient coping skills are major contributors to stress for women (Luthar & Walsh, 1995).

Parenting Dysfunction and Education

Women who are pregnant may have the added stress of child rearing, often with the uncertainty of developmental outcomes for other children who have been exposed to drugs or alcohol in utero. Deficient parent role models, parental psychopathology, and the low frustration tolerance in addicted women increase the potential for child abuse. The use of illegal drugs often results in a deviant lifestyle that is focused on drug seeking to the neglect of parenting responsibilities as well as self-care (Wasserman & Leventhal, 1993). Sexual promiscuity and prostitution are frequently associated with drug use in women, placing them at risk for exposure to violence, sexually transmitted diseases, malnutrition, and medical neglect (Simmons, Havens, Whiting, Holtz, & Bada, 2009). Compared to males, female substance abusers are more likely to have experienced sexual victimization in situations where they perceived their lives to be in danger (Dansky & Brady, 1996). Many alcohol- and drug-using women come from homes where physical and sexual abuse were common occurrences and parenting was poor or nonexistent. As a result, their own parenting behavior may be markedly deficient. These factors in combination potentiate the risk for poor developmental outcomes in alcohol or other drug exposed children who remain in the custody of alcohol and drug using parents (Pedersen et al., 2008). A 1999 report by the National Center on Addiction and Substance Abuse at Columbia University indicated that 82% of the 915 child welfare professionals surveyed nationally cited alcohol in combination with other drugs as a primary factor in 70% to 90% of child abuse and neglect cases (Reid, Macchetto, & Foster, 1999).

Burns and Burns (1988) proposed a four-factor causal pathway for parenting dysfunction in drug using mothers that includes (1) the negative heritage of poor parenting; (2) the behavior of the vulnerable drug exposed child; (3) maternal emotional instability; and (4) absent or deficient social support. In addition to the factors proposed by Burns et al., the intense craving and resulting drug seeking in some users often leads to risk-taking behaviors, which place both mother and child in dangerous situations. For example, the effects of passive exposure to crack cocaine smoke and chemicals used in the manufacture of methamphetamine are a significant cause of injuries and other medical problems in children who spend time in "crack houses" or "meth labs" (Mayes, 1996).

Parenting education and skills training are important components of any treatment program for pregnant women. In a systematic review of the literature on treatment approaches for substance-using parents involved with the child welfare system, Osterling and Austin (2008) identified the following components as contributors to successful outcomes:

1. Women-centered treatment that involves children
2. Specialized health and mental health services
3. Home visitation
4. Concrete assistance

Co-Occurring Disorders

Parental psychopathology may add another dimension to the risk of poor outcomes. Studies that have examined the impact of parental psychopathology on child development have found that the children of depressed or otherwise psychiatrically disturbed parents have a higher prevalence of behavior problems, emotional instability, and academic problems (Goodman, 2007). Parental psychopathology and problems with parent–infant attachment in alcoholic families may help to explain the higher prevalence of behavioral disorders and externalizing behaviors among children of alcoholic parents (Das Eiden, Edwards, & Leonard, 2002).

Addiction problems in both men and women are often accompanied by other forms of psychopathology. Numerous studies have indicated that addicted women, particularly those who are addicted to crack cocaine have a high prevalence of past histories of physical and sexual abuse (Savage & Russell, 2005; Wallace, 1991). As the prevalence of Post-Traumatic Stress Disorder (PTSD) among addicted women is unknown, many clinicians believe it to be a primary factor in both the development and the persistence of drug use in this population (Dansky et al., 1996). Depression, antisocial personality, and other Axis II disorders have also been cited as predictors of treatment outcomes in addicted women (Rounsaville et al., 1987). Although comorbidity within addict populations is widely recognized by both clinicians and researchers, treatment strategies for substance abuse and mental illness have largely developed in isolation from one another. Individuals with concurrent drug addiction and psychiatric illness may require a highly structured treatment environment, at least initially, to allow for a stabilization period. In some cases, they may not be able to assume child care responsibilities until after stabilization occurs. Psychiatrically disturbed addicts may also exhibit a more erratic recovery process than addicts without concurrent psychiatric problems, characterized by movement in and out of treatment programs (Grella, 2006; Greenfield et al., 2007). Programs must be flexible enough to allow these individuals continued access to care. Pregnancy may also make it more difficult to identify psychiatric problems in women, since many symptoms such as low energy levels, sleeplessness, and loss of appetite are also associated with the physical changes that occur during pregnancy.

Programs Designed for Women's Needs

Given the myriad factors that contribute to drug dependence in women, the most successful models of treatment are likely to be those which include comprehensive, gender specific treatment components with aggressive outreach and case management (May et al., 2008). Beginning in the 1980s, the federal government allocated funds for the development and evalua-tion of a new era of drug treatment programs for women, which incorpo-rated strategies and program components that had been identified in the research literature as effective in intervening with pregnant and parent-ing women. There is now a growing body of literature on effective treat-ment models for this population (Barry et al., 2009; Colletti et al., 1995; Greenfield et al, 2007; Magura, Laudet, Kang, & Whitney, 1999).

Much of the data available on treatment outcomes for pregnant and parenting women is based on individuals who are admitted to treatment and intervention programs. However, individuals who enter alcohol and drug treatment programs may be different from those who do not. Studies that have examined differences between treated and untreated addicts have found that untreated addicts may experience fewer or less severe social problems than individuals who seek treatment (Rounsaville & Kleber, 1985). While there have been few studies that have examined fac-tors that motivate pregnant and parenting women, a 1985 Swedish study by Tunving and Nilsson found that concern for children and fear of loss of custody were important factors in the decision to seek treatment. Ironically, these same factors may create barriers to treatment because of lack of child care provisions in treatment programs and fear of being referred to Child Protective Services (Smith, Dent, Coles, & Falek, 1992).

Treatment outcome studies have found that, in general, successful abstinence is linked to retention in treatment; that is, the longer clients remain in treatment, the more likely they are to remain abstinent (DeLeon, Melnick, & Kressel, 1997; Nardi, 1998). Thus, retention in treatment is often used as a marker for effectiveness in evaluations of alcohol and drug treatment programs.

Roberts and Nishimoto (1996) compared outcomes in 369 women who participated in three different treatment modalities: (1) a traditional outpatient program for women (1½ hours a day, once a week); (2) an inten-sive day treatment program (5½ hours a day, 5 days a week); and (3) a coed residential therapeutic community. These researchers found higher reten-tion rates in the intensive day treatment program that was distinguished by gender specific interventions, less confrontation, onsite nursery and child care, on site pediatric care, parent training, and family therapy.

In 1989, in response to growing concern about the consequences of per-enatal drug and alcohol exposure, Congress appropriated funds for a com-prehensive demonstration program for pregnant and postpartum women and their infants (PPWI). The program was jointly funded by the Center for Substance Abuse Prevention (CSAP) and the Maternal and Child Health Bureau (MCHB). Funded program models combined a number of different strategies, ranging from residential treatment to aggressive outreach and referral programs. A total of 147 grants were funded under this initiative.

In 1994, MCHB sponsored a series of focus groups with staff from 22 of the funded projects to identify successful strategies and lessons learned. The focus group discussions identified six factors that were related to successful recruitment and retention of pregnant and parenting women (Laken & Hutchins, 1996):

1. Women who are motivated to seek drug treatment often need tangible and emotional support from others to remain in treatment.
2. The physical and social environments of drug treatment programs play an important role in retention. This includes providing a family-like environment where women are comfortable and can find support.
3. Celebrations and other incentives are useful in rewarding behavior change, which also increases retention.
4. Allowing input into the program design empowers clients and improves the treatment approach and retention.
5. Advocacy on behalf of clients models how clients can negotiate with the agencies and institutions and further strengthens the bond between client and caseworker.
6. Programs must be gender and culturally sensitive to retain women from a variety of racial and ethnic backgrounds.

In 1992, the CSAP was given authorization to fund 11 demonstration projects for comprehensive residential treatment programs that permitted substance-abusing women to live with their children. These grants were subsequently transferred to the Center for Substance Abuse Treatment (CSAT). Programs funded under this initiative addressed service needs in four critical areas (CSAT, 1998):

1. *Biological/physical:* including detoxification, nutrition, medical care, HIV prevention, and treatment
2. *Psychological/social:* including gender specific interventions and treatment for concurrent comorbidity
3. *Support services:* such as housing, child care, advocacy, employment and training
4. *Educational services:* including parenting education, reproductive and preventive health education, and resource development

The programs ranged in length from 6 to 12 months, with aftercare follow-up from 6 to 24 months. Participants spent an average of 20 weeks in treatment. Data aggregated from the individual evaluation studies conducted by these programs indicated that overall 35.2% of participants successfully completed treatment. Preliminary postdischarge outcomes on 338 women who had been served by these projects between January and September 1993 indicated that women who completed treatment were significantly more likely to have decreases in drug use (including use of alcohol), higher levels of employment, and less criminal justice involvement between admission and follow-up (CSAT, 1998).

CONCLUSION

Alcohol and other drug use during pregnancy continues to be a significant risk factor for birth defects and poor developmental outcomes for children. FASD is considered one of the leading preventable causes of birth defects in the United States. There is now overwhelming evidence that universal health promotion strategies such as warning labels and public education have not been sufficient to deter many women from using alcohol, illicit drugs, and tobacco during pregnancy. However, the good news is that over the past 36 years since FAS was first identified, numerous evidence-based approaches to prevention and intervention have been tested and found to be effective in reducing alcohol and potentially other types of drug use during pregnancy.

There are now a number of well-validated brief screening tools to facilitate the identification of women who may be in need of treatment for alcohol or drug problems. Moreover, screening and identification of women can occur in a variety of settings. BMIs are effective, relatively low cost interventions for most women who are pregnant. BMIs have been implemented successfully in community-based primary care facilities, pediatric practices, emergency departments, correctional facilities, drug treatment programs, and other community settings. Research on BMIs has demonstrated that effective intervention can be cost effective, involve minimal staff training, and can be integrated into regular program or clinic activities without posing an undue burden to staff. Manualized BMIs such as Project CHOICES (CDC, 2003) are widely availablse for adoption.

Despite extensive research on evidence-based brief interventions and treatment models for women, there has been only limited translation and dissemination of these models to communities of practice. The most effective approaches to prevention are those that address the complex etiology of alcohol and drug dependence through an ecological approach, taking into account the individual, familial, social, and cultural factors that contribute to persistent alcohol and drug use.

It is becoming increasingly clear that the eradication of FASD and other drug-related developmental problems will require a multiagency, multilevel coordinated effort to translate, disseminate, fund, and implement evidence-based intervention strategies. Education and intervention must extend beyond the limited context of pregnancy to women in other stages of life development. Such strategies must include health promotion/education, early intervention for hazardous alcohol or drug use among young nonpregnant women, and accessible effective treatment for alcohol- and drug-dependent women.

REFERENCES

Abel, E. (1998). Prevention of alcohol abuse related birth defects-I. Public education efforts. *Alcohol Abuse and Alcoholism, 33*(4), 411–416.

Abma, J. M., & Mott, F. L. (1991). Substance use and prenatal care during pregnancy among young women. *Family Planning Perspectives, 23*(3), 117–128.

Anda, R., Felitti, V., Bremner, J., Walker, J., Whitfield, C., Perry, B., et al. (2006). The enduring effects of abuse and related adverse experiences in childhood. *European Archives of Psychiatry and Clinical Neuroscience, 256*(3), 174–186.

Anderson, M. (1986). Personalized nursing: An effective intervention model for use with drug dependent women in an emergency room. *International Journal of the Addictions, 21*(1), 105–122.

Barr, H. M., Bookstein, F. L., O'Malley, K. D., Connor, P. D., Huggins, J. E., & Streissguth, A. P. (2006). Binge drinking during pregnancy as a predictor of psychiatric disorders on the structured clinical interview for DSM-IV in young adult offspring. *American Journal of Psychiatry, 163*(6), 1061–1065.

Barry, K., Caetano, R., Chang, G., DeJoseph, M. C., Miller, L. A., O'Connor, M. J., et al. (2009). *National task force on fetal alcohol syndrome and fetal alcohol effect. Reducing alcohol-exposed pregnancies: A report of the national task force on fetal alcohol syndrome and fetal alcohol effect.* Atlanta, GA: Centers for Disease Control and Prevention.

Bowerman, R. (1997). The Effect of a community supported ban on prenatal alcohol and other substance abuse. *American Journal of Public Health, 87*(8), 1378–1379.

Bradley, K. A., Boyd-Wickizer, J., Powell, S. H., & Burman, M. L. (1998). Alcohol screening questionnaires in women: A critical review. *Journal of the American Medical Association, 280*(2), 166–171.

Burd, L., Klug., M. G., & Martsolf, J. T. (2004). Increased sibling mortality in children with fetal alcohol syndrome. *Addiction Biology, 9*, 179–186.

Burke, B., Arkowitz, H., & Menchola, M. (2003). The efficacy of motivational interviewing: A meta-analysis of controlled clinical trials. *Journal of Consulting and Clinical Psychology, 71*(3), 843–861.

Burns, W., & Burns, K. A. (1988). Parenting dysfunction in chemically dependent women. In I. J. Chasnoff (Ed.), *Drugs, alcohol, pregnancy and parenting.* Chicago: Kluwer.

Centers for Disease Control and Prevention. (2003). Motivational intervention to reduce alcohol-exposed pregnancies- Florida, Texas and Virginia 1997–2001. *Morbidity and Mortality Weekly Report, 52*(19), 441–444.

Centers for Disease Control and Prevention. (2009). Alcohol use among pregnant and nonpregnant women of childbearing age United States 1991–2005. *Morbidity and Mortality Weekly Report, 58*(19), 529–532.

Center for Substance Abuse Treatment. (1998). *Telling their stories: Treating women with substance abuse problems and their children.* Rockville, MD: U.S. Department of Health and Human Services.

Chan, I. W., Wingert, W. A.,Wachsman, I., Schuetz, S., & Rogers, C. (1986). Differences between dropouts and active participants in a pediatric clinic for substance abuse mothers. *Journal of Drug and Alcohol Abuse, 12*(1–2), 89–99.

Chasnoff, I. J., Landress, H. J., & Barrett, M. E. (1990). The prevalence of illicit drug or alcohol use during pregnancy and discrepancies in mandatory reporting in Pinellas County, Florida. *New England Journal of Medicine, 322,* 1201–1206.

Christoffel, K. K., & Salafsky, I. (1975). Fetal alcohol syndrome in dizygotic twins. *Journal of Pediatrics, 87*(6), 963–967.

Coles, C. D., Brown, R. T., Smith, I. E., Platzman, K. A., Erickson, S., & Falek, A. (1991). Effects of prenatal alcohol exposure at school age: I. Physical and cognitive development. *Neurotoxicology and Teratology, 13,* 357–367.

Coles, C. D., Krable, J., Drews-Bosch, C., & Falek, A. (2000). Early identification of risk for effects of prenatal alcohol exposure. *Journal of Studies on Alcohol, 61*(4), 607–616.

Coles, C. D., Smith, I. E., Fernhoff, P. M., & Falek A. (1984). Neonatal neurobehavioral characteristics as correlates of maternal alcohol use during gestation. *Alcoholism, 9*(5), 454–460.

Coletti, S. D., Schinka, J. A., Hughes, P. H., Hamilton, N. I., Renard, C. G., Sicilian, D. M., et al. (1995). Par village for chemically dependent women: Philosophy and program elements. *Journal of Substance Abuse Treatment, 12*(4), 289–296.

Corse, S. J., & Smith, M. (1998). Reducing substance abuse during pregnancy: Discriminating among levels of response in a prenatal setting. *Journal of Substance Abuse Treatment, 15*(5), 457–467.

Craig, A. (1995). The effectiveness of alcohol warning labels: A review and extension. *American Behavioral Scientist, 38*(4), 622–633.

Dansky, B. S., & Brady, K. T. (1996). Victimization and PTSD in individuals with substance use disorders: Gender and racial differences. *American Journal of Drug & Alcohol Abuse, 22*(1), 75–93.

Das Eiden, R., Edwards, E. P., & Leonard, K. E. (2002). Mother–infant and father–infant attachment among alcoholic families. *Development and Psychopathology, 14,* 253–278.

DeLeon, G., & Jainchill, N. (1991). Residential therapeutic communities for female substance abusers. *Bulletin of the New York Academy of Medicine, 67*(3), 277–290.

DeLeon, G., Melnick, G., & Kressel, D. (1997). Motivation and readiness for therapeutic community treatment among cocaine and other drug users. *American Journal of Drug & Alcohol Abuse, 23*(2), 169–189.

Eckardt, M. J., File, S. E., Gessa, G. L., Grant, K. A., Guerri, C., Hoffman, P. L., et al. (1998). Effects of moderate alcohol consumption on the central nervous system. *Alcoholism Clinical and Experimental Research, 22*(5), 998–1040.

Finkelstein, N. (1996). Using the relational model as a context for treating pregnant and parenting chemically dependent women. In B. L. Underhill & D. G. Finnegan (Eds.), *Chemical dependency. Women at risk.* New York: Harrington.

Fleming, M. F., Lund, M. R., Wilton, G., Landry, M., & Scheets, D. (2008). The healthy moms study: The efficacy of brief alcohol intervention in post partum women. *Alcoholism: Clinical and Experimental Research, 32*(9), 1600–1606.

Floyd, R. L., Ebrahim, S. H., & Boyle, C. A. (1999). Preventing alcohol-exposed pregnancies among women of childbearing age: The necessity of a preconceptional approach. *Journal of Women's Health & Gender-Based Medicine, 8*(6), 733–736.

Floyd, R. L., Sobell, M., Velasquez, M. M., Ingersoll, K., Nettleman, M., Sobell, L., et al. (2007). Preventing alcohol exposed pregnancies. *American Journal of Preventive Medicine, 32*(1), 1–10.

Friedman, S. H., Heneghan, A., & Rosenthal, M. (2009). Characteristics of women who do not seek prenatal care and implications for prevention. *Journal of Obstetric and Gynecologic and Neonatal Nursing, 38*(2), 174–181.

Goodman, S. (2007). Depression in mothers. *Annual Review of Clinical Psychology, 3,* 107–135.

Gordon, R. (1983). An operational classification of disease prevention. *Public Health Reports, 98,* 107–109.

Greenfield, S. F., Brooks, A. J., Gordon, S. M., Green, C. A., Kropp, F., McHugh, R. K., et al. (2007). Substance abuse treatment entry, retention, and outcome in women: A review of the literature. *Drug and Alcohol Dependence, 86*(1), 1–21.

Greenfield, S. F., Trucco, E. M., McHugh, R. K., Lincoln, M., & Gallop, R. J. (2007). The women's recovery group study: A stage I trial of women-focused group therapy for substance use disorders versus mixed-gender group drug counseling. *Drug and Alcohol Dependence, 90*(1), 39–47.

Grella, C. E., Hser, Y., & Huang, Y. C. (2006). Mothers in substance abuse treatment: Differences in characteristics based on involvement with child welfare services. *Child Abuse and Neglect, 30*(1), 55–73.

Grucza, R. A., Norberg, K. E., & Bierut, L. J. (2009). Binge drinking among youths and young adults in the United States: 1979–2006. *Journal of the American Academy of Child Adolescent Psychiatry, 48*(7), 692–702.

Harter, S. L., & Taylor, T. L. (2000). Parental alcoholism, child abuse, and adult adjustment. *Journal of Substance Abuse, 11*(1), 31–44.

Jacobson, J. L., Jacobson, S. W., Sokol, R. J., & Ager, J. W. (1998). Relation of maternal and pattern of pregnancy drinking to functionally significant cognitive deficit in infancy. *Alcoholism: Clinical and Experimental Research, 22*(2), 345–351.

Jones, K. L., Smith, D. W., Ulleland, C. N., & Streissguth, A. P. (1973). Pattern of malformation in offspring of chronic alcoholic mothers. *Lancet, 1,* 1267.

Koren, G., Hutson, J., & Gareri, J. (2008). Novel methods for the detection of drug and alcohol exposure during pregnancy: Implications for maternal and child health. *Clinical Pharmacology & Therapeutics, 83*(4), 631–634.

Kosten, T., Gawin, F. H., Kosten, T. R., & Rounsaville, B. J. (1993). Gender differences in cocaine use and treatment response. *Journal of Substance Abuse Treatment, 10,* 63–66.

Laken, M., & Hutchins, E. (1996). *Recruitment and retention of substance using pregnant and parenting women: Lessons learned.* Arlington, VA: National Center for Education in Maternal and Child Health.

Landesman-Dwyer, S., Keller, S. L.,& Streissguth, A. P. (1978). Naturalistic observations of newborns: Effects of maternal alcohol intake. *Alcoholism: Clinical and Experimental Research, 2*(2), 171.

Lex, B. W., Teoh, S. K., Lagomasino, I., Mello, N., & Mendelson, J. H. (1990). Characteristics of women receiving mandated treatment for alcohol or polysubstance dependence in Massachusetts. *Drug and Alcohol Dependence, 25,* 13–20.

Luthar, S., & Walsh, K. G. (1995). Treatment needs of drug-addicted mothers. *Journal of Substance Abuse Treatment, 12*(5), 341–348.

MacKinnon, D. P., Nohre, L., Pentz, M. A., & Stacy, A. (2000). The alcohol warning and adolescents: 5-year effects. *American Journal of Public Health, 90*(10), 1589–1594.

Magura, S., Laudet, A., Kang, S. Y., & Whitney, S. (1999). Effectiveness of comprehensive services for crack-dependent mothers with newborns and young children. *Psychoactive Drugs, 31*(4), 321–338.

Mattson, S., & Riley, E. (1998). A review of neurobehavioral deficits in children with fetal alcohol syndrome or prenatal exposure to alcohol. *Alcoholism: Clinical and Experimental Research, 22*(2), 279–294.

May, P., Gossage, J. P., Marais, A. S., Hendricks, L. S., Snell, C. L., Tabchnick, B. G., et al. (2008). Maternal risk factors for fetal alcohol syndrome and partial fetal alcohol syndrome in South Africa: A third study. *Alcoholism Clinical and Experimental Research, 32*(5), 738–753.

May, P. A., Miller, J. M., Goodhart, K. A., Maestas, O. R., Buckley, D., Trujilio, P. M., et al. (2008). Enhanced case management to prevent fetal alcohol spectrum Disorders in northern plains communities. *Journal of Maternal and Child Health, 12*(6), 747–759.

May, P. H., Hymbaugh, K. J., & Aase, J. M. (1983). Epidemiology of FAS among American Indians of the Southwest. *Social Biology, 30*, 374–387.

Mayes, L. (1996). Exposure to cocaine: Behavioral outcomes in preschool and school age children. *National Institute on Drug Abuse Research Monograph No., 164*, 211–229.

Melnikow, J. A., Alemagno, S. A., Rottman, C., & Zyzanski, S. J. (1991). Characteristics of inner-city women giving birth with little or no prenatal care: A case control study. *Journal of Family Practice, 32*(3), 283–288.

Nardi, D. (1998). Risk factors, attendance and abstinence patterns of low income women in perinatal addiction treatment: Lessons from a 5 year program. *Issues in Mental Health Nursing, 18*, 125–138.

National Institute on Alcohol Abuse and Alcoholism. (1997). *Fetal alcohol syndrome: Report on the 1997 site visit to South Africa.* Rockville, MD: National Institute on Alcohol Abuse and Alcoholism;

Osterling, K. L., & Austin, M. J. (2008). Substance abuse interventions for parents involved in the child welfare system: Evidence and implications. *Journal of Evidence Based Social Work, 5*(1–2), 157–189.

Pederson, C. L., Vanhorn, D. R., Wilson, J. F., Martorano, L. M., Venema, J. M., & Kennedy, S. M. (2008). Childhood abuse related to nicotine, illicit and prescription drug use by women: Pilot study. *Psychological Reports, 103*(2), 459–466.

Petitti, D., Coleman, C., Binsacca, D., & Allen, B. (1990). Early prenatal care in urban black and white women. *Birth, 17*(1), 1–5.

Prochaska, J. O., DiClemente, C. C., & Norcross, J. C. (1992). In search of how people change: Applications to addictive behaviors. *American Psychologist, 47*, 1102–1114.

Ramadoss, J., Hogan, H. A., Given, J. C., West, J. R., & Cudd, T. A. (2006). Binge alcohol exposure during all three trimesters alters bone strength and growth in fetal sheep. *Alcohol, 38*(3), 185–192.

Reid, J., Macchetto, P., & Foster, S. (1999). *No safe haven: Children of substance-abusing parents.* New York: Center on Addiction and Substance Abuse at Columbia University.

Roberts, A., & Nishimoto, R. H. (1996). Predicting treatment retention of women dependent on cocaine. *American Journal of Drug and Alcohol Abuse, 22*(3), 313–333.

Rossett, H., & Weiner, L (1985). Alcohol and pregnancy: A clinical perspective study. *Annals of Review of Medicine, 36,* 73–80.

Rounsaville, B., & Kleber, H. D. (1985). Untreated opiate addicts. How do they differ from those seeking treatment? *Archives of General Psychiatry, 42,* 1072–1077.

Russell, M., Martier, S. S., Sokol, R. J., Mudar, P., Bottoms, S., Jacobson, S., et al. (1994). Screening for pregnancy risk-drinking. *Alcoholism: Clinical and Experimental Research, 18*(5), 1156–1161.

Sampson, P. S., Streissguth, A. P., Barr, H. M., & Bookstein, F. L. (1989). Neurobehavioral effects of prenatal alcohol: Part II. partial least squares analysis. *Neurotoxicology and Teratology, 11,* 477–491.

Savage, A., & Russell, L. A. (2005). Tangled in a web of affiliation social support networks of dually diagnosed women who are trauma survivors. *Journal of Behavioral Health Services and Research, 32*(2), 199–214.

Schempf, A. (2007). Illicit drug use and neonatal outcomes: A critical review. *Obstetrical and Gynecological Survey, 62*(11), 749–757.

Sculpholme, A., Robertson, E. G., & Kamons, A. S. (1991). Barriers to prenatal care in a multi-ethnic sample. *Journal of Nurse Midwifery, 36*(2), 111–116.

Silverman, K., & Schonberg, S. K. (2001). Adolescent children of drug-abusing parents. *Adolescent Medicine, 12*(3), 485–491.

Simmons, L. A., Havens, J. R., Whiting, J. B., Holz, J. L., & Bada, H. (2009). Illicit drug use among women with children in the United States: 2002–2003. *Annals of Epidemiology, 19*(3), 187–193.

Smith, I., & Coles, C. D. (1991). Multilevel intervention for prevention of FAS and effects of prenatal alcohol exposure. In M. Galanter (Ed.), *Recent developments in alcoholism: Treatment issues* (Vol. 9). New York: Plenum.

Smith, I., Dent, D. Z., Coles, C. D., & Falek, A. (1992). A comparison study of treated and untreated post partum cocaine abusing women. *Journal of Substance Abuse Treatment, 9,* 343–348.

Smith, I. E., Lancaster, J., Moss-Wells, S., & Falek, A. (1987). Identifying high risk pregnant drinkers: Biological and behavioral correlates of continuous drinking during pregnancy. *Journal of Studies on Alcohol, 48*(4), 304–309.

Stenius, V. M., Veysey, B. M., Hamilton, Z., & Andersen, R. (2005). Social roles in women's lives. *Journal of Behavioral Health Services & Research, 32*(2), 182–198.

Substance Abuse and Mental Health Services Administration. (1997). *Substance use among women in the United States.* Office of Applied Studies: Health and Human Services Administration.

Substance Abuse and Mental Health Services Administration. (2005). *National survey on drug use and health.* Office of Applied Studies: Health and Human Services Administration.

Substance Abuse and Mental Health Services Administration. (2007, October 4). *Substance use treatment among women of child bearing age. NSDUH Report.* Office of Applied Studies.

Sunil, T. S., Spears, W. D., Hook, L., Castillo, J., & Torres, C. (2008). Initiation of and barriers to prenatal care use among low-income women in San Antonio, Texas. *Maternal Child Health Journal, 14*(1), 133–140.

Teagle, S., & Brindes, C. D. (1998). Substance use among pregnant adolescents: A comparison of self reported use and provider perception. *Journal of Adolescent Health, 22*(3), 229–238.

Walker, D. S., Fisher, C. S., Sherman, A., Wybrecht B., & Kyndely, K. (2005). Fetal alcohol spectrum disorders prevention: An exploratory study of women's use of, attitudes toward, and knowledge about alcohol.*Journal of the American Academy of Nurse Practioners, 17*(5), 187–193.

Wallace, B. (1991). Chemical dependency treatment for the pregnant crack addict: Beyond the criminal sanctions perspective. *Psychology of Addictive Behavior, 5*(1), 23–25.

Warren, K., & Li, T. K. (2005). Genetic polymorphisms: Impact on the risk of fetal alcohol spectrum disorders. *Birth Defects Research, Part A: Clinical Molecular Teratology, 73*(4), 195–203.

Wasserman, D. R., & Leventhal, J. M. (1993). Maltreatment of children born to cocaine-dependent mothers. *American Journal of Disease of Childhood, 147*(12), 1324–1328.

Weiner, L., & Morse, B. A. (1988). FAS: Clinical perspectives and prevention. In I. J. Chasnoff (Ed.), *Drugs alcohol pregnancy and parenting* (pp. 127–143). Boston: Kluwer.

Whitaker, R. C., Orzoi, S. M., & Kahn, R. S. (2006). Maternal mental health, substance use and domestic violence in the year after delivery and subsequent behavior problems in children at age 3 years. *Archives of General Psychiatry, 63*, 551–560.

Wilson, C., Harris, S. K., Sherritt, L., Lawrence, N., Glotzer, D., & Shaw, J. S. (2008). Parental alcohol screening in pediatric practices. *Pediatrics, 122*, 1022–1029.

9

Programs for Young Children With Substance-Abusing Parents

Alissa Mallow

INTRODUCTION

Under the best of circumstances, parenting children presents challenges. When parents are affected by substance misuse the challenges are exacerbated. Substance misuse carries with it, among other complications, financial difficulties, housing problems, family violence, mental illness, and medical difficulties. When the parent is substance involved, the possibility of becoming involved in the child welfare system is enormous. With reports that up to 80% of all child welfare cases in the United States involve a substance-misusing parent, it makes sense that these cases are fraught with psychosocial problems and require a cadre of additional support and service coordination. Additionally, as these youngsters are often in foster care longer, reunification may be problematic as well (Carlson, 2006; Green, Rockhill, & Furrer, 2007; Gruber & Taylor, 2006; Ryan, March, Testa, & Louderman, 2006; Worcel, Furrer, Green, Burrus, & Finigan, 2008).

The number of children experiencing this is staggering. Combined data from Substance Abuse and Mental Health Services Administration's (SAMHSA's) 2002–2007 National Surveys on Drug Use and Health were used to provide average annualized estimates of the number of children under age 18 living with a parent who was involved with alcohol or illicit drugs. It was discovered that over 8.3 million children (11.9%) lived with at least one parent who was dependent upon or abused alcohol or an illicit drug during the past year. Of the children living with a substance-abusing parent, almost 7.3 million (10.3%) lived with a parent who was dependent upon or abused alcohol, and about 2.1 million (3.0%) lived with a parent who was dependent upon or abused illicit drugs.

With such a large number of affected children, the legal system, child welfare professionals, and the substance abuse treatment community realized that rather than working at cross-purposes, they all had the same goals:

1. Assisting the mother in becoming sober;
2. Sustaining recovery and repairing emotionally from the ravages of addiction;
3. Addressing the concomitant and underlying difficulties that may have led to the addiction;
4. Maintaining the sanctity of the family.

This has culminated in a concerted effort by these systems in providing mother–child treatment services. As this partnership was developing, the federal government was becoming increasingly concerned about the length of stay for children in the foster care system. As a result, the National Center on Addiction and Substance Abuse (CASA) began focusing on identifying the types of services required to foster reunification and appropriate treatment. This chapter explores some of the laws and programs concentrating on young children and their substance-misusing parents, with particular attention paid to the Adoption and Safe Families Act (ASFA), and the National Center for Addiction and Substance Abuse report *No Safe Haven: Children of Substance-Abusing Parents*, and will describes several innovative programs across the country working with this population.

ADOPTION AND SAFE FAMILIES ACT OF 1997

The ASFA of 1997 is federal legislation spotlighting the problem of youngsters remaining in foster care for protracted periods secondary to parental inability to provide a safe environment for reunification. The legislation was enacted as a result of the federal government's belief that the states were falling short in their obligation to protect the rights of children. One such example was in the protracted length that children stayed in the foster care system, often "aging out" rather than being placed for adoption (Mapp & Steinberg, 2007; Marsh & Cao, 2005; Ross, 2006).

AFSA has a twofold foci: first, to ensure that children will not return to unsafe homes and that permanent homes are provided with "loving families," and, second, to have states adhere to the 15/22 rule. This provision assumes that after a 15-month period, children whose biological parents are unable or unwilling to rehabilitate are "better off" without them (Ross, 2006). Therefore, when a parent has a youngster in foster care for 15 of the last 22 months, the state is mandated to move toward termination of parental rights and adoption of the child. AFSA stipulates that all state child welfare agencies must be planning to return the child to the parent and, in the event the child cannot be returned, simultaneously must initiate permanency planning so that the child can be adopted. The law does stipulate that the 15-month deadline is not upheld in cases where the child is placed in kinship foster care, if the state has been unable or failed to provide the services "deemed necessary" for reunification, and if the state can show a compelling reason why parental rights should not be terminated (Ross, 2006).

Once a reunification plan has been established, AFSA stipulates that parents have approximately 1 year to comply. For substance-abusing women, this means obtaining and sustaining sobriety immediately without the roller-coaster ride of relapses and failed treatment attempts. For some women this is undoable. Advocates in the areas of child welfare and substance abuse treatment have voiced concern regarding AFSA's 12–15-month time frame as this criterion does not extend enough time for a woman to enter and complete treatment (Rockhill, Green, & Newton-Chris, 2008; Ross, 2006). Without clear intention, the passage of AFSA promoted better coordination of services between child welfare agencies and substance abuse treatment programs, the reduction of barriers to treatment for women, and greater cross-agency training.

NO SAFE HAVEN: CHILDREN OF SUBSTANCE-ABUSING PARENTS

No Safe Haven: Children of Substance-Abusing Parents was a 2-year examination of the intersectionality between chemical dependency and child neglect/abuse. The study was published by the National Center on Substance Abuse and Addiction (CASA) of Columbia University in January 1999 and was based on interviews with child welfare professionals across the United States as to their perceptions about substance abuse problems among their clients. The key findings, although more than 10 years old, remain timely. Briefly, 71.6% of the respondents viewed parental substance abuse as the leading cause for an increase in child abuse cases since 1986. Child welfare professionals reported a substantial portion of their caseloads involved children whose parents were poly–substance addicted and required placement in foster care, and these youngsters were in care longer than children whose parents were not addicted.

Most notable was the finding that over 61% of child welfare professionals were unable to match treatment programs with parental needs, as programs addressing both reunification and substance abuse were not readily available. This results in workers referring clients to "whatever program was available" rather than matching the "program and client." When individuals are referred to programs based solely on availability rather than services provided, establishing the foundation to develop a drug-free lifestyle is compromised. Conversely, treatment, regardless of type, is better than no treatment at all when the individual is seeking to recover from addiction. The CASA report captures this dilemma and underscores the complex relationship between child neglect/abuse and substance abuse and addiction with the concept of "two clocks." CASA describes these clocks as:

- *Clock of child development*: Children are entitled to safe homes and nurturing relationships with their caretakers.
- *Clock of recovery*: Parents entering treatment programs are entitled to the time it takes to overcome the addiction and the processes of recovery characterized by several treatment attempts and relapses before treatment "works." (CASA, 1999, p. 6).

CASA (1999) describes four guiding principles that inform the recommendations. First, children of substance-abusing parents have the right to have their parents receive timely and comprehensive treatment, offering the parent a reasonable attempt at recovery. Second, children are entitled to sober parents. Therefore, they should not be subjected to parents who are either resistant to entering treatment or have difficulty maintaining a drug-free lifestyle. Third, parental recovery cannot take precedence over the child's needs and developmental processes. Finally, child welfare agencies are responsible for supporting families that are nurturing for children. Therefore, if the relationship with the biological family cannot be sustained, a nurturing and supportive adoptive family should be pursued. The recommendations based upon these guiding principles focus on prevention, reform, funding, training, and data collection. The child welfare system as it exists needs reforming. That is, it needs to move toward the capacity to respond more effectively to substance-abusing families. First, each family referred to child welfare agencies needs to be assessed for substance abuse. In addition, the report supports efforts to prevent substance abuse. Prevention is focused on two levels. First, prevent substance abuse. Educational efforts are important toward this goal. Despite prevention, there will be substance abuse. At this point, prevention efforts need to focus on preventing child maltreatment. Second, treatment funding has to be aimed toward comprehensive programming with an emphasis on cross-discipline collaboration and training. A dogmatic approach can only serve to hinder outcomes for children and their parents rather than enhancing them.

TREATMENT SERVICES FOR YOUNG CHILDREN
AND THEIR SUBSTANCE-ABUSING MOTHERS

A myriad of factors effect women when addicted. The severity of addiction rapidly accelerates for women. Women experience more medical difficulties, psychological troubles, and face greater social stigmatization, especially if childbearing. Women are more compromised psychologically secondary to their substance usage and have more failed treatment attempts. Oftentimes, women perceive their difficulties to be a result of depression and anxiety rather than resulting from their substance abuse. In fact, 70% of women in substance abuse treatment have concomitant psychiatric difficulties such as anxiety, depression, and posttraumatic stress disorder (Greenfield, et al, 2007; Jansson & Velez, 1999; Kaufman, 1994).

Nutrition is compromised in addiction, creating amenorrhea or irregular menstruation (REF). Therefore, women may not recognize bodily changes consistent with pregnancy. The belief that a woman will rid her body of toxic substances in preparation for and continuation of pregnancy is a misnomer. For some women, there is a continuation of caffeine intake, for others soda, and for those with addiction difficulties, the continued use of alcohol and other drugs of abuse. Poor prenatal care or inconsistent prenatal care occurs as some women are "afraid" to enter the medical system. The medical risks to the fetus can be compounded, as some substances are tetragenic compromising fetal development. For example, alcohol is a tetragenic. The March of Dimes describes fetal alcohol syndrome as the number one most preventable birth defect (www.marchofdimes.com/professional). Although not described as a tetragenic, the abuse of cocaine and other stimulants while pregnant places the woman at risk for preterm labor, placental abruption, and fetal demise (Jansson & Velez, 1999).

Women-Specific Programs

The history of chemical dependency treatment programs in the United States and in particular women-specific programs are well-documented (Bride, 2001; Greenfield et al., 2007; Kandall, 1996). As women became more visible in treatment programs, established treatment programs began to grapple with low retention rates and poorer outcomes for their female clients. It was discovered that some treatment techniques such as the confrontational model grounding therapeutic communities (TC) were "male oriented" and did not benefit women, in that these techniques served to exacerbate feelings of guilt, shame, and experiences of victimization (Kandall, 1996). The experience gained by these established programs lead to development of modified therapeutic communities (MTC) with gender-specific services that focused on the unique needs of women.

Pregnant substance abusers faced the most stigma. Even among their addicted counterparts, they are seen as most "blameworthy"; after all, many believe women will rid themselves of all toxic substances during pregnancy. The medical complications of prenatal substance abuse and medical staff critical of women who "did this to themselves" (Kandall, 1996), the stigma of being "pregnant and using," coupled with the addicted pregnant woman's own feelings of self-hatred, shame, and guilt increased the tendency to avoid prenatal care. As time progressed, programs began offering women the opportunity to bring their children with them into treatment. This intervention moved beyond "day care" and offered dyadic work to improve mother–child interactions (Kandall, 1996). Many programs began to offer concurrent mental health therapies targeting the children, such as play and art therapy, while their mothers were in their own therapy groups. Parenting groups focused upon "real-time" interactions between the mother and child rather than offering more abstract parenting scenarios. Overall, programs began taking a more family-oriented approach.

The Need for Collaboration: Young Children With Substance-Misusing Parents

Services for children raised by addicted parents need to go beyond "fixing of their mother" (Juliana & Goodman, 2005). Recovery from addiction is complicated, and for some women who are children of substance-abusing parents themselves, there is no road map for appropriate parenting of their own children (Carlson, 2006). Characteristically, women involved with the child welfare system are younger, have less education, have serious mental illness in addition to substance addiction, have more children (some in their custody, some not), and have had previous unsuccessful treatment episodes (Osterling & Austin, 2008). Ideally, families should be preserved. Youngsters need parental continuity. If parental continuity is not possible, they need another adult who can be the "psychological" parent, fulfilling the parental responsibility and instilling in the child a sense of being loved, safe, and protected. In addition, children require therapeutic support and treatment from providers who provide continuity of care rather than offering a disjointed string of services. Osterling and Austin (2008) have noted that collaboration between substance abuse treatment providers and child welfare professions does not mean they "just talk." Their organizational and cultural differences must be addressed in order to remove barriers.

Obstacles such as differing time constraints, differences in education and training of staff, funding streams, confidentiality issues, and the definition of "successful outcomes" require explication in order to have all service providers on "the same page."

When the substance-abusing woman becomes involved in the child welfare system, the collaboration between that system and substance abuse services becomes vital (Carlson, 2006; Glider et al., 1996; Osterling & Austin, 2008). To lessen barriers, it has been suggested that a substance abuse treatment professional be assigned to or hired by child welfare agencies (Carlson, 2006). Treatment planning (substance abuse agencies) and case planning (child welfare agencies) must be done conjointly. Advisory boards or task forces can provide oversight regarding collaborative efforts and assist with problem solving. Training and cross training is important. Confidentiality regulations unique to each provider must be explored in order to allow for the disclosure of pertinent information (Green, Rockhill, & Burns, 2008; Osterling & Austin, 2008; Smith & Mogro-Wilson, 2007). As each agency begins to understand the other, working together improves. When barriers dissolve, the services provided to women and their children are enhanced, thereby promoting the best possible outcomes.

INNOVATIVE PROGRAMS

According to Carlson (2006), best practices for addicted women involved in the child welfare system require programs that provide the following services:

- Gender-specific treatment.
- Education regarding their children's psychological, developmental, and physical needs.
- Opportunities through therapeutic activities to repair the mother–child relationship, including the use of parenting support groups, parenting skills groups, and therapeutic groups, so that the woman can resolve the intrapersonal and interpersonal issues underlying substance addiction.
- Dyadic mother–child groups to improve the relationship and give staff the ability to "correct" parenting as difficulties surface in the group.

Locating programs designed with the above practices are a "click away." The Substance Abuse and Mental Health Services Administration (SAMHSA) of the U.S. Department of Health and Human Services maintains a web-based treatment facility locator (www.findtreatment .samhsa.gov). According to SAMHSA, this is the most up-to-date database of programs around the country. Updated yearly, this user-friendly site allows users to customize their location, services provided, special populations, special language services, forms of payment accepted, and payment assistance. The programs described in this section were found using this search engine. Randomly selected in terms of the services provided, they represent the four regions of the country; this list is not inclusive, nor is it an endorsement of these programs. The information reported comes from the program's website and when noted, personal communication with program leadership. These programs were chosen as they offer the services described by Carlson (2006) and offer a seamless provision of care. All the programs highlight their collaborative efforts with child welfare professionals to ensure continuity of care for both the woman and her child. All programs were clear in their mission statements that women require specialized services to promote a sober lifestyle and should have opportunities to discuss their trauma histories, experiences of domestic violence, and improve their ability to care for themselves and their children in a safe, supportive, and empowering environment. As multiple systems are involved in the lives of addicted females, they require intensive case management to assist them not only in reunification with their children, but also with literacy and job training essential in order to provide a smooth transition back to the community.

CASE EXAMPLES

Odyssey House, Inc., in New York City opened its door in 1967 and today offers services and programs to an array of individuals and families struggling with addiction and mental health disorders. Funding for the entire organization comes from New York City, New York State, and federal agencies, as well as from private foundations and corporate donations. In 1973, Odyssey House became the first residential program in the country to offer a parent–child residential treatment program. The program is credited with being one of the first therapeutic communities to evaluate the impact of admitting children with their mothers to a residential facility and was the parent of the original "Perinatal—20" (Glider et al., 1996; Kandall, 1996; Odyssey House, n.d.; Rahdert, 1996). The MABON Program (Mothers And Babies Off Narcotics) as well as Odyssey House's other Family Center Sites allow the woman to live with her children (up to age 5) and provide, among other services, an on-site nursery, preschool, and "Triangle Time." Triangle Time allows for parenting to be "enhanced" as the parent interacts with her child in the presence of a childcare specialist. Although the length of stay is dependent upon the mother's ability to stay in treatment, generally the average length of stay is between 9 and 12 months. Because of the wide array of services offered, the woman and her children can continue in aftercare services at Odyssey House, Inc. (Odyssey House, Inc., n.d.)

Gaudenzia, Inc., is the largest provider of chemical dependency treatment services in Pennsylvania and has programs in Delaware and Maryland as well. The first of its kind in Pennsylvania, Gaudenzia's Vantage Program is a therapeutic community for women and their children. Gaudenzia offers a continuum of care for women involved in the child welfare system offering intensive case management to help the woman negotiate the system as well as providing counseling services.

Rubicon, Inc.'s website states that they are Virginia's most comprehensive and oldest chemical dependency program. The Women and Children's Treatment Program provides services to women who are in jeopardy of losing custody of their children because of their "limited resources in managing custody" (rubiconrehab.com). Through strengthening the functioning of the family unit, the goal is to keep families intact.

East Coast Solutions in North Carolina maintains a therapeutic home for women and their children. The S.E.A.R.I.S.E. program was designed by CASA and seeks to provide integrated substance abuse treatment services to women and their children, as well as provide vocational training to assist with transition back to the community and ensure self-sufficiency. The strength of this program (as with others like it) is the relationships forged with community agencies. The S.E.A.R.I.S.E. program cites linkages with the Department of Social Services, the Literacy Council, and a domestic violence shelter.

Circle Park Behavioral Health Services, Chrysalis Center, Florence, South Carolina, like the other programs discussed, provides residential treatment services to women and their children, specifically those referred by child welfare agencies. The program is designed to help women recover from substance dependency and improve the ability to care for her children in order to provide family stability.

One of the most innovative programs is in Colorado. The Haven is affiliated with the Division of Substance Dependence, Department of Psychiatry, University of Colorado Denver School of Medicine, Addiction Research and Treatment Services. Addiction Research and Treatment Services (ARTS) has been providing modified therapeutic community services to women and infants since 1992 and is Colorado's first program to accept infants into residential treatment with their mothers. The Haven, similar to other programs mentioned, offers women and their children

residential treatment to improve the quality of parenting abilities underscored by a sober lifestyle. What distinguishes this program from the others is the nationally recognized Haven Doula Program. Briefly, once being
assigned to a mother, the doula provides unparallel support from pregnancy through labor and delivery up until 18 months of age. The doula
will accompany the woman to prenatal visits, help her to develop a birth
plan, educate the mother about the labor and delivery process, assist her
in learning to advocate for herself in the health care system, and help with
her preparation for becoming a parent.

After delivery, the doula assists the mother in bonding with her
newborn, learning to play with her child in a developmentally appropriate manner, accompanies her on medical appointments, and helps to link
the mother and child with support (The Haven Doula Program, n.d.).
The graduates of the program can then themselves be trained as Doulas
to work with pregnant women in the residential program. This adds a
dimension to the treatment and recovery process akin to the 12-step philosophy, as graduates who have improved their parenting abilities then
share with other women seeking to restore their lives, their own experiences, strength, and hope.

Marin Services for Women in California addresses the relationship
between chemical dependency and trauma in their treatment approach.
The program began providing services in 1978 and states that they were
the only program in Marin County designed to address and meet the
needs of chemically dependent women and their families. As with the
other programs, they provide the continuum of care—from residential,
outpatient, and aftercare. Additionally, they offer therapeutic and developmental services for the children in their care.

Haymarket Center, Maternal Addiction Center, opened in 1990 in
Chicago to provide services to women who were pregnant. Women, in
any stage of pregnancy, are offered residential services in order to promote a drug-free lifestyle, drug-free pregnancy, and drug-free delivery.
Haymarket Center also offers a program where referrals come directly
from the state child welfare agency. Providing a day treatment program
for women and their children, the staff of the center provides continuity
between the program and the center by visiting the homes of the clients.

ARC Community Services in Madison, Wisconsin, is a comprehensive program that provides the full continuum of care, from residential
to day treatment to aftercare services for women, women involved in
the criminal justice system, and women with their children. This unique
gender-specific treatment organization maintains 11 programs underscored by strengths-based, women-focused philosophy. Their website
clearly states that they seek to "reduce out-of-home placements" for
women and children in their care.

FAMILY DRUG TREATMENT COURT

The Family Drug Treatment Court system, now comprising roughly 700 courts in the United States, was developed with the philosophy that substance abuse was a legal, social, and public health issue and to ensure compliance with AFSA. The development of this specialized court brings together legal, child welfare, and substance abuse treatment professionals in a concerted effort to promote family stabilization and reunification, to decrease length of stay for children in out of home placements, and to promote recovery and abstinence in the parent (Mirchandani 2005; Worcel et al., 2008). Participation in Family Drug Treatment Court is voluntary; however, one does not "refer" a parent for this type of treatment. The woman either is already involved in the legal system with a drug-related offense, is in jeopardy for losing custody of her children, or has already lost custody because of a child neglect or abuse charge.

Family Drug Treatment Court is a "problem-solving" court and offers court-based case management. Other examples of "problem-solving" courts are Integrated Youth Courts, Community Courts, and Integrated Domestic Violence Courts; these problem-specific courts seek to improve outcomes for those who have entered the legal system (Kluger, 2010). In Family Drug Treatment Court, the case managers monitor treatment compliance, offer referrals for other services, and ensure that random urine toxicology is taken. The woman is required to attend regular (often weekly) court hearings, accept referral to and monitoring of her participation in substance abuse treatment, and allow monitoring of her child's safety.

In a study conducted by Worcel et al. (2008), mothers involved in the drug treatment court system entered treatment faster, stayed longer, and were twice as likely to complete treatment successfully. Additionally, this study and others found that mothers involved in drug treatment courts whose children were removed from their custody had higher rates of reunification than those who did not participate in these court programs. However, court monitored programs show an increased rate of reunification as the mother is closely monitored, and therefore is more compliant in treatment (Green, Rockhill, & Furrer, 2007; Mirchandani, 2005; Worcel et al., 2008).

CONCLUSION

For women who are addicted, their ability to parent and often maintain custody of their children is adversely impacted. For their children, out of home placements for longer than expected periods creates a myriad of difficulties. Although federal legislation attempted to mitigate this difficulty, the obstacles created by the 15/22 rule are counterintuitive in terms of the time it may take to recover from substance abuse. Society tends to demonize women who use drugs, stating that they are uninterested in their children, or undeserving of them. Nonetheless, for those of us who have worked with addicted women, it is known that despite their addictions, they genuinely voice concern for and attachment to their children. The programs highlighted are recognized as providing innovative treatment opportunities for women and their children in order to sustain the family or promote reunification. Services that seek to promote the welfare of the family versus targeting a particular member are paramount. One must remember that parents become involved in the child welfare system because of their children. Young children enter the substance abuse treatment system because of their parent. This creates two competing areas for intervention from agencies that have traditionally focused on one rather than both. As recommended by CASA (1999), the collaboration between child welfare organizations and substance abuse treatment providers is an effort to shift the focus to the family, with each member having their own individualized plan and providing comprehensive services to both. Programs that provide parenting classes in addition to mother–child therapeutic groups realize that one cannot correct deficits and misconceptions about parenting without being in a safe environment to "make the mistakes" and for modification to be made immediately in the context of group support. Tensions between child welfare workers and substance abuse treatment workers can only be eased through conversation, education, and standards for service provision that are clear and succinct, and that embrace the mission of both organizations. This effort can create a culture that supports productive collaboration, minimizes barriers to care, stalls the "playing of one system against the other" by clients, and benefits the children in their care.

REFERENCES

Bride, B. E. (2001). Single gender treatment of substance abuse: Effect on treatment retention, and completion. *Social Work Research, 25*(4), 223–232.

Carlson, B. E. (2006). Best practices in the treatment of substance abusing women in the child welfare system. *Journal of Social Work Practice in the Addictions, 6*(3), 97–115.

Glider, P., Hughes, P., Mullen, R., Coletti, S., Sechrest, L., Neri, R., et al. (1996). Two therapeutic communities for substance abusing women and their children. In E. R. Rahdert (Ed.), *Treatment for drug exposed women and children: Advances in research methodology. National Institute on Drug Abuse.* Retrieved from http://archives.drugabuse.gov/pdf/monographs/monograph166/download.html

Green, B. L., Rockhill, A., & Burns, S. (2008). The role of interagency collaboration for substance abusing families involved with child welfare. *Child Welfare, 87*(1), 29–61.

Green, B. G., Rockhill, A. M., & Furrer, C. J. (2007). Does substance abuse treatment make a difference for child welfare case outcomes? A statewide longitudinal analysis. *Children and Youth Services Review, 29*(4), 460–473.

Greenfield, S. F., Brooks, A. J., Gordon, S. M., Green, C. A., Kropp, F., McHugh, R. H., et al. (2007). Substance abuse treatment entry, retention, and outcome in women: A review of the literature. *Drug and Alcohol Dependence, 86,* 1–21.

Gruber, K. J., & Taylor, M. F. (2006). A family perspective for substance abuse: Implications from the literature. *Journal of Social Work Practice in the Addictions, 6*(1/2), 1–29.

Jansson, L. M., & Velez, M. (1999). Understanding and treating substance abusers and their infants. *Infants and Young Children, 11*(4), 79–89.

Juliana, P., & Goodman, C. (2005). Children of substance abusing parents. In J. H. Lowinson, P. Ruiz, R. B. Millman & J. G. Langrod (Eds.), *Substance abuse: A comprehensive textbook* (4th ed., pp. 1013–1020). Philadelphia: Lippincott Williams & Wilkins.

Kandall, S. R. (1996). *Substance and shadow.* Cambridge, MA: Harvard University Press.

Kaufman, E. (1994). *Psychotherapy of addicted persons.* New York: The Guilford Press.

Kluger, J. H. (2010). *Problem-solving courts.* Retrieved from http://courts.state.ny.us/courts/problem_solving

Mapp, S. C., & Steinberg, C. (2007). Birth families as permanency resources for children in long term foster care. *Child Welfare, 86*(1), 29–51.

Marsh, J. C., & Cao, D. (2005). Parents in substance abuse treatment: Implications for child welfare practice. *Children and Youth Services Review, 27*(12), 1259–1278.

Mirchandani, R. (2005). What's so special about specialized courts? The state and social change in Salt Lake City's domestic violence court. *Law and Society Review, 39,* 379–417.

Odyssey House, Inc. (n.d.). Retrieved from http://www.odysseyhouseinc.org

Osterling, K. L., & Austin, M. J. (2008). Substance abuse interventions for parents involved in the child welfare system: Evidence and implications. *Journal of Evidence-Based Social Work, 5*(1/2), 157–189.

Rahdert, E. R. (1996). *Introduction to the perinatal-20. Treatment research demonstration program. National Institute on Drug Abuse.* Retrieved from http://archives.drugabuse.gov/pdf/monographs/127.pdf

Rockhill, A., Green, B. L., & Newton-Curtis, L. (2008). Accessing substance abuse treatment: Issues for parents involved with child welfare services. *Child Welfare, 87*(3), 63–93.

Ross, C. J. (2006). Foster children awaiting adoption under the Adoption and Safe Families Act of 1997. *Adoption Quarterly, 9*(2/3), 121–131.

Ryan, J. P., Marsh, J. C., Testa, M. F., & Louderman, R. (2006). Integrating substance abuse treatment and child welfare services: Findings from the Illinois alcohol and other drug abuse waiver demonstration. *Social Work Research, 30*(2), 95–107.

Smith, B. D., & Mogro-Wilson, C. (2007). Multi-level influences on the practice of interagency collaboration in child welfare and substance abuse treatment. *Children and Youth Services Review, 29,* 545–556.

The Haven Doula Program. (n.d.). Retrieved from http://www.havenfriends .org/about/program---overview/doula/

The National Center on Addiction, & Substance Abuse at Columbia University. (1999). *No safe haven: Children of substance abusing parents.* Retrieved from http://www.ncsacw.samhsa.gov/files/508/NoSafeHaven.htm

Worcel, S. D., Furrer, C. J., Green, B. L., Burrus, S. W. M., & Finigan, M. W. (2008). Effects of family treatment drug courts on substance abuse and child welfare outcomes. *Child Abuse Review, 17*(6), 427-443.

10

Programs for Adolescent Children of Substance-Abusing Parents in School and Residential Settings

Ellen R. Morehouse

INTRODUCTION

The impact of parental substance use on adolescents varies greatly, is mediated by many factors, and can change over time. Adolescent Children of Substance-Abusing Parents (COSAPs) can be found in all settings that serve young people, including social service agencies, youth programs, residential facilities and schools. This chapter will provide strategies for addressing COSAP-specific issues in schools and residential settings, in addition to providing information useful to other settings that do not specialize in addressing COSAP issues. Barriers to implementation and opportunities for education and intervention will be described.

Adolescence presents a critical and unique window of opportunity for intervention as adolescents become less dependent on their parents and begin to form their own identities. The choices they make in adopting positive or negative social and emotional coping strategies can impact the rest of their lives. Interventions with adolescent COSAPs provide the opportunity to interrupt the potential negative trajectories from childhood to teen delinquency, substance abuse, truancy, under achievement, and problems in relationships (Johnson & Leff, 1999).

Understanding the developmental issues of adolescents is critical to effective interventions with adolescent COSAPs. Specifically, it is important to remember that the prefrontal cortex of the adolescent brain is not fully developed so adolescents do not have a well-developed capacity to control emotions and make good judgments. Yet, the hormonal changes during adolescence impact the amygdala (which controls emotions) causing emotions to be intensified. Someone once described adolescents as "Corvettes without brakes." As a result, it is common for adolescents to experience everything as a crisis, have mood swings, be overly sensitive, lack empathy, be impulsive, and not be able to plan or understand cause and effect. In addition, since emotional separation and identity formation are developmental processes that proceed unevenly and at different rates, ambivalence, pseudo sophistication, self-consciousness, and self-absorption are common.

There are differences among early, mid, and late adolescence and these differences vary among and within adolescents. For example, a 15-year-old can be as physically developed as an 18-year-old but have the cognitive and emotional development of a 13-year-old. Generally, younger adolescents are more dependent upon peers for a sense of identity, more loyal to their family, have less developed verbal skills, and because they have less ability for abstract reasoning, are much more concrete. In contrast, older adolescents' newly developing ability for abstract reasoning make them more able to understand the impact of their parents' alcohol and drug abuse and recovery on their own behavior.

CORE INTERVENTIONS FOR HELPING ADOLESCENT COSAPs

The following interventions could be included in all programs where adolescent children of substance-abusing parents may be found, such as community-based youth serving organizations, faith-based organizations, and health care settings, as well as by clinicians in private practice. COSAP-specific services can be viewed on a continuum with awareness raising activities that can benefit everyone on one end of the continuum to intensive psychotherapy that is only needed by some on the other end. Each type of service has different goals (Morehouse, 1995).

Awareness Activities

Awareness activities, such as public service announcements (PSAs), posters, book displays, and so forth, let COSAPs know they are not alone. These activities help them understand that there are many adolescents with substance-abusing parents, that many of these parents have behaviors similar to that of their parents (i.e., break promises, or embarrass them), that many other teens may feel as they do (i.e., angry, ashamed, scared, etc.), and that there are adults who can help.

Awareness activities in schools and other facilities that involve all students or residents include announcements, assemblies, and artistic or informational displays that are seen or heard by everyone. An effective and very low cost example is a prominent wall display of famous COSAPs. Ideally, this activity should occur during National COA Awareness Week (which is the week of Valentine's Day), during national Alcohol Awareness Month in April, or during national Recovery Month in September. The activity consists of putting pictures of famous COSAPs (entertainers, elected officials, athletes, scientists, etc.) on a wall with a large sign that reads "Famous COSAPs." Pictures should include famous COSAPs who are not known for having had their own problem with alcohol or other drugs, such as former President Clinton, as well as other COSAPs who are known for having had their own problems, such as Drew Barrymore. This display gives young people three important messages: You are not alone; COSAPs can grow up to be very successful; and COSAPs can also develop a problem with alcohol or other drugs.

These activities and messages are critical because they break the "don't talk" rule. In most substance-abusing families, children are told not to talk about the parents' substance use so they are reluctant to tell others about upsetting incidents or their resulting feelings. As a result of the isolation and lack of validation, adolescents often believe that what is happening in their family is unique. School- and facility-wide awareness activities universalize their experience and reduce some of the isolation, shame, and confusion.

Finding ways to integrate new activities that can help COSAPs into existing classroom or other settings becomes a challenge. Participation can be active or passive and include activities that target COSAPs without identifying them in the general population, as well as those designed for identified COSAPs. To maximize participation, interventions and activities can be conducted for large groups that provide no barriers to participation.

Reviewing the lists of books, plays, short stories, and poems that will be read in various English classes can create opportunities to discuss the impact parental drinking or drug use has on teens. Huckleberry Finn, plays by Eugene O'Neill, or novels by Jack London or F. Scott Fitzgerald are just some examples of classics that provide vivid illustrations of how teens can be affected. An in-class or homework assignment that asks students to answer questions such as: "What could Huck Finn have done when his father was drunk and yelling at him?" requires all students in the class to identify coping strategies. A follow-up question such as, "What are the possible benefits and drawbacks of that strategy?" helps students think about the usefulness of that strategy. Compiling a list of all the students' answers with benefits and consequences will provide a menu of options for COSAPs without identifying who in the class needs this information. This academic activity can also provide useful information to the non-COSAPs who may have a COSAP friend or relative, in addition to being a useful exercise in problem solving for other difficult circumstances.

A similar activity can be conducted with an athletic team or with all students participating on teams. A meeting during practice or at another time can discuss sportsmanship, concentration, and distractions from performance. The topic of how fans' behaviors can result in penalties for a team and interfere with the athletes' concentration provides an opportunity to discuss how parents' behavior on the sidelines or in the stands can impact the team. Reasons for inappropriate parental behavior, such as excess enthusiasm, over involvement, substance use, or lack of understanding of the sport's rules can all be discussed along with information on how the coach or school administration will respond. Generalizing about inappropriate parental behavior and explaining that there are reasons for it can help decrease an adolescent's shame by bringing about the realization that parents' behavior can be inappropriate for a variety of reasons and can increase the likelihood that the COSAP will self-identify to a coach. In these examples' COSAPs are "participating" in helpful interventions without stimulating resistance from school staff, without being stigmatized, without needing parental involvement, and without having to self-identify.

Substance Abuse Education

Substance abuse education goes a step further than awareness by explaining why parents break promises, act differently when using substances, feel and act sick when not using substances, forget things, and so forth. To be effective, education must fit the cognitive development and learning style of each adolescent. For example, not considering an adolescent's cognitive and emotional development could have a very negative impact when explaining how alcoholism tends to "run in families." Explaining blackouts as a reason for broken promises and forgetfulness should be done differently for a 13-year-old than for an 18-year-old. For example a 13-year-old can be told that it is possible for a dad and son to go fishing, clean the four fish that were caught, put two fish in the refrigerator and two fish in the freezer, and then 1 hour later have the dad say to his son, "let's clean the fish" not remembering that the fish were already cleaned and put away. The 13-year-old can be told that because the dad was drinking while they were fishing and cleaning the fish, even though he didn't act drunk, he didn't remember cleaning the fish. The son should also be told, "There is no reason the dad wouldn't want to remember cleaning and storing the fish, so people don't have blackouts because they don't want to remember and some people don't have to drink a lot to have a blackout." An 18-year-old can be told the following: "Blackouts can occur for some alcoholics and not for others; they are different from passing out; a person doesn't have to seem impaired to have a blackout; they don't occur because someone wants to forget what they did; they are a neurological response that some people have when certain chemicals (such as alcohol) are ingested and the person is unable to remember what happened during a period of time despite reminders."

When providing education consideration must be given to the fact that some adolescents become highly anxious during this time and may not absorb and integrate the information. Others may have learning difficulties that make it difficult to listen and learn in groups, or even to read booklets or fact sheets.

Just as awareness can help reduce isolation and shame, education can help reduce pain. By understanding that an adolescent is not responsible for the parents' substance use or other behavior, or that substance use can make it difficult for a parent to respond adequately and make a teen feel unloved, the adolescent can separate herself or himself from the parent's problem. The ability to understand these concepts was one of the protective factors identified in a study of resilient children of parents with affective disorders (Beardslee & Podorefsky, 1988). The importance of detaching from the parent's drinking problem has been a long-recognized principle of Alateen. Education about these concepts is provided in Alateen, and in books, booklets, and movies about COSAPs and should be a part of all substance abuse education curriculums and COSAP-specific services. Alateen is a self-help program for teens who have a parent, other relative, or close friend who is an alcoholic. Alateen groups consist of teens who share their experiences, learn from each other how to cope with their situations, and provide support for each other using the 12 steps and 12 traditions from Al-Anon and Alcoholics Anonymous. Alateen is part of Al-Anon and Alateen meetings are led by an adult Al-Anon member.

Support for Specific Concerns of Substance Abuse

Giving COSAPs an opportunity to talk about their situation, listening, and expressing empathy are very important because COSAPs often have no one else to talk to about what is happening with their parents. They may often feel that no one is listening or that no one understands; they even may be told that their feelings are wrong. Statements by non–substance-using family members such as "You shouldn't feel that way," "Grow up," "You don't know what it means to be upset," "Stop crying or I'll give you something to cry about," are common responses to COSAPs when they do express feelings. As a result, they learn it is not safe or wise to express feelings.

To help the adolescent COSAP acquire situation-specific coping skills it is critical for professionals to have a thorough knowledge of alcohol and other drug abuse and dependence, knowledge of child and adolescent development, and developmentally appropriate skills. The professional must be able to explain substance abuse in a way that can be understood by the adolescent. Specifically, it is necessary for the adolescent to understand the following:

1. Why a parent can't just stop using a substance;
2. That the parent's use and resulting behavior do not mean that the parent doesn't love them;
3. That they aren't responsible for the parent's substance use or the parent's recovery;
4. That what the parent says or does while they are impaired or in withdrawal is not necessarily what the parent really thinks, feels, or intends to do;
5. That many parents have memory loss when using and, even when they don't seem impaired, they may have no memory of what they said or did, or what promises they made.

Helping an adolescent understand these dynamics is one of the key tasks in reducing the negative impact of the parent's substance use and in enhancing the resiliency of the adolescent.

Skill Building

The next level of services involves examining how an adolescent is coping with the parent's substance use and resulting behavior, evaluating the efficacy of the strategy, exploring new strategies, and helping the adolescent develop or refine the needed skills. The goal of this level of services is skill development for behavioral change and/or support for maintaining healthy behaviors. Some examples of this are learning not to talk back to an intoxicated parent as a way of avoiding punishment, learning to write or draw as a way of dealing with emotions, contacting a friend when upset, learning how to respond when a parent has been inappropriate or is not able to comply with requests from the school or others, or figuring the best way of leaving home, whether by going to college, getting a job, or joining the armed services after high school.

While coping strategies can be provided in books and booklets, individual or group counseling provide a more effective forum to help adolescents develop and master healthy communication, anger management, and stress reduction skills to better meet their needs.

Counseling for Emotional and Behavioral Issues

Counseling can benefit COSAPs when the parent's substance use has resulted in behaviors that have negative consequences for the adolescent. Examples include a wide range of behaviors such as difficulty concentrating in school, problematic peer relationships, substance use, eating disorders or self-mutilation. For some adolescents with behavioral issues, helping them to explore the relationship between parental substance abuse and these issues will be sufficient. For others, COSAP specific counseling can be incorporated in mental health and/or substance abuse treatment.

Counseling in general is based on the premise that "For me to help you, you need to <u>trust</u> me and <u>talk</u> about your <u>feelings</u>"—three things that are difficult for COSAPs to do (Black, 1982). Therefore, it is necessary to modify standard counseling techniques (Morehouse, 1979). It is suggested that this can be done by having the professional break the "don't talk" rule first by demonstrating an understanding of how parental substance abuse can affect adolescents. This can be done verbally or with reading materials or visual aids. The most common concerns and experiences of COSAPs that need to be addressed include:

1. Feeling responsible, directly or indirectly for their parent's substance abuse;
2. Equating their parent's substance abuse with not being loved;
3. Feeling angry with the nonusing parent for not protecting them or for causing the substance abuser's use;
4. Worrying that the substance abuser will get hurt, sick, or die;
5. Being embarrassed by the parent's inappropriate behavior, which can include criminal or sexual behavior;
6. Not knowing what to expect because of the inconsistency;
7. Being confused by the difference between "sober" behavior and "impaired" behavior;
8. Wanting their parents to use a substance and then feeling guilty when they do so.

By stating, "Here are some of the concerns of other teens that have parents who drink or drug too much" the clinician demonstrates that other adolescents may share similar situations or feelings. This can help the COSAP feel less embarrassed about disclosing parental substance abuse and more confident that they will be understood. In describing the common concerns of other COSAPs, the clinician should take time to provide concrete examples of each concern. The COSAP can then be asked, "Do you have any of these concerns or do any of these situations occur in your family?"

The adolescent should then be given the opportunity to talk. Some may just nod silently, some may ventilate, some may acknowledge they have some of the concerns, while others may deny concerns, and some may become so anxious they are unable to sit still. If the adolescent does share, it is important to listen carefully to what he or she is most concerned about and ask questions that determine the impact of the parent's substance use on them. At this point, a more detailed assessment of the situation can take place, including the current and past severity and duration of the drinking and drug use, the degree of family conflict, the adolescent's relationship with the nonusing parent (if there is one), the presence of violence, the importance of alcohol/drugs in the family, the adolescent's constitutional factors, the presence of other nurturing/care taking adults; the ability of the family to maintain family rituals (Steinglass, Bennett, Wolin, & Reiss, 1987), their friends' attitudes and use of substances, and their own attitudes and use of substances.

After this information has been elicited, it is important to provide education about the issues described previously. This can be done verbally, but articles, books, booklets, and videos are very useful as supplements because COSAPs' anxiety often prevents them from absorbing the information. It is also important to provide skills for coping with the parental substance use and resulting behavior. Since COSAPs often lack exposure to adults who model healthy and appropriate behaviors, they frequently need to learn new social skills and skills for responding to stress. This should include the opportunity to role play difficult situations and evaluate the efficacy of different strategies.

It is also important to examine the adolescents' adaptation to the parents' substance use and the adolescents' comfort or discomfort with their own behavior, and to help them see that they have choices in how they react to the parent. Often COSAPs don't see their "problem behavior" as a reaction to the parent. Once they do, they can begin to choose new ways of responding and then develop alternative ways of coping.

Finally, it is important to examine barriers to healthier functioning. Treatment of COSAPs, when needed, should help them to understand how their past and current family situation affects them and to empower them to develop healthy behaviors to positively influence the future. For example, an adolescent who is always hurt by peer relationships because she/he is looking for the nurturing that is not provided by the parent can understand how she/he has unrealistic expectations of friends, becomes hurt, and then keeps people from getting close. An adolescent who has these problematic relationship patterns can learn to identify what his or her needs are, who can meet them at different times, and skills for how to get the needs met, and then learn what are realistic expectations in different relationships. In addition, by participating in counseling groups, COSAPs can also experience reduced isolation, practice sharing their feelings, and develop increased readiness for Alateen and other 12-step programs (Morehouse, 1986).

Use of Supplementary Resources

Printed material and/or videos can provide valuable assistance in working with COSAPs. These materials often help to reduce the shame by confirming that the adolescent is not the only one with this situation. Workbooks can help both the clinician and the adolescent to assess the family situation and help the adolescent express feelings he or she may not be able to express otherwise. Similarly, movie clips, printed materials, and specialized videos of parental substance use can stimulate individual and group discussion.

There are many free booklets, pamphlets, fact sheets, and posters for adolescent COSAPs. They can be obtained from the Substance Abuse and Mental Health Services Administration (SAMHSA), the National Association for Children of Alcoholics (NACOA), Alateen, and other national, state, and local organizations. Costs can range from minimal to considerable, which should be taken into account when developing a program.

HELPING ADOLESCENTS IN SCHOOL AND RESIDENTIAL SETTINGS

Schools and residential facilities are ideal settings for interventions with adolescent COSAPs because interventions can be provided without parental involvement, there is a "captive audience," and there is minimal risk of stigmatization. Interventions can be provided to the entire school or residential facility or tailored to the specific needs of individual COSAPs. Activities that provide COSAP-specific information to all students or residents have the potential to benefit COSAPs at minimal cost.

While all adolescent COSAPs can benefit from activities that increase awareness about the impact of parental substance abuse, the adolescent's individual need for services should be the primary determinant of what interventions are provided (Morehouse, 1995). Secondary factors to be considered include: the adolescent's availability to participate;

the qualifications, training, comfort, and responsibilities of the staff; the policies and mission of the setting; and fiscal considerations.

Individual and group counseling for COSAPs in schools or residential facilities have the benefit of providing support and new skills for healthy coping strategies. However, there are usually barriers to optimal participation (Morehouse & Tobler, 2000). Participation usually requires that the COSAP participants miss or are "pulled" from another activity that is occurring at the same time. In addition to possible resistance from school and facility staff, the COSAPs themselves may be resistant to participate because they don't want to miss class, lunch with friends, practice, or a recreational activity. Therefore, scheduling is critical for participation. Appointments that rotate times and days so the COSAP doesn't miss the same activity each week will decrease resistance to participation.

In residential facilities there are also legitimate scheduling conflicts to consider. For example, if each unit, cottage, or floor has an assigned day to do laundry and a COSAP counseling group consists of girls from various locations, an after school group at the facility will always conflict with at least one girl's laundry day. If this is the only time the group can be scheduled, the leader will have to build in review time at the beginning of each group so the girl or girls that missed the previous group will be "caught up." The scheduling of "make up" sessions between groups is another alternative to maximize participation.

Staff Qualifications, Training, and Responsibilities

Because COSAPs are both over-represented among teens with academic, emotional, and behavioral problems, and are resilient, professionals need good assessment skills so services can be appropriately matched to the needs of the individual adolescent. Professionals who work with adolescent COSAPs must be knowledgeable about addiction and recovery and their impact on the family, child and adolescent development, adolescent specific intervention strategies, and 12-step programs (such as AA, NA, Al-Anon, Alateen, etc.). Substance abuse treatment professionals who lack knowledge of adolescent development and clinical strategies will be just as ineffective as clinicians serving adolescents who lack knowledge of addiction. Therefore, professionals who intend to provide interventions to adolescent COSAPs must identify gaps in their knowledge and experience and seek training and supervision. Well-meaning professionals who recommend family sessions where the adolescent does not speak because of fear of punishment from the impaired parents and then labels the adolescent as resistant, can do more harm than good. Similarly, the addiction professional who uses 12-step expressions with a 13-year-old who has not yet fully developed abstract reasoning ability will not be understood by this youngster and may encounter resistance to participation in services.

Professionals who themselves come from substance-abusing homes must be able to maintain their objectivity. They cannot assume that they know each COSAP's situation or not listen to the adolescent's painful experiences or feelings because it stirs their own painful memories. Similarly, professionals in recovery from a substance use disorder, or who has a partner with a substance use disorder, may find that anger and painful experiences expressed by the adolescent COSAP may engender guilt about their own parenting.

Parental Consent Issues

Some individual or small group counseling for COSAPs in schools and residential facilities may require parental notification or consent. The reluctance of many adolescent COSAPs to have their parent(s) know that they want to participate in a COSAP specific intervention can prevent their involvement. Professionals need to carefully consider the applicable school policies and state regulations on this issue.

The role, function, title, license, or certification of the professional, the nature and scope of the activity or intervention, the age of the COSAP, and the state regulations and setting are some of the factors that determine the need for parent notification or permission to receive COSAP specific services. For example, a state licensed or certified social worker might need parental permission for 14-year-olds to participate in a COSAP counseling group or individual counseling in a school in some states but not in others. However, the coach or teacher who gives advice each week to that same 14-year-old probably won't need such parental permission. Similarly, if the social worker does a presentation to the 14-year-old's entire English class or team together with the teacher or coach, parental permission will not be needed. Moreover, if that 14-year-old is placed in a group home, juvenile justice, or other residential facility, it is likely that the assigned state certified or licensed social worker will not need permission to provide COSAP specific counseling. In situations where consent is required, professionals need to be creative to minimize parent resistance. For example, a letter to parents asking permission for their teen to participate in a substance abuse prevention group that has the goals of developing effective skills for managing peer resistance, communication, time management, decision making, skills for managing stress and anger and improving school performance will encourage parental permission. In contrast, a letter that mentions parental chemical use will provoke resistance.

School-Based Interventions

Interventions in schools can include: education provided by a teacher in a health class; support from a caring teacher, guidance counselor, and/ or social worker; and individual and group counseling provided by a student assistance counselor. Student assistance counselors are usually master's level social workers or counselors who provide a variety of substance abuse prevention activities in a school as part of a Student Assistance Program (Morehouse & Chambers, 1983; National Institute on Alcohol Abuse and Alcoholism [NIAAA], 1984). COSAP-specific groups are almost always included in Student Assistance Programs.

To maximize participation and decrease resistance to school-wide, classroom, small group, or individual interventions, school staff needs to understand the impact of parental addiction on students. Teachers and administrators know that students cannot learn as well when they are hungry so they support school lunch programs. Similarly, schools need to understand that students do not learn as well when they are worrying that their mom is going to pass out with a lit cigarette and start a fire. School staff needs training on how to detect possible signs of parental substance abuse in students and how to respond appropriately (National Association of Children of Alcoholics [NACoA], 2001).

As adolescents mature they become more aware of appropriate and inappropriate parental behavior and make more of an effort to hide their parents' use to prevent embarrassment and stigmatization. If staff responds nonjudgmentally to parents who come to school impaired and does not cause the adolescent to experience further shame or blame, the student is more likely to accept help.

School staff needs to be knowledgeable about adolescents' rights to confidentiality, which vary by state and setting. When seeking permission from the COSAP to share information for the purpose of advocating on his/her behalf, it can be explained that the parent's alcohol or drug use does not have to be mentioned. For example, a student assistance counselor or school social worker can explain to a teacher who is concerned about a COSAP's drop in grades that, "Emily is having a hard time concentrating in class and on her homework. Things have become stressful at home, and there are some health issues. However, Emily is also concerned about her work and would be willing to do an extra assignment to try to bring up her average." In this example the parent's chemical use isn't mentioned and the teacher receives the necessary information to help Emily. Similarly, parents can be told that Emily is receiving counseling because she is experiencing stress and can use support on how to better meet the demands of the school.

Student Assistance Programs

Student Assistance Programs began in the late 1970s as school-based substance abuse prevention programs for secondary school students. They were modeled after Employee Assistance Programs (EAPs) that were used successfully by employing organizations to identify and help employees with alcohol- and other drug-related problems.

Student Assistance Programs focus on students most at risk for developing substance abuse, specifically children of substance-abusing parents and students who were users of substances. As mentioned, Student Assistance Programs were implemented by master's level professionals called student assistance counselors employed by a community-based agency with expertise in substance abuse prevention, or by the school. In either case, the student assistance counselor needs specific training in substance abuse prevention, including training on the needs and issues of students with substance-abusing parents and students who are using substances as well as effective strategies for identifying, engaging, and intervening with these students. This kind of Student Assistance Program provides an ideal opportunity to help COSAPs.

Today there are many variations of Student Assistance Programs and some no longer include COSAP-specific strategies and interventions or have staff that is knowledgeable about COSAP issues.

Residential-Based Interventions

Many children of substance-abusing parents may find themselves living in residential settings that range from juvenile justice to child welfare to mental health residential facilities. Such facilities can provide a perfect opportunity for offering specialized help for these young people.

Adolescents living in residential settings need to prepare for home visits. Common problems they must deal with are: finding ways to respond to an impaired parent; addressing disappointment that the parent hasn't stopped using; seeking involvement with supportive people (Werner, 1986; Werner & Johnson, 2000); and participating in healthy activities out of the house. In addition, many residential facilities have pressure from funding agencies to return adolescents to the family as soon as possible. This pressure often doesn't allow the adolescent enough time to understand the impact of their parent's addiction and to develop the skills needed to cope with it. Involvement in Alateen while in the residential facility will introduce the adolescent to 12-step programs.

The Residential Student Assistance Program (RSAP)

RSAP is a comprehensive substance abuse prevention program for adolescents living in secure and nonsecure facilities. Residents may attend school at the facility or in the community. RSAP includes all of the core program components described previously (Morehouse & Tobler, 2000). While it is not known exactly what percentage of adolescents in these facilities are COSAPs, some studies estimate the numbers to range as high as 50% to 75% (Booth & Zhang, 1996; Reid, Macchetto, & Foster, 1999). Even if the percentages are not that high, they are probably higher than in the general population. Consequently, COSAP specific services should be provided.

In addition to the COSAP issues previously discussed, COSAPs placed voluntarily or involuntarily in residential psychiatric, child welfare, and juvenile justice settings have additional issues. They usually want to go home and hope that the substance-abusing parent will change while they are away. Therefore, they are often likely to minimize the severity of the parent's drinking, drug use, and related behavior as well as their own reactions. This minimization, coupled with anger at the parents who are viewed as responsible for the adolescent being taken out of the home, make it difficult to accurately assess the impact of the parent's substance use on the adolescent and thus, difficult to provide healthy coping strategies.

Participation in a COSAP counseling group at the facility will help the adolescent learn that he/she is not alone, and that talking to peers can be helpful in learning skills to cope with the parent (Dies & Burghardt, 1991). Discharge planning that includes Alateen and/or a counseling group for COSAPs at school or in the community will provide the time needed to further absorb and integrate the work begun in the residential facility.

GUIDELINES FOR PREVENTION AND INTERVENTION WITH COSAPs' SUBSTANCE USE AND ABUSE

Adolescent COSAPs should be given information on how and why they have a greater risk for developing alcohol and other drug problems and must be told that for every year from age 13 to 20 they delay their initiation of use, they can greatly reduce their risk of developing their own substance abuse problem (Grant & Dawson, 1998), and academic and legal problems (Peleg-Oren, Saint-Jean, Carderas, Tammara, & Pierre, 2009).

For adolescents who have already begun using substances, stopping all use is the goal. A thorough assessment should be done to determine if referral to a licensed substance abuse treatment program is needed.

Adolescent COSAPs who are already substance abusers need to have both their COSAP and substance abuse issues addressed simultaneously. They are also more likely to minimize their use and the negative consequences of their use. As a result they are usually more resistant to treatment (Morehouse, 1984).

Providing COSAPs with information on parental blackouts, parental inability to control use or behavior, and parents not necessarily intending what is said or done under the influence, can be seen as applying to the parent but also applying to the adolescent. As adolescents understand more about addiction, they feel less guilty about their own use. With less guilt, it is more likely that the adolescent will be honest about the extent of their use and the resulting behaviors and consequences.

A complete list of substance abuse prevention programs for adolescents can be obtained through SAMHSA's National Registry of Evidence-based Programs and Practices (NREPP, www.nrepp.samhsa.gov). Currently, the four programs on the NREPP list that include adolescent COSAP specific interventions are: Celebrating Families, Project SUCCESS (Schools Using Coordinated Community Efforts to Strengthen Students), Residential Student Assistance Program, and Strengthening Families.

CONCLUSION

Adolescent COSAPs can benefit from a variety of service approaches to improve their functioning and reduce their risk of developing their own substance abuse problems. While adolescent COSAPs are found in any setting, the decision to provide services involves a number of factors including the availability of participants, staff qualifications, training and responsibilities, parent involvement and consent, the mission of the organization, and fiscal considerations. If the decision is made to provide service to this population, procedures must be in place to prevent stigmatization, provide assessment of substance use, and provide referral for substance abuse treatment when necessary. Schools and residential facilities will be better able to accomplish their goals by providing a full range of services in their building.

REFERENCES

Beardslee, W., & Podorefsky, D. (1988). Resilient adolescents whose parents have serious affective and other psychiatric disorders: Importance of self-understanding and relationships. *The American Journal of Psychiatry, 145,* 63–69.

Black, C. (1982). *It will never happen to me.* Mac Printing and Publications Division.

Booth, R. E., & Zhang, Y. (1996). Severe aggression and related conduct problems among runaway and homeless adolescents. *Psychiatric Services, 47*(1), 75–80.

Dies, R., & Burghardt, K. (1991). Group interventions for children of alcoholics: Prevention and treatment in the schools. *Journal of Adolescent Group Therapy, 1*(3), 219–234.

Grant, B., & Dawson, D. (1998). Age of onset of drug use and its association with DSM-IV drug abuse and dependence: Results from the national longitudinal alcohol epidemiologic survey. *Journal of Substance Abuse, 10,* 163–173.

Johnson, J., & Leff, M. (1999). Children of substance abusers: Overview of research findings. *Pediatrics, 103*(5), 1085–1099.

Morehouse, E. (1979). Working in the schools with children of alcoholic parents. *Health and Social Work, 4,* 144–162.

Morehouse, E. (1984). Working with alcohol abusing children of alcoholics. *Alcohol Health and Research World, 8,* 14–19.

Morehouse, E. (1986). Counseling adolescent children of alcoholics in group. In R. J. Ackerman (Ed.), *Growing up in the shadows* (pp. 125–142). Pompano Beach, FL: Health Communications.

Morehouse, E. (1995). Matching services and the needs of children of alcoholic parents: A spectrum of help. In S. Abbott (Ed.), *Children of alcoholics: Selected readings* (pp. 153–176). Rockville, MD: National Association for Children of Alcoholics.

Morehouse, E., & Chambers, J. (1983). A cooperative model for preventing alcohol and drug abuse. *National Association of Secondary School Principals Bulletin, 67*(459), 81–87.

Morehouse, E., & Tobler, N. (2000). Preventing and reducing substance abuse among institutionalized adolescents. *Adolescence, 35*(137), 1–28.

National Association of Children of Alcoholics (NACoA). (2001). *A kit for educators.* Rockville, MD: NACoA.

National Institute on Alcohol Abuse and Alcoholism (NIAAA). (1984). *Preventing alcohol problems through a student assistance program: A manual for implementation based on the Westchester County* (DHHS Publication No. [ADM] 84–1344). New York, Model: U.S. Government Printing Office.

Peleg-Oren, N., Saint-Jean, G., Carderas, G., Tammara, H., & Pierre, C. (2009). Drinking alcohol before age 13 and negative outcomes in late adolescence. *Alcohol: Clinical and Experimental Research, 33,* 1–7.

Reid, J., Macchetto, P., & Foster, S. (1999). *No safe haven: Children of substance-abusing parents.* New York: Center on Addiction and Substance Abuse at Columbia University.

Steinglass, P., Bennett, L., Wolin, S., & Reiss, D. (1987). *The alcoholic family.* New York: Basic Books.

Werner, E. (1986). Resilient offspring of alcoholics: A longitudinal study from birth to age 18. *Journal of Studies on Alcohol, 47*(1), 34–40.

Werner, E., & Johnson, J. (2000). The role of caring adults in the lives of children of alcoholics. *Children of Alcoholics: Selected Readings, 2,* 119–141.

11

Interventions With College Students With Substance-Abusing Parents

David F. Venarde and Gregory J. Payton

INTRODUCTION

Jessie, an undergraduate in her junior year at a 4-year college, has always been a good student. However, lately she has found herself increasingly distracted and worried. Her father's drinking has increased, and he was recently arrested for driving under the influence. Jessie receives frequent panicked phone calls from her mother and feels responsible for helping both her mother and her father. Socially, she is confused about how to cope with drinking in the campus environment. Jessie has avoided drinking in college out of concern for developing a problem like her father's, and she finds herself very anxious when her friends drink, especially when they get drunk. She has become more withdrawn and unsure how she fits in socially. She feels additionally anxious that she is not keeping up with her school work, the one area in which she has always felt a sense of mastery.

College students face a myriad of developmental challenges across academic, social, and health domains. Students who live at home while attending college must balance family relationships with their new social and academic world away from home. Students who reside on campus are adapting to a new-found independence and new patterns of communication with family members. Whether learning to navigate social life with less support from family, or adapting to a less-structured academic routine, college students face major changes—and opportunities—in their transition to university life. For sons and daughters of parents with

223

substance use disorders, the adjustments can be significantly more complex, as opening vignette suggests. Such students are facing major developmental milestones while also coping with the impact—historic and/or
current—of substance use in the family.

In this chapter, we will focus on the particular challenges college students face in managing the impact of parental substance use disorders, and
we will discuss interventions and supports colleges and universities can provide for these students. The chapter includes the following sections: (1) a brief
introductory section on epidemiology; (2) a review of the literature on effects
of parental substance use disorders on sons and daughters; (3) an overview
of substance use on U.S. college campuses; (4) a discussion of campus supports and interventions for the college student population; (5) a brief review
of community and internet resources; and (6) a description of the Sons and
Daughters group run in the New York University Student Health Center's
Counseling and Behavioral Health office and key themes that emerge in
this group.

EPIDEMIOLOGY: A BRIEF OVERVIEW

This chapter, consistent with the larger volume, casts a broad net by addressing students of parents who are abusing a range of substances. Though
much of literature on children of substance-abusing parents (COSAP)
focuses on children of parents with alcohol use disorders—Adult Children
of Alcoholics (ACOA)—we will also examine epidemiology of other substance use disorders to make reasonable estimates about the overall impact
of parental alcohol and other drug use on college students.

One study of ACOA's estimates that 15% of children in the United
States are currently exposed to alcohol abuse or dependence by an adult
in the family (Grant, 2000). This percentage addresses current exposure,
suggesting the percentage of children who have been exposed to parental
alcohol problems at some time during the course of childhood would be,
of course, higher. The estimates on the number of ACOAs in attending colleges and universities range from 17% to 33% (Fischer et al., 2000). These
estimates include children of parents who are actively using as well as parents who are in recovery. Given the estimate of 19 million students enrolled
in colleges and universities in the United States during 2009–2010 (U.S.
Census Bureau, 2009), even at the low end of the range, 17% represents over
3 million affected students. Moreover, studies show a past-year prevalence
of alcohol use disorders in the United States ranging from 4.4% to 9.7%, with
a lifetime prevalence ranging from 13.5% to 30.3% (Ross, 2008). Therefore,
even by very conservative estimates, at least 15 out of 100 college students
have coped with a parental alcohol use disorder at some point in their lives.

Little epidemiological data exist for children of parents with substance use disorders involving drugs other than alcohol. However, by examining some of the data on prevalence of other substance use disorders, we get a sense of the potential impact on children of substance abusing parents (COSAPs) in this country. The National Comorbidity Survey reports lifetime prevalence rates for illicit drug abuse (7.9%) and dependence (3.0%) (Kessler & Merinkangas, 2004). The National Survey on Drug Use and Health (NSDUH) reports a past-year prevalence of adult illicit drug dependence of 2.0% (Substance Abuse and Mental Health Services Administration [SAMHSA], 2006). In addition, the recent National Epidemiological Survey on Alcohol and Related Conditions included misuse of prescription medications, with lifetime prevalence rates for prescription stimulants (2.0%), opioids (1.4%), sedatives (1.1%), and tranquilizers (1.0%) (Huang et al., 2006). Though these data do not differentiate between parents and nonparents, or between parents of children who do or do not attend college, they provide some context for the use of illicit drugs and the misuse of prescription medications in the United States. While both the lifetime and past-year prevalence rates for alcohol use disorders are higher than any of the other substances noted above, it is clear that many college students will be affected by parental abuse of illicit drugs and, increasingly, the misuse of prescription medications.

This research suggest the critical importance of a thorough review of family substance use histories for clinicians working in the college mental health setting. Without such a history, it is difficult for clinicians to properly identify and respond to potential risk factors among the students they are treating. Though some students present at counseling services with parental substance use as an identified concern, most present for other reasons (e.g., stress, relationship problems, and depression) and may not initially identify family substance use disorders. And certainly, although many students grow up in the presence of parental substance use disorders, they may not have the language to discuss this: They may consider their experience "normal" or "the way it is," even if a parent has clearly struggled. And while some students may not be ready to discuss this topic in treatment, others will find relief at finally being able to talk about this family secret and may also be open to other options, such as a group that could be helpful.

RISK FACTORS FOR COSAPs IN COLLEGE

The genetic and psychosocial risk factors for COSAPs are addressed in more detail in Chapter 1. In this section, we provide a brief review of these risk factors, with emphasis on the particular vulnerabilities for college students. As the earlier review of the literature suggests, it is evident that COSAPs are a far from homogeneous group sharing universal characteristics, personality styles, or patterns of interpersonal relationships. As one might expect, COSAPs are a diverse group in other ways as well, representing a range of ethnic/racial, geographic, and socioeconomic backgrounds. However, two main factors require emphasis in our consideration of this student group: (1) The evidence on genetic heritability of substance use disorders is compelling, and therefore biological sons and daughters are at higher risk for developing substance use disorders themselves (Gelertner & Kranzler, 2008; Tsuang et al., 1998). (2) A review of the empirical literature on psychosocial adjustment of COSAPs suggests that these college students are at increased risk for a range of negative outcomes in addition to substance use disorders (Fischer et al., 2000; Harter, 2000; Sher, Walitzer, Wood, & Brent, 1991).

As noted, the evidence for genetic factors in the development of substance use disorders is now substantial. Based on twin, family, and adoption studies of alcohol dependence, heritability estimates range from 50% to 60%, indicating that half, or over half, of the risk for alcohol dependence is genetic (Gelertner & Kranztler, 2008). Other research indicates similar genetic risks for other substances, including opioids, cocaine, and nicotine, plus the finding that genetic factors work across substances (Tsuang et al., 1998). Thus, as sons and daughters are exposed to substances during their college years, they are at greater risk of developing an unhealthy relationship with substances than their peers who do not have a parental history of a substance use disorder. Plus, the evidence suggests that heritability is not substance-specific: In other words, a son or daughter of a parent with an alcohol use disorder is at greater risk of developing any substance use disorder, not just an alcohol use disorder. In short, the sons and daughters of parents with any substance use disorder represent a population highly vulnerable to substance use disorders themselves.

Though findings in the empirical literature on psychosocial adjustment of adult children of substance users (again, this is primarily literature examining ACOAs) are not wholly consistent (Rodney, 1996), much of the literature indicates increased risks for the COSAP population. In a review of the empirical literature on the psychosocial adjustment of adult children of alcoholics, Harter (2000) concluded that ACOAs are at increased risk for a variety of negative outcomes, including substance abuse, antisocial or undercontrolled behaviors, depressive symptoms, anxiety disorders, low self-esteem, difficulties in family relationships, and generalized distress and maladjustment. In addition, Harter's review also notes that "studies with college students have suggested increased distress and pathology across most dimensions" (Harter, 2000, p. 319). Also of note is research with college students suggesting lower levels of academic achievement among college ACOAs (Sher et al., 1991), challenging the stereotype of COSAPs as high achievers.

In her review, Harter (2000) stresses that the risks are not uniformly found in ACOAs, nor are any of the identified risks specific to ACOAs. Some of the literature suggests that family dysfunction, rather than the parental alcohol use itself, is the more relevant risk factor for ACOAs. In a study of 549 college students, Fischer et al. (2000) examined ACOA status alongside family dysfunction, finding that both ACOA status and level of family dysfunction were predictors of stress for college students, with family dysfunction appearing to be the better predictor. Other studies (Fewell, 2006; Mothershead, Kivlingham, & Wynkoop, 1998) have also examined parental attachment as a variable alongside family dysfunction, and psychological or interpersonal distress in the ACOA population, with results suggesting that quality of parental attachment, too, plays a role in college student adjustment. Thus, it is important for clinicians working with COSAPs to be mindful of family functioning and the quality of the parent–child relationship in addition to the details of parental substance use.

Lacking in the empirical literature is convincing evidence of maladaptive interpersonal relationships (apart from relationships with family members) among college students, though more research is needed in this area, given the anecdotal clinical data on this topic. As discussed later in this chapter, struggles in relationships are a frequent theme in the Sons and Daughters group at New York University.

Another area requiring further investigation and understanding is the variation of risk factors across racial, ethnic, and socio-economic dimensions. In her discussion of collegiate African American ACOAs, Rodney (1996) suggests that clinicians may be well served by noting protective factors more specific to the African American community, including religious socialization and racial identity.

Notably missing from the empirical literature is clear support for a uniform profile of ACOAs or COSAPs (Rodney, 1996; Harter, 2000). Though COSAPs are at higher risk for substance use disorders and difficulties in psychosocial adjustment, they do not fit neatly into personality types or categories. Despite the popular and clinical literature regarding personality types or codependency among ACOAs (Black, 1981; Woititz, 1983), the empirical support for these descriptions is lacking.

As discussed below, despite the paucity of empirical support for the unique characteristics described in the clinical and popular literature, some students do find the clinical descriptions of family roles and styles of relating to others to be helpful. Clinicians are best served, therefore, by balancing an awareness of the empirical literature with use of clinical judgment and the application of interventions that students find most immediately understandable and helpful.

THE COLLEGE ENVIRONMENT: SUBSTANCE USE ON CAMPUS

College students navigate a period of increased independence from family, heightened self-reliance, consolidation of identity, and progress toward mature friendships and romantic relationships. These students are making sense of their worlds through a wider lens, incorporating input from a broader range of sources, including an expanded peer group, college faculty and staff, and coworkers in their year-round internships or summer jobs. In addition, they are entering into a social world in which substances may play a significant role. As we strive to understand the psychosocial risks factors for COSAPs, it is also helpful to examine what is known about substance use on college and university campuses in the United States.

Alcohol remains far and away the substance of choice on college campuses in the United States, and its misuse is linked to greater negative consequences for college students than any other substance. However, the use of some illicit drugs and the misuse of prescription medications have risen on campuses in the past decade (Johnston, O'Malley, Bachman, & Schulenberg, 2006, 2008). Thus, sons and daughters, who, as discussed above, are at greater risk for developing substance use disorders, are pursuing their educations in contexts where alcohol and other substances may be readily available and frequently used by their peers.

The tradition of heavy drinking on college campuses dates back centuries, and colleges and universities have attempted to mitigate the harm caused by alcohol misuse on campuses for almost as long, with mixed results. The recent data indicate that in many categories, alcohol use has changed little on college campuses over the past several decades. Approximately 83% of college students report that they consume alcohol (Johnston et al., 2008). The majority of undergraduates are underage drinkers, though by their senior year in college, students are often celebrating their 21st birthdays. With the exception of a small minority of "dry" campuses (mainly religious-based campuses on which alcohol and other substances are not permitted), the general trends in alcohol use are fairly consistent, across large or small, rural or urban campuses.

Of students who drink, a significant percentage of students drink heavily and with negative effects. Though the percentage of students who "binge drink" (typically defined as four or more drinks per episode for women, five or more drinks per episode for men) varies widely from school to school, on average 40% of college students report binge drinking within the past 2 weeks (Johnston et al., 2008). A wide range of consequences— including hangovers, blackouts, sexual assaults, unprotected sex, missed classes—are related to alcohol use on campuses. Approximately four to five alcohol-related deaths occur each day among college students in the United States (Hingson, Heeren, Winter, & Wechsler, 2005). The majority of these deaths involve motor vehicle accidents, though college students also die secondary to acute intoxication and other forms of accidental death.

Marijuana is the most commonly used illicit drug on college campuses, with approximately 33% of college students reporting marijuana use within the past year (Johnston et al., 2006). Though the percentage of students using marijuana is far smaller than the percentage drinking alcohol, we also have some indications that marijuana use is increasing on campuses (Johnston et al., 2006; Mohler-Kuo et al., 2003; National Center on Addiction and Substance Abuse [CASA], 2007). Other illicit substances are used with less frequency than marijuana, with the following estimates of past year use among college students for the year 2005: cocaine (5.7%), hallucinogens (5%), ecstasy (2.9%), inhalants (1.8%), and heroin (0.3%) (Johnston et al., 2006).

As noted above, misuse of prescription medications on campuses has risen significantly in the past decade. A variety of prescription medications—including psychostimulants, opioids (mainly prescription pain medications), tranquilizer/anxiolytic medications, and sedatives—are susceptible to misuse by college students. The psychostimulants (primarily Ritalin and Adderall, used in the treatment of attention deficit hyperactivity disorder) are used both as study drugs and as recreational stimulants. Opioid medications (including Oxycontin, Vicodin, Demerol, Percocet) are potent synthetic opiates that have become much more widely prescribed in the United States over the past decade. Students also misuse tranquilizer/anxiolytics (including Xanax, Ativan, Valium) and sedatives (Nembutal and Seconal), sometimes using medications prescribed to friends or family members, sometimes purchasing from local dealers, or on the Internet. From 1993 to 2005, the increases in misuse of prescription medications are striking: past year use increased for opioids from 2.5% to 8.4%; for stimulants from 4.2% to 6.7%; for tranquilizers from 2.4% to 6.4%; and for sedatives, from 1.5% to 3.9% (CASA, 2007). An additional concern is the combination of multiple substances at once, often with little understanding of the potential risks of interactions among the substances, or interactions with other prescribed medications a student may be taking.

Thus, college students enter an environment in which they are likely to be exposed to a range of substances. And, as noted above, as a group COSAPs are at increased risk for misuse of these substances. And whether or not they choose to use alcohol or any other substance, they are navigating an environment that may be particularly stressful for them, as seeing their peers intoxicated may stir intense feelings, and provide clear reminders of family experiences.

CAMPUS SUPPORT FOR COSAPs

Many colleges and universities nationwide endeavor to meet the needs of the substantial number of college students who identify as adult children of alcohol or substance-abusing parents. To this end, colleges and universities have developed formal outreach programs, primary care screenings, campus trainings and consultation services, referral networks, and individual or group treatment services. From the dormitory residences to the consulting rooms of mental health professionals, many campuses provide interdisciplinary support mechanisms to address the needs of this student population.

One facet of university programming for COSAPs is preventive programming and outreach. Wellness programs or Health Promotion programs often address the psychosocial and behavioral risk factors for college students with substance-abusing parents. Akin to public health education, wellness or health promotion programs work throughout campus environments—student centers, residences and classrooms—to reach a broad range of students. Through psychoeducational programming, these campus services identify the effects of growing up with a substance-abusing parent on relationships, mood, personal substance use, and transition into adulthood (Kadison, 2004; McMillen, 1986; Spencer-Thomas, 2009).

A review of university websites indicates that wellness efforts often include the following educative elements: (1) the risk factors and developmental outcomes that typify COSAPs; (2) familial dynamics and resulting relational styles of COSAPs; and (3) coping strategies and potential stressors within the campus environment. Specifically, wellness programming may educate students about the increased propensity of COSAPs toward substance abuse, the roles that COSAPs may play in their familial or romantic relationships, or the ways in which students of substance-abusing parents often struggle with issues of self-esteem or self-worth. Moreover, these programs address typical reactions amongst this population to life on campus, including social withdrawal and aversion to substance-using environments, interpersonal conflict with peers around issues of substance use, increased risk for substance abuse behaviors, and increased difficulty balancing familial role with a burgeoning independent identity.

Psychoeducation and outreach efforts may include referrals to individual or group treatment on campus (Landers & Hollingdale, 1989). Numerous colleges and universities nationwide identify COSAPs as a specific population that may benefit from campus counseling services, often citing staff expertise or specialized treatment services. Students may choose to meet with campus mental health professionals for numerous reasons: affordability, ease of access, lack of familiarity with off-campus community services, and a positive transference to the student health service office.

Individual counseling may be most appropriate for those students who have recently become aware of parental substance abuse or who are acutely impacted by a parent's chronic use. Additionally, individual treatment may be indicated for students who react with shame, denial or silence to their parent's substance use, or who fear the judgment of peers. Due to the significant stressors associated with parental substance abuse, co-occurring mood, relational and familial problems may necessitate individual treatment. Once engaged in counseling, treatment may be tailored to the student's developing awareness of how parental substance abuse has impacted his or her life over time, while aiding the student's efforts at coping with campus life and current stressors (Landers & Hollingdale, 1989).

Group treatment may be appropriate for those students who wish to better understand their experiences as COSAPs and connect with supportive peers. Group counseling creates an atypical environment in which students' experiences can be shared, understood, and honored. While students may be reluctant to disclose details about parental substance abuse with peers, support groups can allow for this candor. Moreover, students learn from one another through the reciprocity involved in group treatment: students often appropriate fellow group members' successful coping strategies and build upon fellow members' insights. Group treatment may involve features of the aforementioned psychoeducational programming, connecting thematic content from group sessions with research or resources to support students (Vannicelli, 1989).

COMMUNITY AND INTERNET RESOURCES

Due to the short-term treatment models of most college counseling centers, individual and group treatments often result in referrals for continued care. While resources vary by community, the needs of COSAPs are regularly addressed by private practitioners, national organizations, and internet communities. Referrals should be provided only after careful consideration of the student's current level of functioning, preferences for treatment modality, and any salient cultural values or identities.

College students are often referred to community groups, particularly 12-step groups such as Al-Anon, and other organizations that broadly serve children of alcoholics or other drug abusers. Additionally, students may be referred to substance abuse and recovery programs that provide ancillary services to family members.

While community groups offer valuable services and resources, college students of substance-abusing parents may not readily engage with these organizations or perceive them to be a good fit. Students may prefer to participate in programs or support groups with peers, due to a higher level of anticipated comfort in addressing their concerns in the campus context. Moreover, some college students may find that the theoretical underpinnings of 12-step groups conflict with personal values or beliefs. For instance, Al-Anon and other peer-led programs typically draw from Judeo-Christian tenets and incorporate theistic language into their meetings. College students who do not identify as religious or spiritual may experience these groups as unsuitable for their needs. Thus, referrals to off-campus community services, particularly 12-step groups, must follow a substantive exploration of students' values and developmental identity.

Additional resources for college students of substance-abusing parents include private practitioners. College counseling centers typically refer to local clinicians who have consistently demonstrated professionalism and competency in their response to referrals from colleges or universities. However, in some communities there may be a paucity of mental health professionals who specialize in issues related to COSAPs. Moreover, accessibility—both in terms of cost and transportation—may be an obstacle to obtaining competent off-campus care. To address these concerns, college counseling centers can build partnerships with local mental health professionals to cultivate low-cost and convenient treatment options, including support groups and on-site consultations.

As an adjunctive approach, virtual communities and internet resources offer innumerable means of psychoeducation and support. From identifying local resources, to detailing the long-term effects of parental substance abuse on personal coping strategies, to moderating listservs or chats that reinforce healthful behaviors and normalize students' experiences, Web resources can address students' needs in an engaging, creative manner. Furthermore, websites and virtual communities are syntonic with college students' increasingly technological means of communicating and socializing. Students may be more inclined to peruse a websites or contribute to a dialogue thread than visit a community group meeting. As an anonymous means of gathering information and interacting with fellow COSAPs, internet resources allow for students with varying degrees of comfort or readiness to engage with this material. However, clinicians should shepherd students toward those sites or virtual communities that are developed through research and expert guidance.[1]

---

[1]In addition to the general Web resources often provided to students, the following are examples of college-specific sites that provide information and psychoeducation about adult children of substance-abusing parents: University of Illinois at Urbana-Champaign: http://www.counselingcenter.illinois.edu/?page_id=144; Binghamton University State University of New York: http://www2.binghamton.edu/smart-choices/but-is-it-a-problem/when-i-was-kid.html; University of California, Los Angeles: http://www.counseling.ucla.edu/library/aca.html; University of Rochester: http://rochester.edu/ucc/help/info/abuse.html

SONS AND DAUGHTERS OF ALCOHOL- AND DRUG-USING
PARENTS SUPPORT GROUP: A CASE STUDY

As noted above, group interventions can provide valued support to COSAPs on campus. The following case example describes the Sons and Daughters group at the New York University Student Health Center's Counseling and Behavioral Health service. In this section, we describe the structure and guidelines for the group; the key themes and topics that routinely emerge in the group; and potential benefits of this group format to student COSAPs.

Sons and Daughters of Alcohol and Substance-Abusing Parents is a support group for undergraduate and graduate students who identify with the eponymic group title. To advertise the group, outreach efforts are made through Residential Education, the Office of Student Activities, and the Health Promotion office. In addition, students are regularly referred by staff clinicians throughout the student health system, and the group is publicized in brochure material and internet content related to student health services. The group is offered each term, with a typical size of six to eight members. Synchronized with the academic calendar, group sessions typically commence within the first month of the term (Fall, Spring, and Summer) and continue, weekly, until the end of the semester. This typically results in a total of ten to twelve group sessions, each an hour in length.

Potential members are screened by the group facilitator—typically a psychology fellow specializing in substance abuse treatment—prior to their participation. Screening affords the group facilitator the opportunity to educate students as to the group's purpose, structure and format as well as evaluate appropriateness of fit. Broad inclusion criteria include the following: (1) identifying as a son or daughter of an alcohol or drug abusing parent; (2) interest in exploring the impact—both acute and chronic—of parental substance use; and (3) the capacity to support other students in their efforts to cope with the effects of an alcohol or other drug abusing parent. Screening clinicians also consider current stability of mood, personality style, and level of functioning when admitting students into the support group.

Beyond comporting with the aforementioned inclusion criteria, group facilitators evaluate the student's level of preparedness for focused exploration of these issues. Students who are severely distressed by parental substance abuse or who have suffered recent traumas associated with their parent's abuse may best be served through individual treatment. Moreover, students with rigid attitudes toward substance abuse or the coping styles of other students may be inappropriate group members. Lastly, group facilitators evaluate the student's availability and level of commitment, as consistent attendance is an essential element of mutual support.

Once formed, the facilitator initiates the first session by reviewing the purpose of the group, as well as the structure and calendar of sessions. Within this prologue, the obligation of confidentiality is reviewed, and students are asked to maintain confidentiality for all information disclosed to the group. Moreover, students are asked to bring external discussions about the group (e.g., between two friends within the group who socialize outside the group) to the subsequent session so as to minimize outer/inner group dynamics.

Utilizing a support group approach, students typically generate the content of each session. While the facilitator may choose to carry over themes from week to week, the Sons and Daughters of Alcohol and Substance-Abusing Parents support group relies significantly on member-generated content. In recent years, content has constellated around the following themes: familial relationships and roles, relational styles, defensive styles, and personal substance use.

Family Relationships and Roles

As might be expected, group discussions often address family dynamics and the students' functioning within the family system. Students often use the group as a chance to grapple with their level of responsibility for the substance-abusing parent, questions regarding setting boundaries/limits with family members, and roles they have developed within their family system.

Many students feel a tremendous sense of responsibility to care for the unwell parent, and experience guilt when they focus on their own responsibilities as students, friends, or employees. The group can serve as a chance for students to discuss this sense of responsibility and manage both its practical and emotional implications. The group's format provides the opportunity to discuss the very painful sense that the substance-using parents will suffer, or even die, if the student is not available for consistent caregiving.

Related to this sense of responsibility, students discuss ways of setting limits with family members, establishing boundaries that may be necessary for the students to succeed in their own pursuits. Students discuss frequency of contact with family, type of contact (phone, in-person, email), and explore options for best managing their relationships within the family. While some students express desire for maximum distance from family members or have had little or no recent contact with the substance-abusing parent, many students discuss the desire for maintaining meaningful contact with family without falling into the role of ultimate responsibility for the substance-abusing parent.

Some of the students in the group read the popular literature on ACOAs and may identify with roles described in these texts. For example, students describe various iterations of the hero, adjuster, placater, and scapegoat roles (Black, 1981). While not exhaustive or prescriptive, these identities frequently capture the developmental experiences of COSAPs.

As the hero, students speak to the early, positive reinforcement they received for academic excellence or exceptional performance in a sport or talent. The hero served to distract and uplift the family, creating what students describe as a positive façade or mask of familial stability and success. As the adjuster, students speak to their chameleon-like capacity—their ability to quickly adapt to an unstable environment and unpredictable outcomes in relationships. They describe the necessary coping strategy they developed early in life to weather both emotional and physical tumult at home. As the placater, students describe a tendency to give unconditionally in relationships, placing others' needs ahead of their own and avoiding conflict at all cost. Students describe developing the placater role as a means of soothing substance-abusing parents and other family members affected by the substance abuse. As the scapegoat, students typically describe a role in which they have assumed responsibility for parental substance abuse, either as a means of interpreting the abuse or due to direct blame from caregivers. Students connect their role as the scapegoat to both the familial and personal need for excusing substance abuse behavior in the home.

Though discussion of these family roles may emerge in the content of group work, it is important to note that students relate to these identities in highly variable ways. It is common for students to embody characteristics of all four identities and report occupying different positions within the family dynamic over time. Through identifying and exploring family roles, group members reportedly experience a normalizing effect. Moreover, after participation in the group, students frequently report that insights gained in the support group foster increased role flexibility within family dynamics.

Relational Styles

Relational styles—characterized by interpersonal skills, roles in relationships with nonfamily members, and corresponding levels of intimacy and trust—are frequently described by students in the Sons and Daughters group as directly resulting from coping strategies and familial roles developed as a reaction to parental substance abuse. Students at times draw unambiguous connections between early developmental experiences within their families to current relational styles. Specifically, students frequently identify the following features of interpersonal relationships: mistrust, tendency toward caregiving, withdrawal/isolation, and porous boundaries.

Characteristics of mistrust are frequently reported, influencing the early development of a bond and continuing through a long-term relationship. Students in the Sons and Daughters group describe feeling suspicious of the intentions of friends or romantic partners, anticipating the "inevitable disappointment" or dejection that historically accompanied their relationships. Moreover, students describe mistrusting friends' or partners' abilities to effectively care for them; instead, students forecast their solitude and self-reliance, preferring to rely on themselves rather than rely on the capricious nature of intimate relationships.

Another salient feature of relationships, described by college students of substance-abusing parents, is a tendency toward caregiving. Having regularly assumed caregiver responsibilities so as to contain the effects of substance abuse in their family, students frequently fulfill similar roles in romantic and platonic relationships. Love, intimacy, and affection are understood through acts of doing for others, often sacrificing personal needs or minimizing feelings so as to attend to the other. Their relationships recapitulate familial dynamics, both attracting and reinforcing roles as caregivers.

In addition, students in the group often describe struggles with social withdrawal and isolation. Within the campus community, students with a history of familial substance abuse often feel uncomfortable relating to their peers around issues of alcohol and drug use—common features of collegiate life and the developmental period students occupy, as noted earlier in this chapter. As a result, students regularly describe feeling "different" or "strange" within the campus environment. Support groups may be the only environment in which these students feel comfortable voicing their reactions to alcohol and substance use on campus without fear of judgment or rejection.

A final feature of relational style typically reported by college students of substance-abusing parents can be roughly described as porous boundaries. This population describes difficulty with establishing and maintaining boundaries in relationships—struggling to set limits, safeguard their emotional needs, and to maintain an individuated identity. Students frequently report "feeling consumed" by a relationship, consciously and unconsciously giving themselves over the other. As children, the students quickly learned to give in to the needs of others as a means of survival. Thus, porous boundaries are ego-syntonic and comport with aforementioned relational styles.

Defensive Styles

Students of the Sons and Daughters of Alcohol and Substance-Abusing support group manifest defensive coping styles similar to those employed by anyone contending with severe and chronic psychosocial stressors. Humor, denial, and avoidance are themes throughout group sessions. In addition, students may employ the defense of "splitting" the substance-abusing parent (viewing the parent as "all good" when sober and "all bad" when intoxicated).

Humor is a regular feature of students' efforts at effectively coping with the effects of parental substance abuse. Personal memories of one's parent—as well as the image constructed by the family system—may constellate around comic episodes involving substances. The substance-abusing parent may be portrayed as the "lovable clown" or the "life of the party" as an individual or systemic reaction-formation to the negative effects of substance abuse.

However, students who regularly rely on humor as a strategy describe negative effects of the defense. For instance, group members report that their comic portrayals of substance-abusing parents often dilute the noxious effects of the abuse and unintentionally collude with stereotypes of "the fun drunk." As a result, students perceive friends, family members, and significant others as confused by the student's negative reactions, due to their assumptions that the student was unharmed by the comical, substance-abusing parent.

Denial and avoidance are common defenses employed by families coping with substance abuse (Vannicelli, 1989). Students often describe feeling pulled to deny or avoid their parent's substance abuse so as to preserve idealized images of a mother or father figure. In these systems, students pretend "not to know what I know" so as to collude with the tacit mechanisms of containment and family functioning. However, students in the group generally seek out treatment as a means of supporting their efforts at confronting parental substance abuse, both in their lives and within their families. Thus, while denial and avoidance may have served historic functions in their relationships with parents and other family members, students in the Sons and Daughters group tend to rely on the space as a consistent opportunity to process their struggles and move forward with a different coping style.

Splitting the substance-abusing parent is frequently reported as a defense mechanism employed throughout childhood. Students often report splitting the substance-abusing parent in two, referring to "drunk mom/sober mom" or "drunk dad/sober dad." For instance, several group members reported calling their substance-abusing parent by their first name when relating to them while intoxicated. These members reserved "mom" or "dad" for sober exchanges. Group members frequently report memories in binary language, with positive experiences associated with moments when their parent was sober juxtaposed with negative experiences when their parent was intoxicated. The dichotomy serves as a means of preserving attachment to a positive parental object while rejecting the qualities associated with the substance abuse.

The group allows for discussion of ways in which these defensive styles may have been necessary and adaptive for the students. And, when these defenses are no longer serving them well, students have the opportunity to discuss new and more productive ways of coping.

Personal Substance Use

A final, common theme of the Sons and Daughters of Alcohol and Substance-Abusing Parents support group is group members' struggles with substance use in their lives. Due to a lack of role-modeling with moderation, students frequently report "struggles with the extremes." At one end of the spectrum, students report strong aversion to and even repulsion by alcohol or drug use—to the extent that the smell, sight, or suggestion of the substances evokes strong reactions. At the other end of the spectrum, students report previous and current substance abuse, resulting in deleterious financial, relational, and health effects.

Students who report abstinence and strong aversion to alcohol or drug use often describe accompanying negative mood states, such as fear and anger. These students state that the "mere sight or smell" of a substance induces both emotional and physiologic responses that include nausea, anxiety, or sadness. To cope with such reactions, students typically avoid substance-using contexts and peers—often resulting in the aforementioned experiences of social withdrawal and isolation. Many students report losing or severely straining relationships on campus due to their abstinence and aversion to substances.

Students who report personal struggles with substance abuse often describe feeling "destined to drink"—portraying their substance use as a direct consequence of their parent's substance use. Whether the attribution is made to a genetic predisposition or learned behavior, students understand their substance abuse as following a direct line of cause and effect. Others report a more subtle understanding of their substance abuse, interpreting their behavior as a manifestation of poor coping strategies—pointing out that their substance abuse is akin to other, unhealthy means of self-soothing, such as bingeing and purging.

Students often struggle with disclosing personal substance abuse within the group context for numerous reasons. First, these students may fear negative reactions of abstinent group members. Second, substance-abusing students worry that their substance use is merely another iteration of the group's raison d'etre, evoking feelings of guilt and shame. Finally, substance-abusing students may feel the need to compartmentalize their struggles with substances, preferring to focus on their identities as collateral damage of parental substance abuse rather than active users.

Between these extremes of strong aversion and substance abuse is an alternate identity within the group: moderate substance user. Most students describe persistent struggles to moderate their substance use, relating strongly to the sense of "all or nothing." Themes of immoderation carry over from week to week, applying to a range of topics that extend beyond substances. Students regularly explore their relationship with substances so as to craft a more moderate approach, often with the hope that this moderation will translate into effective moderation in other areas. Thus, the group serves as an opportunity for all students—abstinent or abusing—to develop awareness and new skills of moderation.

Reported Benefits of the Group

Student reports multiple benefits from participation in the Sons and Daughters group. Perhaps the most frequently voiced benefit is the normalization effect. Students commonly report feeling comforted by the knowledge that others are struggling with similar familial histories and can readily relate to their experiences. This sense of shared identity can be particularly powerful for those who have long felt isolated or unsupported in their efforts at coping. Moreover, for college students navigating an environment of substance use and increasingly complex interpersonal relationships, the echo effect of this shared identity can be very reassuring.

Another common benefit described by the majority of students attending the support group is the opportunity to learn from others and develop new means of coping. Students regularly utilize group sessions as an occasion to present an acute or chronic challenge to the group and solicit feedback. Students commonly report "carrying the voices of group members" into the familial context and incorporating the experiences of others into their coping styles.

Last, group members often describe benefiting from the nurturance of fellow members and relying on this emotional support as a safeguard against the struggles they face. For many students, the Sons and Daughters support group is a rare experience of understanding and encouragement within a broader landscape of self-sufficiency and tumult. Group members react to one another in remarkably intuitive, gentle ways that allow for vulnerability rarely experienced in their daily lives. These group members often characterize the group as an hour of solace that they would typically not seek out or allow for, given their propensity toward attending to others' needs or maintaining a capable façade.

CONCLUSION

Although the large number of COSAPs on college campuses represent a heterogeneous population rather than a unique collective with narrowly defined needs, as a whole this is a group at increased risk for substance use disorders and for psychosocial difficulties. Thus, college campuses are well served by providing ready access to supports for students with these concerns. University and college campuses can serve this population through outreach, psychoeducation, and through direct clinical services. As noted above, the group format may be a particularly potent form of treatment for students who have long felt isolated in their efforts to cope with substance-abusing parents. Overall, interventions with COSAPs at colleges can be based on the existing literature on this topic with a flexible clinical approach guided by the unique needs of each college student who presents with concerns about a substance-abusing parent.

REFERENCES

Black, C. (1981). *It will never happen to me*. New York: Random House.

Fewell, C. H. (2006). *Attachment, reflective function, family dysfunction, and psychological distress among college students with alcoholic parents*. Unpublished doctoral dissertation, New York University.

Fischer, K. E., Kittleson, M., Ogletree, R., Welshimer, K., Woehkle, P., & Benshoff, J. (2000). The relationship of parental alcoholism and family dysfunction to stress among college students. *Journal of American College Health, 48*, 151–156.

Gelertner, J., & Kranzler, H. R. (2008). Genetic of addiction. In M. Galanter & H. D. Kleber (Eds.), *Textbook of substance abuse treatment* (pp. 17–28). Washington, DC: American Psychiatric Publishing.

Grant, B. F. (2000). Estimates of U.S. children exposed to alcohol abuse and dependence in the family. *American Journal of Public Health, 90*(1), 112–115.

Harter, S. L. (2000). Psychosocial adjustment of adult children of alcoholics: A review of the recent empirical literature. *Clinical Psychology Review, 20*(3), 311–337.

Hingson, R., Heeren, T., Winter, M., & Wechsler, H. (2005). Magnitude of alcohol-related mortality and morbidity among U.S. college students ages 18–24: Changes from 1998 to 2001. *Annual Review of Public Health, 26*, 259–279.

Huang, B., Dawson, D. A., Stinson, F. S., Hasin, D. S., Ruan, W. J., Saha, T. D., et al. (2006). Prevalence, correlates, and comorbidity of nonmedication prescription drug use disorders in the United States: Results of the National

Epidemiological Survey on Alcohol and Related Conditions. *Journal of Clinical Psychiatry, 67*, 1062–1073.

Johnston, L. D., O'Malley, P. M., Bachman, J. G., & Schulenberg, J. E. (2006). *Monitoring the future: National survey results on Drug Use, 1975–2005: Volume II: College students and adults ages 19–45* (NIH Publication No. 06–5584). Bethesda, MD: National Institute on Drug Abuse.

Johnston, L. D., O'Malley, P. M., Bachman, J. G., & Schulenberg, J. E. (2008). *Monitoring the future: National survey results on Drug Use, 1975–2007. Volume I: Secondary school students* (NIH Publication No. 08–6418A). Bethesda, MD: National Institute on Drug Abuse.

Kadison, R. D. (2004). The mental-health crisis: What colleges must do. *The Chronicle of Higher Education, 51*(16), B. 20.

Kessler, J. C., & Merikangas, K. R. (2004). The National Comorbidity Survey Replication: Background and aims. *International Journal of Methods in Psychiatric Research, 13*(2), 60–68.

Landers, D., & Hollingdale, L. (1989). Working with children of alcoholics on a college campus: A rationale and strategies for success. *Journal of College Student Psychotherapy, 2*, 3–4, 205–222.

McMillen, L. (1986). Colleges finding 'wellness programs cut absenteeism, boost productivity and morale of their staff members. *The Chronicle of Higher Education, 31*(23), 20.

Mohler-Kuo, M., Lee, J. E., & Wechsler, H. (2003). Trends in marijuana and other illicit drug use among college students: Results from four Harvard School of Public Health college alcohol study surveys (1993–2001). *Journal of American College Health, 52*, 17–24.

Mothershead, P. K., Kivlingham, D. M., & Wynkoop, T. F. (1998). Attachment, family dysfunction, parental alcoholism, and interpersonal distress in late adolescence: A structural model. *Journal of Counseling Psychology, 45*, 196–203.

National Center on Addiction and Substance Abuse (CASA) at Columbia University. (2007). *Wasting the best and the brightest: Substance abuse at America's colleges and universities.* New York: CASA at Columbia University.

Rodney, H. E. (1996). Inconsistencies in the literature on collegiate adult children of alcoholics; factors to consider for African Americans. *Journal of American College Health, 45*, 19–25.

Ross, S. (2008). The mentally ill substance use. In M. Galanter & H. D. Kleber (Eds.), *Textbook of substance abuse treatment* (pp. 537–554). Washington, DC: American Psychiatric Publishing.

Sher, K. J., Walitzer, K. S., Wood, P. K., & Brent, E. E. (1991). Characteristics of children of alcoholics: Putative risk factors, substance use and abuse, and psychopathology. *Journal of Abnormal Psychology, 100*, 427–448.

Spencer-Thomas, S. (2009). Top 10 strategies for bolstering students' mental resilience. *The Chronicle of Higher Education, 55*(36), A. 26.

Substance Abuse and Mental Health Services Administration. (2006). *2004 National survey on drug use and health: Detailed tables.* Retrieved May 15, 2009, from http://www.oas.samhsa.gov/nsduh/2k4nsduh/2k4tabs/LOTSect5pe.htm

Tsuang, M. T., Lyons, M. J., Meyer, J. M., Doyle, T., Eisen, S. A., Goldberg, J., et al. (1998). Co-occurrence of abuse of different drugs in men: The role of drug-specific and shared vulnerabilities. *Archives of General Psychiatry, 55*, 967–972.

U.S. Census Bureau. (2009). *Facts for features: Back to school: 2009–2010.* Retrieved September 30, 2009, from http://www.census.gov/Press-Release/www/releases/archives/facts_for_features_special_editions/013847.html

Vannicelli, M. (1989). *Group psychotherapy with adult children of alcoholics: Treatment techniques and countertransference considerations.* New York: Guilford Press.

Woititz, J. G. (1983). *Adult children of alcoholics.* Orlando, FL: Health Communications.

12

Programs for Children of Parents Incarcerated for Substance-Related Problems

Audrey L. Begun and Susan J. Rose

INTRODUCTION

Children whose parents abuse substances are subject to many challenges, as explored throughout this book and elsewhere (e.g., Ackerman, 2000; Levy & Rutter, 1992; Straussner & Fewell, 2006). It is assumed by professionals that the increased vulnerability and risk factors these children experience result in an increased probability of developing substance use disorders themselves in the future. In addition, children of substance-abusing parents are exposed to many concomitant and co-occurring challenges that affect their behavioral, learning, social, physical, and mental health outcomes. Because parental substance abuse often results in contact with federal, state, or local criminal justice systems, their children incur additional risks and vulnerabilities during periods of parental incarceration in jails and prisons, as well as during community reentry.

This chapter concerns the population of children who experience a parent's incarceration for offenses related to alcohol and other substances. Following a brief definition of terms, the chapter includes discussions of (1) the population of parents incarcerated for substance-related offenses; (2) how children's caretaking needs are met while parents are incarcerated; (3) how parental incarceration might affect other aspects of child well-being; and (4) practice implications.

DEFINITION OF TERMS

For purposes of this review, the term "substances" designates alcohol and any other drugs that may be secured or used illegally by adults, including illicit or "street" drugs and illegally used or acquired prescription drugs. "Incarceration" refers to several distinct forms of criminal justice system supervision, including jail detention following an arrest but prior to sentencing, a jail term to serve a sentence, serving a prison sentence, and assignment to a residential or transitional setting to complete terms of a sentence.

The primary differences between prisons and jails are jurisdiction, length of stay, prisoner status, and location. Jails are most often administered by local sheriffs or county governments, whereas prisons are operated either by federal or state government entities, although some are private facilities with state or federal contracts. Individuals detained in jails either are awaiting trial and sentencing, or are serving a jail sentence. People leave jail under several conditions: They may be able to finish awaiting trial and sentencing while residing in the community, they may have finished serving a jail sentence, or they may be moved to prison to satisfy their sentencing requirements. People in prison are serving a sentence: Prison sentences are typically longer than jail sentences and typically involve more serious offenses. Finally, jails are usually more locally situated and more easily accessible to family members than most prisons which are regionally located and often situated further away from large population centers. Following their time spent in jail or prison, individuals may or may not continue living under specific supervision requirements as they transition back to life in the community, including assignment to transitional residential settings, home detention, electronic monitoring, work release programs, day reporting, weekender programs, community service, mandated treatment programs, and other options involving varying degrees of restraint and supervision (Minton & Sabol, 2009).

The types of substance-related offenses for which a parent might be arrested and incarcerated vary by state and municipality, but generally include offenses which are (1) directly related to substance possession, use, production, and distribution; (2) crimes committed to obtain drugs; (3) illegal activities that occur while under the influence of alcohol or other drugs; and (4) child maltreatment or endangerment due to substance use, including use of substances during pregnancy, neglect of a child during periods of substance use, and failure to protect a child from accidental ingestion or poisoning by substances (Brendel & Soulier, 2009).

The primary focus of this chapter is parents of children under the age of 18 years. Throughout this chapter, "parents" refers to both mothers and fathers; however, the emphasis is on incarcerated mothers. Though the overwhelming majority of prisoners in the United States are men, and most parents in prison (92%) are fathers (Glaze & Maruschak, 2008), an emphasis on incarcerated mothers recognizes that (1) mothers are more likely to have been their children's primary caregiver prior to incarceration; (2) women have disproportionately higher rates of incarceration for substance-related offenses; (3) incarcerated women have disproportionately higher rates of substance abuse and dependency problems; (4) incarcerated women have disproportionately lower access to treatment services for addressing substance abuse and other mental health challenges; and (5) a mother's incarceration is likely to have a greater disruptive potential for a child (Begun, Rose, LeBel, & Teske-Young, 2009; Parke & Clarke-Stewart, 2002).

INCARCERATED PARENTS

On June 30, 2008, over 2.1 million individuals were being held in state or federal prisons and local jails (West & Sabol, 2009). Local jails admitted about 13 million persons during the 12 months prior to that mid-year measurement, and prisons admitted approximately three-quarters of a million more (Sabol & Minton, 2008; Sabol, Minton, & Harrison, 2007). Well over half of prison inmates at mid-year 2007 were parents of children under the age of 18 years (Glaze & Maruschak, 2008).

Jails Versus Prisons

The impact on families and children of a parent's incarceration in a local jail *versus* a state or federal prison can be significant, especially as it relates to visitation and maintaining a relationship. Jail stays are typically measured in hours, days, weeks, and months, whereas prison terms are measured in months and years. Jails are typically found in the community, whereas state and federal prisons are typically centralized institutions, making them more geographically difficult for family members to visit. Specialized prison facilities for women tend to be even more geographically centralized, concentrating the comparatively smaller population of women prisoners (Belknap, 2003).

In some communities, however, "local" jail facilities may be equally inaccessible for visitation by family members. Individual family resources, such as having or lacking independent, reliable means of transportation may render visitation virtually impossible. Institutional demands, such as minimal facility and personnel resources, as well as security concerns and administrative policies may also act as barriers precluding parent–child visits that are sufficiently frequent, of sufficient duration, and/or of the "contact" types that promote positive family relationships and are most beneficial to the children. Social work professionals working with prisoners and in criminal justice environments often face unique challenges in the clash of their intervention goals with those of the institution, creating a potentially "hostile environment" for practice (Mazza, 2006). The goal of fostering ongoing contact between incarcerated parents and their children can lie in conflict with security goals. For example, in the Milwaukee metropolitan area, neither the centrally located short-term criminal justice facility nor the longer-term jail permits children under the age of 18 years to visit their incarcerated parents (www.county.milwaukee.gov/VisitingInformation.htm).

Parents as Prison Inmates

The U.S. Department of Justice, through the Bureau of Justice Statistics, routinely collects and reports a wide range of criminal justice system data. Glaze and Marushcak (2008) provided the most current statistical information available regarding the status of parents in prison and their minor children. They reported that on a single day at mid-year 2007, an estimated 809,800 of prison inmates were parents to over 1.7 million minor children. The number of children with parents in prison has increased every year since such data were first reported in 1991, and the numbers have grown disproportionately for mothers versus fathers: the number of children with mothers in prison has increased by 131% compared to a 77% increase of children with fathers in prison. Compared to White children, Black and Hispanic children were 7.5 and 2.5 times more likely, respectively, to have a parent in state or federal prisons (Glaze & Maruschak, 2008).

Prison inmates are more likely than not to be parents of multiple children: During 2004, just under a quarter reported having only one child, 39% of federal and 29% of state prison inmates had more than one child, with an average of two children each, and the remainder did not have children (Glaze & Maruschak, 2008). Considerable numbers of these children are relatively young in age. Among the children of state and federal prisoners, 22% and 16%, respectively, were aged 4 years or less; 30% and 34%, respectively, were aged 5–9 years; 32% and 35%, respectively, were aged 10–14 years; and 16% and 15%, respectively, were between 15 and 17 years of age. The ages of children of women in prison was skewed slightly higher than for men, with 53% compared to 47% in the 10–17 age range (Glaze & Maruschak, 2008).

A considerable majority of prisoners incarcerated in state (62%) and federal (70%) prisons for repeated drug offenses were parents, and drug offenders in prison were more likely to be parents than not: 59% in state prisons were fathers and 63% were mothers; 69% in federal prison were fathers and 55% were mothers (Glaze & Maruschak, 2008). Regardless of the offenses for which these parents were serving prison sentences, over 67% in state prisons and 56% in federal prisons met clinical criteria (Diagnostic and Statistical Manual of Mental Disorders, 4th ed.) for substance abuse or dependence (Mumola & Karberg, 2006).

Parents in Jails: One Study

It is unclear how many of the 785,556 adults incarcerated in the nation's local jails at mid-year 2008 were parents, or how many of the more than 12 million admitted annually have minor children (Minton & Sabol, 2009; Stojkovic, 2005). Data from one community provide a general picture, but must be carefully interpreted as the samples were neither uniformly nor randomly generated. These data are derived from an intervention study entitled *Supporting Jails in Providing Women with Substance Abuse Services*, primarily designed to deliver treatment preparation in-reach services to jailed women with substance-related problems (Begun, Rose, LeBel, & Teske-Young, 2009; Begun, Rose, & LeBel, in press).

Among the 1,199 women participants from two jail facilities (the Criminal Justice Facility for women at the presentencing stage, and the House of Correction for women serving sentences), 80% were mothers who reported having anywhere up to 11 minor children, with the mean number of minor children falling between two and three. The children of these women ranged in age from infants to 41 years, with a mean child's age of 12 years. The majority of mothers (52%) reported their oldest child as being under the age of 18 years. Among the subset of 628 mothers with minor children, the mean of their children's ages was 9 years and the median age of their firstborn children fell between 8 and 9 years of age. At least 79% of mothers participating in this jail study had at least one minor child living with them during the year prior to incarceration, and over 60% had two or more children with whom they had been living.

Incarcerated Parents and Their Substance Problems

Clear evidence links substance use problems and criminal activity among individuals in jails and those released back into the community. In 2002, among the nation's state prisoners, 19.2% of men and 30.8% of women were incarcerated for drug-related offenses, and 24% of all jail inmates were incarcerated for drug offenses (Glaze & Maruschak, 2008; Harrison & Beck, 2003). At the time they committed the offenses for which they were incarcerated, 40% of women and 32% of men in prison reported being under the influence of alcohol or other substances; half of all jail inmates during 2002 reported being under the influence of alcohol while committing their offenses (Greenfield & Snell, 1999; Harrison & Beck, 2003). Among individuals jailed for property and drug offenses, 25% reported committing offenses to get money for drugs (Karberg & James, 2005).

High rates of clinically significant substance abuse or dependence have been reported among jailed inmates convicted of burglary (85%), driving while intoxicated (81%), weapons violations (79%), and drug possession (75%) (Karberg & James, 2005). Anywhere from 10% to 60% of women in prisons are substance dependent, compared to about 6% of women in the general population (Fazel, Bains, & Doll, 2006; Substance Abuse and Mental Health Services Administration [SAMHSA], 2007).

Among the women who volunteered to participate in brief screening for alcohol and other drug problems through the *Supporting Jails in Providing Women with Substance Abuse Services* intervention project, 66% scored "positive" on the AUDIT-ID measure (also called the AUDIT-12; Maggia et al., 2004). More significantly, more than half of the women who scored positive reported very high risk scores, indicating greater dependence and harm from their substance use. These scores were consistent with their later scores on the TCU Drug Screen (Knight, Simpson, & Hiller, 2002; Peters, Strozier, Murrin, & Kearns, 1997). Such high scores suggest that the severity of drug use by many of these women resulted in their experiencing significant difficulties in fulfilling their roles as parents, and their children likely suffered on an ongoing basis from these parenting difficulties.

Substance Abuse Services in Jails and Prisons

It is generally understood that a child's well-being is closely tied to the parents' functioning, and often the best way to help children is to help their parents first. Parents who leave jail or prison settings with untreated substance use disorders, compared to those who are successfully treated during incarceration, are more likely to experience health, behavioral, and continued or relapsed substance abuse problems at community reentry (Aos, Miller, & Drake, 2006; Inciardi, Martin, & Butzin, 2004; Prendergast, Farabee, & Cartier, 2004; Springer, McNeece, & Arnold, 2003). Unfortunately, significant discrepancies exist between the numbers of incarcerated individuals who need substance abuse–related services *versus* those actually receiving such services. Despite the high incidence and prevalence rates of substance abuse and dependence among prison and jail inmates, only 15–17% of them receive substance abuse treatment while incarcerated (SAMHSA, 2000).

Few criminal justice facilities offer any type of drug and alcohol treatment services. If offered at all to incarcerated individuals, such programs are more commonly offered at state or federal prison facilities than in jails, particularly for incarcerated women (Hill, 2004; Messina & Prendergast, 2004). However, the use of these types of programs at state and federal institutions is not high either (SAMHSA, 2000). Among state prisoners who used drugs in the month before their offense, only 39% reported taking part in drug treatment or other drug programs since admission (Mumola & Karberg, 2006). Moreover, the percentage of recent drug users taking part in substance abuse treatment programs with a trained professional was reported by only 15% of state prisoners, although 34% of state prisoners reported taking part in self-help groups, peer counseling, and drug abuse education/awareness programs. Essentially, most drug treatment services (such as therapeutic communities) including those focused on developing skills to manage drug use, are less likely to be provided (Belenko & Peugh, 2005; Mumola & Karberg, 2006; Taxman & Cropsey, 2007).

A number of recent research studies have identified the critical elements of substance abuse treatment needed for effective intervention with criminal justice populations. For example, retention in treatment has been positively associated with an individual's motivation to change and elements of an individual's motivation to change have been positively associated with the strength of the therapeutic alliance that is established (Brocato & Wagner, 2008). These results suggest that the establishment of a positive working relationship between the inmate and practitioner and the practitioner's skill at helping increase and maintain motivation to change are more important than the specific components of intervention protocols.

Due to the high prevalence of substance use dependence and abuse among prisoners, available alcohol and other drug treatment services are not sufficient or appropriately designed to address the needs of this population (Belenko & Peugh, 2005; Mumola & Karberg, 2006). The sheer number of individuals in need of substance abuse treatment services, coupled with under-resourced budgets for health and human services, hamper the ability of jail administrators to deal with these needs, particularly among women inmates (Begun et al., in press; Golder et al., 2005; Stojkovic, 2005). Furthermore, though the duration of prison terms may be sufficient for meaningful and effective intervention, the comparatively brief duration of jail incarceration limits the number and nature of intervention goals that might reasonably be achieved (Begun et al., in press; Solomon, Osborne, LoBuglio, Mellow, & Mukamal, 2008).

Offenders released with untreated substance problems are more likely to continue use or relapse to substance abuse after their release, as well as to participate in criminal behaviors that contribute to recidivism

(Begun et al., in press). Many incarcerated parents have long histories of substance abuse—averaging 13 years or more (Smith, Krisman, Strozier, & Marley, 2004). As a result, they may require collateral interventions that help retrain many social, economic self-sufficiency, parenting, cognitive, and other behavioral functions (Smith et al., 2004).

Inmates who engage in effective substance abuse treatment during incarceration evidence lower rates of behavioral problems and disciplinary actions while incarcerated and higher levels of successful discharge from parole without negative impact on public safety (Messina & Prendergast, 2004; Springer et al., 2003; Taxman, Byrne, & Young, 2002; Weinman, Dignam, & Wheat, 2004). Furthermore, inmates who seek treatment soon after release are also more likely to engage and remain in treatment longer than nontreatment seekers at reentry (Worcel, Furrer, Green, Burrus, & Finigan, 2008). Women who receive treatment for their substance abuse and who utilize other social services during community reentry following jail stays are significantly less likely to be rearrested during the year following release than are women not provided with these types of postrelease services (Freudenberg, Wilets, Greene, & Richie, 1998). Reduced recidivism would presumably be positive for their children, allowing for more stable home lives, with fewer disruptions in where they will live and go to school.

Although evidence supports the desirability of participating in appropriate substance abuse treatment closely following incarceration, accessibility, eligibility, availability, and financial resources all can interfere with efforts to develop continuity of care initiated during incarceration (Bhati, Roman, & Chalfin, 2008). In the *Supporting Jails in Providing Women with Substance Abuse Services* project, women identified barriers to treatment at reentry using the Allen Barriers to Treatment Inventory (ABTI; Allen, 1994). The most strongly endorsed barriers included inability to pay for services and lack of health insurance for treatment; no program openings/wait lists; no transportation to programs; and not knowing where services were available. These barriers were more commonly endorsed than were the items suggesting that they did not want to quit using substances (Begun et al., in press).

In short, the type, intensity, and duration of alcohol and other drug treatment intervention currently delivered to incarcerated parents or those recently released from jails and prisons are seldom adequate for achieving the goals necessary for successful parenting or regaining custody of children in the child welfare system (Begun et al., in press; Golder et al., 2005; Krebs, Brady, & Laird, 2003). Many substance abuse treatment services offered to prison inmates have empirical support for positive outcomes when they are made available and delivered with good fidelity (National Institute on Drug Abuse [NIDA], 2006). Substance abuse treatment effectiveness studies are beginning to identify the elements of intervention that are most critical to positive outcomes with populations of individuals who are incarcerated and abuse substances. These elements include positive parenting, anger management, providing treatment for co-occurring psychiatric disorders, and posttraumatic stress symptoms in conjunction with treatment to address alcohol and other drug problems (Ford, Moffitt, Steinberg, & Zhang, 2008; Kerridge, 2009).

Although prison settings may be more likely to dedicate a portion of budget, staff, and space resources to human service, health, and substance abuse treatment services, jails may better serve these parents by delivering interventions designed to prepare individuals for treatment at community reentry (Begun, Rose, LeBel, & Teske-Young, 2009; Windell & Barron, 2002). Treatment preparation is a viable form of intervention with individuals preparing for community reentry, particularly when accompanied by efforts to coordinate the systems with which the individuals will be interacting (Windell & Barron, 2002). All too often, however, former inmates lack access to the services needed for maintaining their recovery gains achieved during incarceration. About 24–28% of adults on parole or other supervised release from prison became or remained active users of illicit drugs, a rate considerably higher than the 7–8% rate among adults in the general population (SAMHSA, 2007).

ADDRESSING NEEDS OF CHILDREN WITH INCARCERATED PARENTS

Children of incarcerated parents can experience a wide array of developmental challenges and negative outcomes that may differ across the periods of initial arrest, incarceration, and reentry to community life (Brazzell, 2008; Dallaire, 2006; Myers, Smarch, Amlund-Hagen, & Kennon, 1999; Parke & Clarke-Stewart, 2002). Observed mid- and long-term effects include but are not limited to child antisocial behavior; child offending; poor school performance, truancy, and school phobias; social withdrawal and poor social skills; depression, trauma, anxiety, guilt, shame, and fearfulness; sleep disturbances; attention deficits; low self-esteem; and misuse of drugs and alcohol (Murray & Farrington, 2008; Nesmith, 2008; Snyder, Carlo, & Mullins, 2001). The mechanisms through which parental incarceration contributes to these negative outcomes are not fully understood; however, likely candidates include separation trauma, exposure to environmental risks and social disadvantages resulting from parental incarceration and absences, strain expressed by substitute caregivers, and family stigma associated with the parents' offenses and incarceration histories (Murray & Farrington, 2008). In addition, the children of incarcerated women often experience repetitive cycles of parental incarcerations and relapsing substance problems which have been associated with greater risks for adjustment problems (Moos, Finney, & Cronkite, 1990).

Very young children of incarcerated mothers bear an especially difficult burden. Infants born to incarcerated mothers face lifelong emotional development risks as maternal separation can interfere with attachment relationships and can result in other adverse cognitive and emotional developmental delays. These children are more vulnerable than average to developmental delays and later substance abuse or involvement in the criminal justice system (Rebecca Project for Human Rights, 2006; U.S. Department of Justice [USDOJ], 2000).

Children who enter substitute care while their mothers are incarcerated may never return or achieve a permanent home. Community jails do not have the resources to coordinate the care needed to keep family bonds intact and provide case management alongside child welfare authorities. Furthermore, jails and prisons do not routinely provide services for addressing women's problems with alcohol and other drugs during incarceration and in the process of community reentry. The result is women who have limited personal and financial resources to address their substance use after release, children who languish in substitute care, and the likelihood that these children will encounter difficulties with social institutions (i.e., with schools and criminal justice systems) and substances themselves (Gabel, 1992; Johnston, 1995).

Pregnant Mothers and Substance-Related Incarceration

Significant inconsistencies exist across states in their criminal prosecution of women who abuse substances while pregnant (Brendel & Soulier, 2009). Some state laws leading to prosecution may specify harm to a fetus or child resulting from consumption or use of alcohol and other drugs, whereas others are based on generic child abuse and criminal endangerment criminal laws (Alcohol Policy Information System [APIS], 2008). In addition to civil commitment or loss of custody following birth, criminal prosecutions of women who used substances during pregnancy have included such charges as child endangerment, illegal drug delivery to a minor, and manslaughter, although the number of convictions and decisions upheld in higher courts are relatively small nationally (Brendel & Soulier, 2009).

States may or may not mandate treatment for the mother with an identified substance use disorder (APIS, 2008). An unfortunate consequence of women's awareness concerning the possibility of commitment or incarceration for using substances during pregnancy is that some of the very women most in need of good prenatal care for themselves and their babies avoid seeking it for fear that screening and early detection efforts may lead to legal consequences, loss of custody of the baby and/or other children they may already have, civil commitment, or incarceration difficulties (Brendel & Soulier, 2009).

Regardless of the reason for incarceration, the birth outcomes associated with incarceration during pregnancy are not consistent across populations of women defined by race and ethnicity (Howard, Strobino, Sherman, & Crum, 2009). For example, in Texas prisons, White women are more likely to have positive outcomes (greater gestational age and birth weight at delivery) associated with incarceration early during pregnancy than Black or Hispanic women. This finding is partially explained by White women being more likely to have a positive history for preincarceration use of tobacco, alcohol, and other drugs for which the prison setting may present a more "protective" environment, including prenatal care, than existed in the communities from which this women were incarcerated (Howard, Strobino, Sherman, & Crum, 2009).

Some institutions have experimented with allowing mothers and their infants or very young children to remain together during a portion of the incarceration period (Parke & Clarke-Stewart, 2002). Prison nurseries are designed to permit mothers who deliver infants while in custody to remain with the infant for at least the first year of life. Parenting programs may or may not be offered to these mothers, as well (Parke & Clarke-Stewart, 2002). Although "codetention" has measurable benefits for parent–infant bonding and mothers' behavior while incarcerated, there are significant concerns related to the infants' development considering the relative impoverishment found in prison environments that have not been intentionally enriched to meet these special needs (Parke & Clarke-Stewart, 2002). Intensive intervention has tentatively demonstrated effectiveness in improving mother–infant relationships and child development outcomes among substance-abusing mothers whose infants are born during incarceration and who attempt reunification at community reentry (Kubiak, Young, Siefert, & Stewart, 2004).

Caring for the Children of Incarcerated Parents

Among the issues facing incarcerated parents are how their children's caretaking needs will be met; if, when, and how visitation will occur; and, whether or not their parental rights are at risk of being permanently terminated (Lewis, 2004). Who meets and how well a child's caretaking needs are met represent key factors in a child's adjustment to having a parent incarcerated (Parke & Clarke-Stewart, 2002). A single mother's parental rights may be court-terminated for failure to pass drug testing throughout a predetermined period, such as 18 months, and there are historical and between-state inconsistencies as to whether the period of incarceration has been included or excluded in their permanency planning timelines (Tebo, 2006; Zimmerman, 2005).

Parental Caretaking Disrupted by Incarceration

During the month prior to arrest or to incarceration, 48% and 56% of parents in state and federal prisons, respectively, had lived with at least one of their children; this represents a total of more than 351,270 parents (Glaze & Maruschak, 2008) and well over 2 million minor children (Tebo, 2006). Mothers were particularly likely to have been living with one or more children prior to arrest or incarceration: 64% of mothers in state prisons compared to 46.5% of the fathers, and 81% of mothers in federal prisons compared to 55% of the fathers (Glaze & Maruschak, 2008). Just prior to incarceration, the majority of the daily care was provided to minor children by inmate mothers (77% and 83% for state and federal prisoners), inmate fathers (26% and 31% for state and federal prisoners), or the inmate sharing care with someone else (18% and 14%, respectively, for state and federal prison mothers; 63% and 59%, respectively, for fathers). In only about 10% of families were the children's daily care needs being primarily met by someone else.

Family cohesion and parental monitoring are recognized protective factors in the prevention of substance abuse by adolescents and young adults, and can attenuate other vulnerability and risk factors such as exposure to community violence (Kliewer et al., 2006; Robertson, Baird-Thomas, & Stein, 2008). Parents who are incarcerated have a diminished ability to protect their children through active monitoring, and concern about the well-being and whereabouts of their minor children is often the "most stressful" aspect of a mother's incarceration (Belknap, 2003).

Who Provides Substitute Care

During the month before arrest, 42% of the mothers in state prison and 52% of mothers in federal prisons reported living in a single parent headed household; this was less true for fathers where about 19% lived in a single parent headed household before arrest. While parents were in state prison, mothers most commonly reported that their children were being cared for by grandparents (45%), followed by the other parent (37%), other relatives (23%), foster care systems (11%), or friends/others (8%), although mothers with multiple children may have had multiple childcare arrangements (Glaze & Maruschak, 2008). Fathers most often relied on the children's mothers to provide care (88%), otherwise they relied on the children's grandparents (12.5%), other relatives (5%), foster placement (2%), or friends/others (2%). Women often attempt to avoid formal placement of their minor children during a period of incarceration for fear of permanently losing custody (Mumola, 2000). In one study of incarcerated parents with addiction problems, the maternal grandmothers were most likely to be identified as the preferred caregiver for raising the children (Smith, Krisman, Strozier, & Marley, 2004).

In some cases when a parent is incarcerated, the relationship between the child's parents often becomes strained and the incarcerated parent has serious concerns related to the child being brought for visits and to the child's welfare while in the other parent's care (Lewis, 2004). In other cases, all adults in a household may be arrested and incarcerated for drug-related activities, resulting in significantly changed and more complicated arrangements for meeting the caretaking needs of minor children (Tebo, 2006). Separations between children and mothers are often the result of substance abuse rather than incarceration which may occur subsequently to the separation (Moses, 2009; Phillips, Burns, Wagner, & Barth, 2004). Whether or not children will be reunited with their mothers following incarceration depends upon factors such as the length of her sentence, nature of her offenses, her participation and progress in rehabilitation programs, the ages of the children, the quality and strength of mother–child relationships, and attitudes held by caseworkers and foster parents toward the mother (Smith, 2002). Maintaining or regaining custody of children has been identified as a motivation for seeking substance abuse treatment by 44% of women with children under the age of 18 who participated in a 5-year National Treatment Improvement Evaluation Study (NTIES) concerning the impact of drug and alcohol treatment in the United States (Substance Abuse and Mental Health Data Archive [SAMHDA], 1997). However, in many cases parents face barriers to reunification resulting from the "multiple clocks" phenomenon by which the different systems with which they are engaged (e.g., child welfare, substance treatment, child development, housing, and income maintenance) endorse incompatible timelines related to required behavior changes (see Sun, 2009, p. 397).

PRACTICE IMPLICATIONS

Meeting the Parental Contact Needs of Children During Parental Incarceration

Maintaining connections between incarcerated parents and their children can facilitate children's coping and improve the chances for successful family reunification following the parents' release (Parke & Clarke-Stewart, 2002;

Zimmerman, 2005). A child's "best interests" are most often served by maintaining contact with an incarcerated parent, as well as through accurate information concerning the parent's whereabouts and time to release (Tebo, 2006). Contact between parents in state prison and their children most commonly occurs in the form of letters (70%), by telephone (53%), or personal visits (42%), and more than three-quarters of parents have had some form of contact with their children since prison admission (Glaze & Maruschak, 2008). Weekly contact is difficult to achieve, and only occurs with 56% of incarcerated mothers and 39% of incarcerated fathers; as many as 54% of parents never see any of their children during incarceration, although infrequent contact occurs through phone, mail, or visitation with mothers (60%) more than fathers (40%) (Hairston & Rollin, 2006).

Because parent–child visitations are recognized as correlates of successful reunification upon release (Sharp, 2003), prison settings have experimented with a variety of child- and family-friendly visitation options, designed with the goal of minimizing negative developmental outcomes in the children of incarcerated mothers and fathers (Tebo, 2006). These experiments have included full physical contact visitations (versus no contact visits), family visiting areas with facilities and parent–child interactive materials, overnight visitation, cohabitation during infancy, and greater flexibility in visitation schedules (Tebo, 2006). In addition, some programs have emphasized parent education programs in preparation for reunification, as well as health education that includes the use of contraception for family planning and HIV risk reduction (regardless of substance abuse history) and the effects of drugs on pregnancy and infant outcomes (Sun, 2009).

Programs for Children/Families With Incarcerated Parents

The stigma associated with parental incarceration can be an overwhelming burden for children, one that often masks their needs for care. It is important to recognize the secondary positive effects on child well-being that are potentially associated with formerly incarcerated parents and their children receiving services characterized as nurturing, nonstigmatizing, and culturally competent (Mazza, 2006). Conversely, children can experience overwhelming negative impacts when their parents serve long sentences for substance abuse or its related criminal behavior (Mazza, 2006).

Family involvement during adults' incarcerations has been associated with decreased chemical dependency and several other positive outcomes (Smith, Krisman, Strozier, & Marley, 2004). For example, Dependency Drug Courts (DDCs) or family treatment drug courts have emerged as a promising option for addressing parental substance problems and promoting family unification following a parent's arrest for substance-related offenses. In Sacramento, the children of DDC participants had considerably higher rates of being reunited with parents than was observed among non-DDC families (42% vs. 27%) after 24 months of follow-up and the parents who participated in the DDC had higher rates of treatment participation (Boles, Young, Moore, & Dipirro-Beard, 2007). The DDC is a model for communities to meet requirements of the Federal Adoption and Safe Families Act (the ASFA Act of 1997, PL 105-89) with regard to parents of minor children who have been arrested for drug-related offenses (Boles et al., 2007). Through this mechanism, drug treatment and case management services can be provided to court-involved families affected by both child welfare and substance problems.

Similarly, Restrictive Intermediate Punishments combined with drug and alcohol treatment (RIP/D&A), when completed, has shown effectiveness in reducing the risk of adults' rearrest compared to offenders serving traditional jail sentences and specifically to probation offenders. These results were reported for jail programs in Pennsylvania with follow-up measurement at 1, 2, and 3 years postrelease among drug-dependent offenders who were deemed eligible for intermediate punishment programs (Warner & Kramer, 2009). RIP/D&A was less effective when the offenders failed to complete the program and was also less effective than state prison incarceration. Approaches such as this may be worth considering as a means of preventing the retraumatizing of children whose parents are rearrested and reincarcerated.

Practitioners who work with children of parents incarcerated for substance-related offenses might consider utilizing evidence-supported interventions designed for treating addicted parents alongside their sons and daughters. On one hand, this conjoint approach may serve as a preventive/early intervention strategy for children and adolescents who are, by definition, at relatively high risk for developing substance use disorders themselves (Kelley & Fals-Stewart, 2007). The approach also may support children in developing a better understanding of their parents' substance-related problems, which in turn may provide elements of relief for them (Kelley & Fals-Stewart, 2007). Conjoint strategies may also serve the parents as a treatment motivator and as a source of support for the parents' ongoing sobriety efforts.

Intervention Impact Factors

One factor which appears to be relevant to child outcomes is the child's age or developmental stage at the time of family intervention for a parent's substance-related problems: when treatment leads to improved parental functioning of alcohol abusing/dependent fathers and their partners during the children's preadolescence, the impact across the children's behavioral outcome domains is significantly better than when it is delayed until adolescence (Kelley & Fals-Stewart, 2007). These results were observed with outpatient family treatment populations, and it remains to be seen if the same conclusions apply to children whose parents are incarcerated. Specifically, it is important to consider the possibility that intervening early with these children will prove more cost-effective than delaying intervention until adolescence. Furthermore, it may be important to create opportunities during and following incarceration for engaging preadolescent children in the type of collaborative intervention measured in this study where children work along with their parents in learning to maintain sobriety.

Although conjoint family strategies may represent a "gold" standard for practice, the reality is that many parents with identified substance abuse problems refuse, avoid, or reluctantly permit interventions involving their children (Fals-Stewart, Kelley, Fincham, & Golden, 2004). However, it is not unusual for these children to be referred for services on the basis of their own behavioral or mental health issues. One family intervention strategy with positive outcomes in several efficacy tests involving adolescents who abuse substances is embodied in the BEST and BEST-Plus programs (Bamberg, Findley, & Toumbourou, 2006). This strategy involves parents and siblings along with target adolescents as a means of improving the family environments that encourage responsible behavior and recovery. Applicable in a variety of community settings, the approach may be adaptable in situations where parents who have been incarcerated express concerns over emergent substance abuse in their sons and daughters, either during their incarceration or during community reentry.

One barrier to parent–child visitation is the inability of child welfare, foster families, and other case workers to accompany minor children to the facilities for visitation to occur. Lack of financial resources needed to secure services, lack of transportation to aftercare services, and long waiting lists for limited publicly funded substance abuse treatment slots are all barriers to family reunification following a parent's release from jail or prison.

One innovation that can help in overcoming these barriers is the use of "parent advocates" who can promote the mental health and welfare of these children. Parent advocates, who have personal experience in the mental health delivery system, help families navigate systems, access traditional and nontraditional services, and believe they are able to communicate with families in ways different from professionals and case managers (Munson, Hussey, Stormann, & King, 2009). These parent advocates rely on their having "been there" to relate to families and help them translate professional processes into more user-friendly concepts, provide direction and support during professional meetings, and link parents with others going through similar experiences.

CASE EXAMPLE: Kendra and Kenny

On Halloween, Kendra (10 years) and Kenny (9 years) came home from school in their party costumes to an empty apartment. This was not unusual since their mother, Ms. Lynch, worked an irregular part-time schedule in the stockroom of a nearby discount clothing store. The evening became unusual when their mother did not come home and they did not hear from her. The children fed themselves cereal and fell asleep watching television. Their mother was still not home the next morning when they woke up. Together the children got themselves fed (cereal again), dressed, and off to school. The day became increasingly unusual when Kenny got into a fight during lunch recess when he tried to steal food from another student and Kendra could not stop crying after seeing him taken to the principal's office. The lunchroom supervisor took her to the office infirmary.

The school social worker quickly learned about the acute source of the siblings' anxiety for their mother. She soon discovered that Ms. Lynch was being held in the local jail pending charges being filed. Ms. Lynch was arrested at the store where she was employed when security cameras recorded her stealing three cartons of clothing and hiding them in an accomplice's car. Together the women had been stealing merchandise over a period of months and either "returning" it to other stores or selling it at resale outlets in the area. The women then used the cash to pay for alcohol and cocaine that they used with their boyfriends. During the initial intake period Ms. Lynch was not allowed access to a telephone and had failed to inform the police or jail staff about her minor children at home. Later she informed the school social worker that this was because she feared losing her children to "the system" and believed that she would be home soon to care for them herself.

The school social worker called a colleague at Child Protective Services and together they were able to arrange temporary care for the children with their maternal grandmother. Ms. Lynch was unable to post bond and remained in jail for 2 months while awaiting trial and sentencing for multiple offenses. During this time, the children were not permitted visits to the jail and their grandmother refused to accept telephone calls from their mother because she felt it was important for her daughter to "really suffer as a punishment to make her realize the wickedness of her actions." The children were permitted to write letters to their mother, which they did several times a day, and received letters back from Ms. Lynch about once per week.

After several weeks, Ms. Lynch sent a packet of the children's letters to the school social worker because she was desperately concerned about their welfare. The letters from Kendra to her mother raised the social worker's concern about anxiety, depression, and suicidal thinking. Kendra was having a very difficult time managing her fears about what was happening to her mother in jail, which she saw as a very dangerous place based on television and movie depictions of prison violence, and what was going to happen to her and her brother in the future. She was also suffering from being ostracized and becoming the target of mean-spirited gossip and jokes as schoolmates learned about what was happening in her family. Though she tried to keep the secret, telling people her mother was in the hospital for heart condition, classmates in the neighborhood found out when eviction notices appeared at their apartment. The family was losing their residence as a result of the mother not being able to pay rent while incarcerated and having let it slide during many months before her arrest as her problems with substance abuse were escalating. Both Kenny and Kendra began struggling with school work, despite their grandmother's best efforts to make them keep up with homework. They found it difficult to concentrate on lessons and, as they began failing, they began referring to themselves as "the Double Ls—the Loser Lynches."

As their mother's legal situation evolved and she began serving a sentence in the county jail, it became evident that the children were in need of longer-term living arrangements. Their grandmother admitted that she was not up to the challenge over the long haul, and the children's birth father was contacted. The mother became terrified of the children being placed with their father because their family situation had fallen apart when his abuse of her became severe and she began to fear for her children's safety. The children had little contact with him during the past 4 years as he lived in another city that was 2 hours distant. This father was uncertain about whether or not he would be able to "handle" taking care of the children. He was worried about a number of issues, including whether or not he could be a "good parent" and the impact of this dramatic change on his own tenuous recovery from marijuana addiction. He expressed a great sense of guilt regarding the possibility that he had "ruined his children's chances for a normal life" by possibly passing along his own "weakness" for drugs, "failing to be a good father figure," and having played a role in encouraging their mother's abuse of substances during their (stormy) 8 year relationship. He also continued to be angry with Ms. Lynch about the crippling legal expenses resulting from his past domestic violence charges which he continued to pay off.

While she served her sentence, Ms. Lynch was offered an opportunity for evaluation of her need for substance abuse treatment and other services likely to arise during community reentry. She scored very high on screening instruments for alcohol and other drug problems, indicating that treatment for substance-related problems should be a high priority for her. The jail did not have budget dedicated to providing these services to women during incarceration. However, the assessment program led to Ms. Lynch being enrolled in a jail in-reach program by which a case manager from a community-based behavioral health agency was assigned to meet with her in jail to prepare her for reentry. Together they began developing detailed plans for what Ms. Lynch would do about seeking substance abuse treatment services, as well as meeting her family's child welfare needs and securing housing so that she did not leave jail and become homeless. Significant concerns remained as to how Ms. Lynch would reenter the workforce following her conviction for retail theft.

Meanwhile, the school social worker began searching the Family & Corrections Network for information in their National Resource Center on

Children and Families of the Incarcerated (http://fcnetwork.org). As a result, she was able to help Kendra and Kenny find information from the library resources created for families and children whose mothers or fathers are in prison or jail. The school social worker helped the grandmother understand the importance of these visits to both the children and her own daughter's efforts to change, and the grandmother began to facilitate monthly visits and regular telephone contacts. The children were enrolled in a community-based mentoring program for children of incarcerated parents; although the program was designed for families of a parent in prison, they were able to assign a mentor to the Lynch children as part of their pilot initiative to prevent children from becoming involved in drugs and crime themselves. The mentoring program, along with a church-based after school program, provided enough respite for the grandmother that she became willing to continue as the primary caretaker for Kendra and Kenny.

Though the children continued to experience periods of intense anxiety and sadness, and their future remained unpredictable, their school performance gradually improved. Their mentor helped them invent a new label for themselves: "the Double Ls: the Likeable Lynches" and helped them find a few friends that they could enjoy without suffering from the stigmatization of their parents' difficulties with incarceration and substance abuse.

Case Analysis

The case of the Lynch family demonstrates a number of significant elements. These include (1) substance abuse contributes to people committing crimes that lead to both drug and nondrug offenses; (2) a variety of emotional, social, and other vulnerabilities are manifested by children whose parents are incarcerated for substance-related problems—including the children's concerns regarding their parents' safety and well-being; (3) the difficulty of finding services for individuals and families in jail as opposed to prisons, and the poor coordination of programs and services across administrative systems; (4) the multigenerational nature of the challenges faced by these families; (5) the broad scope and "domino effects" of problems that erupt in families when a parent is incarcerated for substance-related offenses; (6) the need for compassionate, creative, and persistent social work practice on behalf of these families; and (7) the need for advocacy on behalf of the children of incarcerated individuals.

CONCLUSIONS

The children of parents incarcerated for substance-related offenses face the same challenges experienced by any child of a substance-involved parent, compounded by the difficulties associated with parental incarceration in jail or prison. These children must not only deal with their own sense of loneliness, fear, anxiety, and abandonment brought on by parental incarceration, but with the societal stigma of a parent who has done something "bad"; that is, abused substances. They require increased sensitivity by social workers and other caregivers who appreciate that they want and need an ongoing relationship with their parent. An integrated and coordinated array of "wraparound" intervention services to meet the needs of the parents, children, and substitute caregivers are necessary to help achieve a more hopeful and successful life for themselves and their families.

REFERENCES

Ackerman, R. J. (2000). Alcoholism and the family. In S. Abbott, *Children of alcoholics: Selected readings* (Vol. II, pp. 265–287). Rockville, MD: National Association for Children of Alcoholics.

Alcohol Policy Information System. (2008). *APIS analysis of alcohol and pregnancy policies.* Bethesda, MD: National Institute on Alcohol Abuse and Alcoholism (NIAAA), US Department of Health and Human Services (DHHS), National Institutes of Health (NIH). Retrieved June 17, 2009, from http://www .alcoholpolicy.niaaa.nih.gov/

Allen, K. (1994). Development of an instrument to identify barriers to treatment for addicted women, from their perspective. *International Journal of Addictions, 29*(4), 429–444.

Aos, S., Miller, M., & Drake, E. (2006). *Evidence-based adult corrections programs: What works and what does not.* Olympia, WA: Washington State Institute for Public Policy.

Bamberg, J., Findley, S., & Toumbourou, J. (2006). The BEST plus approach to assisting families recover from youth substance problems. *Youth Studies Australia, 25*(2), 25–32.

Begun, A. L., Rose, S. J., & LeBel, T. P. (in press). How jail partnerships can help women address substance abuse problems in preparing for community reentry. In S. Stojkovic (Ed.), *Managing special populations in jails and prisons* (Vol. 2). Kingston, NJ: Civic Research Institute (CRI).

Begun, A. L., Rose, S. J., LeBel, T. P., & Teske-Young, B. (2009). Implementing substance abuse screening and brief motivational intervention with women in jail. *Journal of Social Work Practice in the Addictions, 9*(1), 113–131.

Belenko, S., & Peugh, J. (2005). Estimating drug treatment needs among state prison inmates. *Drug and Alcohol Dependency, 77,* 269–281.

Belknap, J. (2003). Responding to the needs of women prisoners. In R. Muraskin (Series Ed.) & S. F. Sharp (Vol Ed.), *Prentice hall's women in criminal justice series: The incarcerated woman: Rehabilitative programming in women's prisons* (pp. 93–106). Upper Saddle River, NJ: Prentice Hall.

Bhati, A. S., Roman, J. K., & Chalfin, A. (2008). *To treat or not to treat: Evidence on the prospects of expanding treatment to drug-involved offenders.* Washington, DC: Urban Institute Research Report.

Boles, S. M., Young, N. K., Moore, T., & Dipirro-Beard, S. (2007). The sacramento dependency drug court: Development and outcomes. *Child Maltreatment, 12*(2), 161–171.

Brazzell, D. (2008). *Using local data to explore the experiences and needs of children of incarcerated parents. Urban Institute Research Report.* Washington, DC: The Urban Institute. Retrieved from http://www.urban.org/UploadedPDF/411698_incarcerated_parents.pdf

Brendel, R. W., & Soulier, M. F. (2009). Legal issues, addiction, and gender. In K. T. Brady, S. E. Back & S. F. Greenfield (Eds.), *Women & addiction: A comprehensive handbook* (pp. 500–515). New York: Guilford Publications.

Brocato, J., & Wagner, E. F. (2008). Predictors of retention in an alternative-to-prison substance abuse treatment program. *Criminal Justice and Behavior, 35*(1), 99–119.

Dallaire, D. H. (2006). Children with incarcerated mothers: Developmental outcomes, special challenges and recommendations. *Journal of Applied Developmental Psychology, 28,* 15–24.

Fals-Stewart, W., Kelley, M. L., Fincham, F., & Golden, J. (2004). Substance-abusing parents' attitudes toward allowing their custodial children to participate in treatment: A comparison of mothers versus fathers. *Journal of Family Psychology, 18,* 666–671.

Fazel, S., Bains, P., & Doll, H. (2006). Substance abuse and dependence in prisoners: A systematic review. *Addiction, 101*(2), 181–191.

Ford, J. D., Moffitt, K. H., Steinberg, K. L., & Zhang, W. (2008). *Breaking the cycle of trauma and criminal justice involvement: The Mothers Overcoming and Managing Stress (MOMS) study.* Rockville, MD: National Criminal Justice Reference Service. Retrieved from http://www.ncjrs.gov/pdffiles1/nij/grants/222910.pdf

Freudenberg, N., Wilets, I., Greene, M. B., & Richie, B. E. (1998). Linking women in jail to community services: Factors associated with rearrest and retention of drug-using women following release from jail. *Journal of the American Medicine Women's Association, 53,* 89–93.

Gabel, S. (1992). Behavioral problems in sons of incarcerated or otherwise absent fathers: The issue of separation. *Family Process, 31,* 303–314.

Glaze, L. E., & Maruschak, L. M. (2008). *Parents in prison and their minor children* (Bureau of Justice Statistics Special Report No. NCJ 222984). Washington, DC: U.S. Department of Justice. Bureau of Justice Statistics. (Revised 3/30/10, Retrieved July 5, 2009, from http://bjs.ojp.usdoj.gov/content/pub/pdf/pptmc.pdf.)

Golder, S., Ivanoff, A., Cloud, R. N., Besel, K. L., McKiernan, P., Bratt, E., et al. (2005). Evidence-based practice with adults in jails and prisons: Strategies, practices, and future directions. *Best Practices in Mental Health, 1*(2), 100–132.

Greenfield, L. A., & Snell, T. L. (1999). *Women offenders* (NCJ 175688). Washington, DC: U.S. Department of Justice, Bureau of Justice Statistics, Special Report.

Hairston, C. F., & Rollin, J. (2006). Prisoner reentry: Social capital and family connections. In R. Immarigeon (Ed.), *Women and girls in the criminal justice system: Policy issues and practice strategies* (pp. 1–6). Kingston, NJ: Civic Research Institute.

Harrison, P. M., & Beck, A. J. (2003). *Prisoners in 2002* (NCJ 200248). Washington, DC: Bureau of Justice Statistics.

Hill, H. A. (2004). *The special needs of women with co-occurring disorders diverted from the criminal justice system.* Delmar, NY: The National GAINS Center. Retrieved March 20, 2011, from http://gainscenter.samhsa.gov/pdfs/courts/WomenAndSpects.pdf

Howard, D., Strobino, D., Sherman, S., & Crum, R. (2009). Timing of incarceration during pregnancy and birth outcomes: Exploring racial differences. *Maternal & Child Health Journal, 13*(4), 457–466.

Inciardi, J., Martin, S., & Butzin, C. (2004). Five-year outcomes of therapeutic community treatment of drug-involved offenders after release from prison. *Crime & Delinquency, 50*(1), 88–107.

Johnston, D. (1995). Effects of parental incarceration. In K. Gabel & D. Johnston (Eds.), *Children of incarcerated parents* (pp. 59–88). New York: Lexington Books.

Karberg, J. C., & James, D. J. (2005). *Substance dependence, abuse, and treatment of jail inmates, 2002* (Bureau of Justice Statistics Special Report No. NCJ 209588). Washington, DC: US Department of Justice, Bureau of Justice.

Kelley, M. L., & Fals-Stewart, W. (2007). Treating paternal alcoholism with learning sobriety together: Effects on adolescents versus preadolescents. *Journal of Family Psychology, 21*(3), 435–444.

Kerridge, B. T. (2009). Sociological, social psychological, and psychopathological correlates of substance use disorders in the U.S. jail population. *International Journal of Offender Therapy and Comparative Criminology, 53*(2), 168–190.

Kliewer, W., Murrelle, L., Prom, E., Ramirez, M., Obando, P., Sandi, L., et al. (2006). Violence exposure and drug use in Central American youth: Family cohesion and parental monitoring as protective factors. *Journal of Research on Adolescence, 16*(3), 455–478.

Knight, K., Simpson, D. D., & Hiller, M. L. (2002). Screening and referral for substance abuse treatment in the criminal justice system. In C. G. Leukefeld, F. M. Tims, & D. Farabee (Eds.), *Treatment of drug offenders: Policies and issues* (pp. 259–272). New York: Springer Publishing.

Krebs, C., Brady, T., & Laird, G. (2003). Jail-based substance user treatment: An analysis of retention. *Substance Use & Misuse, 38*(9), 1227–1258.

Kubiak, S. P., Young, A., Siefert, K., & Stewart, A. (2004). Pregnant, substance-abusing, and incarcerated: Exploratory study of a comprehensive approach to treatment. *Families in Society: The Journal of Contemporary Social Services, 85*(2), 177–186.

Levy, S. J., & Rutter, E. (1992). *Children of drug abusers.* New York: Lexington Books.

Lewis, P. (2004). Comment: Behind the glass wall: Barriers that incarcerated parents face regarding the care, custody and control of their children. *Journal of the American Academy of Matrimonial Lawyers, 19*(1), 97–115. Retrieved from http://www.aaml.org/sites/default/files/Journal_vol_19-1-6_Incarcerated_Parents_and_Custody.pdf

Maggia, B., Martin, S., Crouzet, C., Richard, P., Wagner, P., Balmes, J. L., et al. (2004). Variation in AUDIT (Alcohol Use Disorder Identification Test) scores within the first weeks of imprisonment. *Alcohol & Alcoholism, 39*(3), 247–250.

Mazza, C. (2006). Children of incarcerated parents. In N. K. Phillips & S. L. A. Straussner (Eds.), *Children in the urban environment: Linking social policy and clinical practice* (pp. 191–215). Springfield, IL: Charles C. Thomas, Publisher, Ltd.

Messina, N. P., & Prendergast, M. L. (2004). Therapeutic community treatment for women in prison: Assessing outcomes and needs. In K. Knight & D. Farabee

(Eds.), *Treating addicted offenders: A continuum of effective practices* (Chap. 18, pp. 1–12). Kingston, NJ: Civic Research Institute.

Minton, T. D., & Sabol, W. J. (2009) *Jail inmates at midyear 2008—Statistical tables* (Bureau of Justice Statistics Report No. NCJ225709). Washington, DC: U.S. Department of Justice, Bureau of Justice Statistics.

Moos, R. H., Finney, J. W., & Cronkite, R. C. (1990). *Alcoholism treatment: Context, process, and outcome.* New York: Oxford University Press.

Moses, M. C. (2009). Does parental incarceration increase a child's risk for foster care placement? *National Institute of Justice Journal, 255,* 12–14. Retrieved August 7, 2009, from www.ojp.usdoj.gov/nij/journals/255/parental_incarceration.html

Mumola, C. (2000). *Incarcerated parents and children. Bureau of Justice Statistics Special Report.* Washington, DC: Bureau of Justice Statistics. Retrieved from http://bjs.ojp.usdoj.gov/content/pub/pdf/iptc.pdf

Mumola, C. J., & Karberg, J. C. (2006). *Drug use and dependence, state and federal prisoners, 2004. Bureau of Justice Statistics Special Report.* Washington, DC: US Department of Justice. Retrieved from http://bjs.ojp.usdoj.gov/content/pub/pdf/dudsfp04.pdf

Munson, M. R., Hussey, D., Stormann, C., & King, T. (2009). Voices of parent advocates within systems of care model of service delivery. *Children & Youth Services Review, 31*(8), 879–884.

Murray, J., & Farrington, D. P. (2008). The effects of parental imprisonment on children. *Crime and Justice: A Review of Research, 37,* 133–206.

Myers, B. J., Smarsh, T. M., Amlund-Hagen, K., & Kennon, S. (1999). Children of incarcerated mothers. *Journal of Child and Family Studies, 8*(1), 11–25.

National Institute on Drug Abuse. (2006). *Principles of drug abuse treatment for criminal justice populations: A research-based guide* (No. 06-5316). Bethesda, MD: National Institutes of Health (NIH). Retrieved August 7, 2009, from http://www.drugabuse.gov/PODAT_CJ/

Nesmith, A., & Ruhland, E. (2008). Children of incarcerated parents: Challenges and resiliency, in their own words. *Children and Youth Services Review, 30*(10), 1119–1130.

Parke, R., & Clarke-Stewart, K. A. (2002). *Effects of parental incarceration on young children. Urban Institute Research Report.* Washington, DC: US Department of Health and Human Services. Retrieved August 7, 2009, from http://aspe.hhs.gov/HSP/prison2home02/parke&stewart.pdf

Peters, R. H., Strozier, A. L., Murrin, M. R., & Kearns, W. D. (1997). Treatment of substance-abusing jail inmates: Examination of gender differences. *Journal of Substance Abuse Treatment, 14*(4), 339–349.

Phillips, S., Burns, B. J., Wagner, H. R., & Barth, R. P. (2004). Parental arrest and children involved with child welfare services agencies. *American Journal of Orthopsychiatry, 74,* 174–186.

Prendergast, M., Farabee, D., & Cartier, J. (2004). Corrections-based substance abuse programs: Good for inmates, good for prisons. In K. Knight & D. Farabee (Eds.), *Treating addicted offenders: A continuum of effective practices* (Chap. 30, pp. 1–8). Kingston, NJ: Civic Research Institute.

Rebecca Project for Human Rights. (2006). Retrieved from http://www.rebeccaproject.org

Robertson, A. A., Baird-Thomas, C., & Stein, J. A. (2008). Child victimization and parental monitoring as mediators of youth problem behaviors. *Criminal Justice and Behavior, 35*(6), 755–771.

Sabol, W. J., & Minton, T. D. (2008). *Jail inmates at midyear 2007* (Bureau of Justice Statistic Bulletin No. NCJ221945). Washington, DC: U.S. Department of Justice, Bureau of Justice Statistics. Retrieved June 17, 2009, from http://bjs .ojp.usdoj.gov/content/pub/pdf/jim07.pdf

Sabol, W. J., Minton, T. J., & Harrison, P. M. (2007, June). *Prison and jail inmates at mid-year 2006* (NCJ 2177675). Washington, DC: U.S. Department of Justice, Bureau of Justice Statistics. Retrieved from http://bjs.ojp.usdoj.gov/ content/pub/pdf/pjim06.pdf

Sharp, S. F. (2003). Mothers in prison: Issues in parent-child contact. In R. Muraskin (Series Ed.) & S. F. Sharp (Vol. Ed.), *Prentice Hall's Women in Criminal Justice Series. The incarcerated woman: Rehabilitative programming in women's prisons* (pp. 151–166). Upper Saddle River, NJ: Prentice Hall.

Smith, A., Krisman, K., Strozier, A. L., & Marley, M. A. (2004). Breaking through the bars: Exploring the experiences of addicted incarcerated parents whose children are cared for by relatives. *Families in Society—The Journal of Contemporary Human Services, 85*(2), 187–195.

Smith, N. (2002). Reunifying families affected by maternal substance abuse: Consumer and service provider perspectives on the obstacles and the need for change. *Journal of Social Work Practice in the Addictions, 2*(1), 33–53.

Snyder, Z. K., Carlo, T. A., & Mullins, M. M. C. (2001). Parenting from prison: An examination of a children's visitation program at a women's correctional facility. *Marriage and Family Review, 32*(3–4), 33–61.

Solomon, A. L., Osborne, J. W. L., LoBuglio, S. F., Mellow, J., & Mukamal, D. A. (2008). *Life after lockup: Improving reentry from jail to the community.* Washington, DC: Urban Institute.

Springer, D. W., McNeece, C. A., & Arnold, E. M. (2003). *Substance abuse treatment for criminal offenders: An evidence-based guide for practitioners.* Washington, DC: American Psychological Association.

Stojkovic, S. (2005). Placing special correctional populations in the context of larger issues of jail and prison management. In S. Stojkovic (Ed.), *Managing special populations in jails and prisons* (pp. 1–12). Kingston, NJ: Civic Research Institute.

Straussner, S. L. A., & Fewell, C. H. (2006). *Impact of substance abuse on children and families: Research and practice implications.* Binghamton, NY: Haworth Press.

Substance Abuse and Mental Health Data Archive. (1997). *National Treatment Improvement Evaluation Study (NTIES). Final report.* Rockville, MD: U.S. Department of Health and Human Services, Substance Abuse and Mental Health Services Administration (SAMHSA), Center for Substance Abuse Treatment (CSAT). Retrieved from http://www.icpsr.umich.edu/ SAMHDA/NTIES/NTIES-PDF/ntiesfnl.pdf

Substance Abuse and Mental Health Services Administration. (2007). *Results from the 2007 National Survey on Drug Use and Health: National findings* (Publication No. SMA 07-4293). Rockville, MD: Office of Applied Studies NSDUH Series H-32, Department of Health and Human Services (DHHS). Retrieved June 16, 2009, from http://www.oas.samhsa.gov/ NSDUH/2k7NSDUH/2k7results.cfm

Sun, A. P. (2009). *Helping substance-abusing women of vulnerable populations: Effective treatment principles and strategies.* New York: Columbia University Press.

Taxman, R. S., Byrne, J., & Young, D. (2002). *Targeting for reentry: Matching needs and services to maximize public safety.* College Park, MD: Bureau of Governmental Research. Retrieved from http://www.ncjrs.gov/pdffiles1/nij/grants/196491.pdf

Taxman, F. S., & Cropsey, K. L. (2007). Women and the criminal justice system: Improving outcomes through criminal justice and non-criminal justice responses. *Women & Criminal Justice, 17*(2/3), 5–26. DOI: 10.1300/J012v17n02_02.

Tebo, M. G. (2006). A parent in prison: States slowly beginning to help inmates' children, and advocates say it's overdue. *American Bar Association Journal, 92,* 12. Retrieved from http://www.lexisnexis.com/us/lnacademic

U.S. Department of Justice. (2000). *Report on minor children who have a mother or father in prison.* Washington, DC: U.S. Department of Justice, Bureau of Justice Statistics.

Warner, T. D., & Kramer, J. H. (2009). Closing the revolving door? Substance abuse treatment as an alternative to traditional sentencing for drug-dependent offenders. *Criminal Justice and Behavior, 36*(1), 89–109.

Weinman, B. A., Dignam, J. T., & Wheat, B. (2004). Lessons learned from the Federal Bureau of Prisons' drug abuse treatment programs. In K. Knight & D. Farabee (Eds.), *Treating addicted offenders: A continuum of effective practices* (pp. 1–11). Kingston, NJ: Civic Research Institute.

West, H. C., & Sabol, W. J. (2009). *Prison inmates at midyear 2008—Statistical tables* (Bureau of Justice Statistic Bulletin No. NCJ225619). Washington, DC: U.S. Department of Justice, Bureau of Justice Statistics.

Windell, P. A., & Barron, N. B. (2002). Treatment preparation in the context of system coordination serves inmates well. *Journal of Psychoactive Drugs, 34,* 59–67.

Worcel, S. D., Furrer, C. J., Green, B. L., Burrus, S. W. M., & Finigan, M. W. (2008). Effects of family treatment drug courts on substance abuse and child welfare outcomes. *Child Abuse Review, 17,* 427–443. DOI: 10.1002/car.1045

Zimmerman, A. M. (2005). Note: Home alone: Children of incarcerated mothers in New York City under the Rockefeller drug laws. *Cardozo Journal of Law & Gender,* (12), 445. Retrieved March 20, 2011, from https://litigation-essentials.lexisnexis.com/webcd/app?action=DocumentDisplay&crawlid=1&doctype=cite&docid=12+Cardozo+J.L.+%26+Gender+445&srctype=smi&srcid=3B15&key=4d704ad1f25192dd013ab47a52eca7cf

IV. Conclusion

13

Stories From the Inside: Life as the Child of a Substance-Abusing Parent

Anonymous, Christopher H. Acker, Claudia Narváez-Meza, and Peter X

INTRODUCTION

This chapter provides a vivid glimpse of the conflict and emotional distress experienced by social workers who grew up with substance-abusing parents. We are grateful to the four authors for sharing their personal stories with us, and believe that their narratives illustrate many of the dynamics and treatment issues discussed throughout the book. These poignant narratives provide us with a glimpse inside the hearts and minds of social work colleagues who have struggled to make sense of their own pain. All identifying details have been changed to protect the identities of family members.

ROBERT: SHAME, DENIAL, AND THE FAMILY SECRET

Robert's story clearly illustrates the confusion that COSAPs experience in not being able to openly discuss "the family secret." While growing up, Robert observed his mother's inexplicable, shame-inducing behaviors that he could not attribute to their correct source, the effects of mood-altering drugs. As is so often the case, the non–substance-abusing parent, in this case

---

Editors' Note: "Anonymous" is a well-known individual and we are deeply appreciative of her contribution to this chapter. "Peter X" is a licensed social worker who is currently working in an urban housing program. Although he prefers to remain anonymous, we thank him very much for his contribution as well.

his father, participated in the denial and unwillingness to openly recognize the problem. Consequently, Robert felt that his perceptions were wrong and he adopted the caretaking role of being a responsible child who should not rock the boat. Robert's description of his family reflects the dynamics of substance-abusing families described by Lam and O'Farrell (Chapter 3), and the healing process he experienced in therapy points to some of the techniques described by Dayton (Chapter 7) in her discussion of the effects of trauma and how they can be ameliorated by attention to body states.

Robert's Story

Having the opportunity to read my writing in a published book should be a momentous occasion to share with my family. However, when my writing centers on my childhood experiences with my mother's struggle with substance abuse, I don't think sharing this story with them is an option at this point. The reason for this reluctance is that 3 years after I moved out of my parents' house at the age of 24, they still deny the existence of addiction. It has taken me nearly 10 years to accept that my mother has had a problem with substance abuse, and this is because of the power of denial. Denial not only affects the substance abuser but also the children in the home. Even when evidence is insurmountable, denial erases the possibility of addiction. To the outsider, certain events I experienced when I was in middle and high school clearly reek of addiction, but to the child who lives within the world of denial, I did not see the world that way. My mother suddenly "quit" her well-paying job as a registered nurse and had me pick up her last paycheck at the hospital where she worked. Her behavior at home started to change; every so often she seemed to be in a daze where she couldn't speak clearly without slurring her words, and she had trouble keeping her eyes open and maintaining her balance as she walked. She frequently told us she was sick with a stomach virus or that her sinus infection was acting up, while my father backed up these ludicrous stories. I began finding multiple prescription bottles (Percocet being the name on one of the bottles) in her purse and bedroom; in fact, I consistently drove to the drugstore to pick up her medications and was confused when the pharmacist asked me how my mother was feeling.

I truly believed my mother's sinuses acted up and that she needed the medication for her "congestion." When she sprawled out on the couch during family get-togethers, clearly out-of-it, my family constantly went along with her story, which further added to my accepting a physical illness to explain her unusual behaviors. I knowingly got in the car with my mother when she was in one of her dazes; she ran countless red lights and stopped short constantly. My father would also let her drive when she was under the influence without any fear of the deadly consequences he could have been responsible for. Not once did I ask to get out of the car or refuse a ride with her. Doing so meant admitting something was wrong with my family.

The feelings I experienced as a teenager when in presence of my intoxicated mother were the most intense, unpleasant, and relentless emotions I've ever felt. I can recall countless incidents—usually at the dinner table, at restaurants, or at other confining, inescapable places—where I watched my mother roll her eyes back into her head, doze off with a fork in her mouth, or chew on a napkin she mistook for lettuce. To try to put this indescribable feeling into words, "anger" or "discomfort" doesn't do it justice. The feeling can be best compared to either wanting to throw up or wanting to break a table in half. Everything in my body would tell me to scream my lungs out and make my pain known to my family. But I never did. Instead of acting upon my feelings by causing havoc or by speaking to my parents about what I felt, I kept quiet despite the reliability of the information my feelings tried to give me. Emotions became so far out of reach that accessing them seemed nearly impossible.

In reading about ACOAs in the typical academic literature, the discussion of family roles is a common topic. I fit into the role of the "responsible one" as snugly as the last piece to a jigsaw puzzle. From middle school throughout college, my friends used to kid me I was "16 going on 40." Although meant as a joke, that statement contained a great deal of truth. I didn't drink, smoke, do drugs, or get in trouble either at school or at home. Looking back at my childhood, I never really experienced your typical adolescent rebellion and I attribute this to what I experienced at home. The way I coped with my mother's addiction and the feelings it provoked in me was by devoting myself to schoolwork. Studying was a way to channel my turbulent emotions; in a way, I learned to repress my feelings by stuffing myself into my textbooks and homework. Achievement in school replaced any success I could achieve within the home. I was also the responsible one at home. I cleaned parts of the house when no one wanted to, took the dogs out when everyone else forgot, and when my parents were short on money for the week, I lent them as much as they needed. Around the time my mother's addiction started to emerge, she desperately wanted a second dog to fulfill whatever void she felt. When she asked to "borrow" $400 for a beagle, what choice did a 15-year-old have but to give her money with no questions asked?

Family dynamics in a substance-abusing household make it difficult for a child to question or discuss the "family secret." I confronted my mother on two separate occasions, both of which occurred during my late adolescence. The second occasion, which exemplifies the unwavering vigor of denial, took place 3 days before Christmas. After leaving a restaurant, where my mother was completely under the influence of her prescription medication, I couldn't suppress my feelings anymore. I let the floodgates open in the backseat of the car. My parents freaked out, and once we arrived at the bookstore we were going to, my mother frantically ran inside. Her arms waved about as she screamed at me. Her wedding ring somehow managed to slip off her finger and dropped into the flowerbed outside the bookstore. While my father and I sifted through the dirt, he berated me for not only accusing my mother, but doing so 3 days before Christmas. I thought I was wrong for bringing up what I said. I blamed myself for having those damning thoughts and feelings; if both of my parents didn't agree with the information I brought up, then perhaps I was mistaken.

I didn't seek therapy as a young adult solely for the purpose of addressing my mother's addiction; although the denial slowly loosened up as I separated from my family by entering college, it still had an influence over me during those years. Applying to graduate schools for social work brought upon me a generalized anxiety due to my necessary return to living in my parents' basement. It didn't take long for my therapist to explore my anxiety and discover that the root of the issue was dealing with my mother's substance abuse. As luck would have it, my therapist was roughly the same age as my mother. To say that she provided me with a maternal figure to help me reprocess my childhood experiences is an accurate statement. Through her gentle support and sharp therapeutic interventions, I slowly came to accept my mother's struggle instead of fighting reality. She continually asked me detailed and sometimes bizarre questions, such as "Where in your body are you feeling that?" "What color is that feeling?" "What shape does that feeling have?" and other questions that caused me to access those feelings that I suppressed for so long. My therapist's expertise in eye movement desensitization and reprocessing (EMDR) further assisted me along the ACOA journey; simple lateral eye movements with verbal prompts to hone in on the feelings associated with the past incident under scrutiny was a tonic, an elixir, that forced me to face my anger at my parents, and to reprocess my faulty cognitions and replace them with more positive beliefs. But the biggest miracle of all was her ability to help me examine my family's struggle in a nonjudgmental and empathetic fashion. Taking one's parent off the idealized pedestal is a tricky process, but the support I received from my therapist allowed me to accept my parents' flaws instead of blaming them for my inner struggle. Externalizing the problem away from my mother and onto the separate entity of addiction didn't solve everything; however, it made me less spiteful of my parents.

Was therapy a magical cure? Hardly. The fact that I still cannot share with my parents the accomplishment of becoming a published writer reveals that the work of an ACOA is a long, arduous process. But coming to the end of this personal narrative, I've come to realize something—I feel a tremendous pride in myself for obtaining this professional accomplishment. Although a pat on the back from my father or mother never hurts, I don't need their approval as much as I did as a child and teenager. I don't need to sacrifice some of my needs in order to satisfy theirs. I'm very much along the path to healing knowing that feeling a sense of acceptance toward my past has replaced the power of denial. One day, I hope to share this chapter with my parents, but until that day arrives, I think I'll be okay.

SONIA: AN IMMIGRANT'S PERSPECTIVE ON PARENTAL SUBSTANCE ABUSE AND DOMESTIC VIOLENCE

Sonia's story describes the horror of growing up in family where alcoholism is coupled with domestic violence. In addition, being a child in an immigrant family living in impoverished circumstances amplifies the feelings of difference and isolation she depicts. Also evident are the longing and hope that underscored moments of trying to connect with her father whenever it was possible. Many of the insights she describes relate to intergenerational attachment issues as described by Fewell (Chapter 2) and her stance in describing them points to the usefulness of mentalization for managing painful affects.

Sonia's Story

In the beginning there was laughter, but to hear a woman's laughter one must first hear her sorrow…

—MARCIA DOUGLAS

Coming from a myriad of struggles has allowed me to process and grow from these places: Immigrant, Latina, Lesbian, Nicaraguan, Social Worker, Buddhist. *These are the journeys of which I speak; no one supersedes the other in importance. Taking from my experiences as a child survivor of domestic violence and parental substance abuse, I have learned that when one yields to struggle, it can become integral to a healing process that fosters self-awareness and a continuum of strength. Before coming to this place of acceptance I had to wrestle with the painful remembrance of witnessing my father seamlessly destroy the fragile beginnings of our young family in a new country. It wasn't until I took postgraduate courses in family systems, attachment theory, object relations, substance abuse and addictions, as well as trauma-focused interventions that I was able to weave together my own fragmented narrative with openness and compassion. As I constructed my genogram, in the process of learning how to help other families construct their own, I learned of how families can easily inherit legacies of suffering. I began to ask my own family members in an effort to (re)member my story. I learned of the multiple losses my father experienced as a child growing up in Nicaragua's rural poverty, without a father, working by age nine, witnessing the daily violence of alcohol and physical abuse among his family members. My father had been raised by many hands, many of which had been unkind to him. These were the hands he remembered when he sat in the dark, in an alcohol-induced stupor, nodding off at a table crowned with shot glasses and empty bottles. I understand now how early traumas and a string of disrupted attachments contributed to his alcoholism and the subsequent battering of my mother. The loss of country, culture, family, language, and status were all variables in his propensity to recreate the violence he had been raised with. The underpinnings to every family's story can be wrought with these difficulties and help give weight to the importance of knowing one's family, their histories, their struggles, and how people inevitably come to be. My work as a trauma recovery clinician continues to arm me with renewed commitment to the children and families healing from intergenerational cycles of violence and abuse. Like many of my clients who have encountered unimaginable suffering and loss, the courage to speak helps one to make meaning in the presence of another. The following narrative of survival is woven from a mixed genre of truth-seeking.*

I am fortunate enough to come from a nation of storytellers. I learned early on that compassion, prayer, and fable become the nectar of a people.

Longing to grasp the unpredictability of adults and feel safe despite the chaos, I would lie in the dark waiting for light. This became my creed, born on the chin of a moon that never failed to be.

Pestle and Verse

I am told the story of my beginnings, often in my mother's kitchen with my cheek to her apron. However, before I came to be I needed to know how my parents came to be. I imagine my young father on his first motorcycle smudging the air black for miles. My mother hums over her naked newborn who sits quietly in a basin of soapy water. I became that child toddling with a head full of lice in rural sun yards as I hung from my mother's hip. I played with green-bellied salamanders under the shutters of my grandmother's watch. I remember how she wore a braid down the center of her back. I loved the color of pumpkin vines and the cool sweetness of tamarind juice on rainy days. My first melodies came from the hollow of a green coconut shell while in the background a choir of old hands were husking corn. These are the first memories of a country I left at two. I am kicking shells into ant hills on the beach. I pocket a tattered photograph where my father's face is eclipsed from the shoulders up. He is a dim halo uncoiling against a sepia sky. He had fled before I came to exist. I imagine the footfalls of a new man just arrived to an American shore. Sun and sawdust crease his shirt as he sits in a cramped room writing postcards. His boots are cracked at the soles and betray his weight in the snow. He is orphaned by my mother's nation, leaving behind an inheritance of family tragedies. I am told that during the first winter of my birth he stopped sending money. With two young children in her arms my mother boarded a one way flight to go find him.

Child Eclipsed

Fast forward to the pavement where I jumped rope and climbed over wire fences. They bordered off the forbidden backside of the local library where films and puppetry pulled yarn from my child's mind that sequenced last night's terror. The sleepy giant, my father laughs as I dance to the sound of his warm change in my pockets. I am wearing his doorman's cap and his uniform shirt hangs large from my small shoulders. I perform despite the rising bile in my throat as I watch him sit and take shot after shot of Black Label. Suddenly my sky is unhinged and they are locked and gasping, the phone line is snapped from a wall. No badge shows at the rusty peephole where I dragged a chair to reach for the bolt that would free me from this tenement nightmare. My mother's screams pounced down the hallways where neighbors hid in silence. I wiggled and pushed my breathless body through the space between the chain and door. I took a blind swan dive down a pitch black stairwell stung with piss and crack vials. I skinned my knees. I arrive at the midnight ledge of a neighbor's home. She stands there amused, her son, my classmate, jeering and pointing at me. I stand trembling in my father's snakeskin boots, his large black tie hangs like a brute tongue from under my chin, strangling my soundless words. The neighbor's stunned silence covets my terror as my father's hands scale my mother's throat. I collapse against my playmate, she finally calls the police.

The Giant Awakens

Then there were three who waited in silence for the doorjamb to shake, their staccato pulse line hemmed in by the moon. Courage and childhood meshed beneath the thin cotton of pink pajamas. Blackness undulates, dips and tickles the back of my knee. My sister and I are curled like two fists beneath the same cover. She was scared awake again, with sheets stinging her following the bed wetting. I help her rake the bed clean, tiptoe down the hall to dump the evidence. My father's snore echoes in the dark. I remember how earlier he had thundered past my mother's watch. After going missing for 3 days, he arrived with a hefty bag of toys that were unloved and discarded by the well-to-do residents he labored for in Riverdale. My father was suddenly a tower where we went scrambling for his shoulders. We are three flown sparrows, sky-bound and reaching. Clad in blue, with the smell of whisky on his chin, the sleepy giant is suddenly awake and overjoyed with our play. My own small fingers trace the letters of his name stitched over the right chamber of his chest. My mother watches in silence. I watch too as he marches us over to where he keeps his liquor. He is telling jokes and winking at my mother. My heart begins a slow gallop and my throat tightens. She disappears into her kitchen.

Litany for My Mother...

I plead to follow you under the late Brooklyn sun, past the menace of rust. The factory owner always held your lateness suspect. I am bent over math equations in the third grade, quietly sitting on a cardboard box spilling with vinyl zippers. Steel grids wheeze over your graying head. The sewing needle plunges to feed your young tribe of three. How did you multiply the quota of one pair of panicked hands within the hour? I add the red apples in my workbook and watch you brush colored threads from inseams. I collect them from around your feet and learn to weave mosaics for your staggered mind. At rest break I plead to follow you. I shuffle my small body behind you, watch as you furtively balm the violent indigos of a new wound. The inebriated husband and your hidden children knew the creed of denim work shirts and crippled beer cans. The spit of promise hissed while love songs played in the darkened living room where his fists almost split you. I learned thunder before words. This daughter, your first earth, remembered sandboxes spilling with children, schoolyard hide-n-seek, sneakers squeaking, and colors of rain against bricks. Grief undulates in the remembering, it coils around my throat. I had existed for only eight summers when he began to peddle your life before my eyes. Dark church pews gleam where I knelt for penance, tides of my hidden pulse anchored the hours. Murmurs of prayer mist over my head. My father kneels beside me. I learned to invent solace, so I won't see where he knuckled the blue crescent beneath your eye. The only time I saw you cry was that evening when he left us for good. Two in the morning, I am crouched behind the sofa. Your shoulders weep quietly, silhouetted against the streetlight and a full moon. It took the fort you became to teach us the namesake of our survival, we were spring reeds at dusk—we were finally safe.

ANDREW: EFFECTS OF SUBSTANCE ABUSE ON THE FAMILY SYSTEM ACROSS GENERATIONS

Andrew is a 24-year-old social worker whose story highlights a number of themes touched on in the book. In addition to intergenerational effects of trauma and substance abuse that he traces back to his grandfather's experiences in World War II (WW II), he recounts the absence of his grandfather in his father's life, the secrets that could not be spoken of, and the subsequent alcoholism of his father. This speaks to intergeneration attachment issues as discussed by Fewell (Chapter 2). As Dayton describes in Chapter 7, trauma without words can be stored in the body and erupt in other symptoms. Andrew speaks of his father running marathons as a way to cope with cravings, and his own use of food as a way to deal with his emotions following his father's death. His sister continued the pattern of using substances as a way to deal with her feelings. Many of the family dynamics reflect issues raised by Lam and O'Farrell (Chapter 3). Andrew also had the experience of finding that a treatment program for COSAPs, as well as a few caring teachers were helpful in giving him the skills he needed for a healthy development (see Chapter 10).

Andrew's Story

When initially asked to write about my experience as the child of a substance abuser, I remember almost falling into the same dynamic that occurs every time I bring up my family and my past—I leap head first into the unpleasant, stereotypical, and painful parts of my development as an individual, and I focus on the sorrow and guilt of living with a substance abuser. Now, as I graduate from social work school with a Substance Abuse and Co-occurring Disorders specialty, I am able to take a different, activist approach to my past and my future development as an empowered clinician, practitioner, and member of society who understands the ramifications that substance abuse has on families and children. I hope to convey to whoever reads this that I did grow up "differently," but that I am continuing to grow and change and will continue to do so. I was born and raised in Staten Island, New York in a lower middle class neighborhood that quickly developed after the construction of the Verrazano-Narrows Bridge. My parents were both Polish; my mother was raised on a little farm outside of Warsaw and my father was raised by Polish immigrants who fled as WWII ravaged Poland by emigrating to Australia.

My theory about the intergenerational issues affecting my family goes like this: My grandfather survived some unspecified, traumatic incident during WWII (something always held as a secret from the younger members in the family), and by the time my father was born, my grandfather was drinking, partying, and basically having a good time—as a way of coping with his trauma. He was not present for much of the time my father was growing up, and this culminated in his disappearance when my grandmother was diagnosed with cancer. My father was then 24, the age I am now. He took care of his mother until her death from cancer. My father began using alcohol as his own coping mechanism. When he met my mother and was courting her he remained sober by engaging in another intoxicating activity—running marathons. Consequently, my mother never observed his drinking until the night they were married, when he actually chose to drink with his friends instead of celebrating their marriage together.

This ties into my story in a very interesting way, because my father was diagnosed with cancer when I was 17 and died during my sophomore year of college. His diagnosis was preceded by a sober period of about 2–3 years because my mother decided, "enough was enough" when I was in 7th grade and left my father. During this time, my father started attending 12-step groups and took up running again to stay away from drinking. Tragically, after receiving his diagnosis of cancer, the same kind that his mother died from, he relapsed and remained actively drinking for the rest of his life.

The true tragedy of this story and the inspiration for my desire to focus on substance abuse in my social work career is what happened to the next "rung" of the generation when my father passed away. After his death, I experienced an emotionally turbulent time, gained 100 pounds, almost flunked out of college, and went into a deep depression whose ramifications I am still dealing with today. This pales in comparison to the fact that my sister, who was 17 at the time of our father's death, actively began using substances in a desperate attempt to cope with her own emotional suffering. Like my father she dove into not only alcohol and experimental use of cocaine, but went straight for a chemical cocktail of every possible substance imaginable. In the end, she stole hundreds of thousands of dollars from my mother, flunked out of three colleges, and crashed two cars. Now, to add salt to an already open wound, let's take a look at the next step on the generational ladder—while my sister was using drugs she became pregnant, and during my summer semester at graduate school (the most difficult for 16 month students) she gave birth to my niece.

Thankfully, my sister calmed down considerably after my niece was born. Do not mistake that for being in recovery, which my sister is not in. As of right now, there is a juggling act in the family for my niece's safety and well-being, with a combination of my sister, mother, and myself raising the child. Time will tell how this "next generation" develops, but I can guarantee that I will have my say.

What I want to impress by writing about myself is the fact that there are things that can be done by and for individuals who survive in families of substance abusers and that people can be coached and led to others who will be supportive of their growth and development. Something I feel immense gratitude for is the fact that I have found people who live by a "different rule set." I choose to get to know people who have had no substance abuse in their lives, or who actively choose to combat the effects of their own traumatic history. I have been inspired and moved by several important people in my life, including my mother, my teachers, several mentors, and even a social worker in my youth. I now move to become one of those people to others, with gratitude to those who have done so for me. Ironically, I actually had the experience of interning at an agency that focuses on substance abuse prevention work, and which I attended for 3 years when I was in 6th, 7th, and 8th grade. It is evident that the goals and strategies that this agency uses to support its clients are effective. The program gave me a type of consistency that I was unaccustomed to in my childhood, leading me to be inspired to believe in myself and continue developing. This counteracted the messages that life was not worth living and there was no use trying to change.

I suspect that if you are reading this in a textbook as a case example that it would benefit you to remember that every step you take toward aiding the development of an individual who has lived with a substance abuser is a step toward both stopping their own substance abuse and potentially stopping the substance abuse of the next generation. Any such intervention will change the family dynamics for all involved, since engaging in self-care disrupts the unhealthy family dynamics that exist in families with a substance-abusing member. I am inspired by the example of my mother going to college after my father's death, because he did not allow her to go to school out of a fear that she would become educated and leave him. My mother has finally finished her bachelor's degree in Social Work and is looking at Master's in Social Work programs as I write this, which is something that warms my heart. She was able to take an extremely negative experience, the loss of her alcoholic husband, and with the support of the social workers and counselors at her college was able to create a productive and pleasant life for herself.

To finish my story, I invite you again to not look at the families of substance abusers as people who are tied to their tragic histories, but rather as individuals who can take those histories and write their futures in any way that they wish. This worked for me, and if you authentically do your best to attempt to support your client it can work for them as well.

EMILY: POVERTY, CHAOS, AND FEAR OVERCOME BY RESILIENCE

Emily is a successful 70-year-old social worker who clearly describes the chaos and fear of growing up with a father whose alcoholism caused him to subject her and the family to poverty, danger, and fear. Her story reflects the theme of growing up before one's time, of having to be rational when one's parents are not able to be so (as described by Johnson, Gryczynski, and Moe in Chapter 5). Her story also reflects the pain of not having the non–substance-abusing parent, her mother, be able to mitigate the effects of the drinking of her husband. Emily embodies the face of the resilient COSAP, who succeeds against all odds. Her dedication to hard work and education helped her to achieve a very successful outcome despite a painful childhood.

Emily's Story

The American Dream is often preceded by a nightmare.

At 70 years of age, I have the luxury of feeling calm enough to look back. Calm in my youth was not a given. I was born in a very rural part of the United States to folks that should not have been married in the first place.

My mother was a beautiful woman, uneducated, and timid. My father was a strong, handsome alcoholic who had been so from the age of 15. He was one of nine. All nine became alcohol addicted.

My first memories were of fear and blood ... lots of it. I believe that the bleeding came from my father's brother who had been bar fighting. (Some find the Fighting Irish funny ... believe me, they are not). In later times, my father was responsible for the death of two. One caused by a highway accident while drunk and another in an infamous bar fight. These fighting times were frequent. My stronger memories came from the fact that my father, who I adored as a young child, never came to my "stuff." By that I mean my school plays, art shows, and the like. I have looked out many windows for the invisible man. We also hid a lot. We were afraid that someone might see Daddy sick. I never invited other children to our house. My mother always had a headache and cried. It scared me. I was afraid that she would die. (Today she is 100 years old! ... much stronger than I knew). At the age of eight after having a car accident (I had to drive my father to the store. He lay sleeping in the back seat while I drove sitting on a huge pillow with the seat pulled up to the steering wheel), my father took me to the local newspaper telling me that since he badly needed his medicine and had no money that I would have to work. Work I did. I became the youngest newspaper "boy" in town.

Fast forward ... years of work went by ... bakery, department store, truck store, airline rep., actress, student, therapist—social worker, psychoanalyst, director of training, adjunct professor at a major university, university Trustee.

I married a wonderful, funny, kind man. We have been together for over 50 years. He does not drink.

My father died 26 years ago. I only tried to kill him once after he injured my mother while drinking. I hit him with a plumbers wrench. The day of his funeral, as he lay in his coffin, I inserted my Ph.D. card in his pocket. My last words to him were not pleasant: "I am here and you are not." I cried days after as I found the 30 odd bottles of liquor he had hidden in old shoes, the toilet tank, and in hollow logs. How he must have suffered as he made us suffer. I returned to my home in New York.

Part of the question I am attempting to address is how the effects of an alcoholic parent are felt at 70 years of age, considering that I have achieved the American Dream. As an aside, the Dream entails: four homes, great health for self and family, ok looks, wonderful career, fantastic husband, three well-loved dogs, the best friends and cousins anyone could have, and the great good fortune to be able to pledge dollars to support a wonderful university. As a psychoanalyst, I know the effects. Some are slightly more positive than others because they work. Some don't.

The effects are easily seen by me: I am a worker. I do all that I can to succeed. "What makes Sammy Run?" Perhaps someone will find out my dirty secret. I must make sure that I am perfect so that others will want to see me and invite me to lunch. I love to eat. I had terrible pin worms as a child ... for years. I am a caretaker par excellence. I took a lot of care of both mom and dad. Despite throwing out gallons of booze, I guess I didn't do such a great job with dad.

I have boundless energy and require little sleep. Many a night I was on the street looking for dad. I always found him. Getting him home was the hard part. I have NO alcoholic friends. I see anyone have more than two glasses of wine and I am gone to the world. After some painful trial and error, I flatly refused to work with alcoholic clients. I was aware of my growing anger toward them and referred them to other fine therapists. I really did them a favor.

I still dream of constant hunger ... referring to both the real thing and the emotional hunger of the children of alcoholics. A typical dream might look like: I am all excited going to the new brightly lit bakery. It is called the Yummery. I take my time looking in, wanting to choose the very best thing in the window. I know that I have just enough money to buy one of whatever I want. Should I buy the lemon cake, the apple tart, the chocolate brownie with no nuts, the Danish pastry with almond paste, or perhaps the jelly-filled donut or even a strawberry turnover? I can't decide. I'll spin around and point! OK! The jelly donut it is. I can't wait. I run to the door, grab the knob and nothing happens. The Yummery has just closed!! Let me in!! "Sorry kid, not today for you."

I often have long conversations with my mother about her past. She is very rational until speaking of my dad. She told me recently that he had died in WWII. "He was shot by a firing squad as a traitor." Later that day, I heard her telling a nurse that he was killed in Mexico. "He got sick with a bad Mexican disease and never came home." The latest story told to a priestly visitor was something about a car accident in which he was killed. She was driving. In truth, my dad died of a massive heart attack. One doesn't have to be a psychoanalyst to understand my mother's feelings about her long dead husband. In her case, headaches solved some of her problems.

In closing, it will suffice to say that I have survived nicely. I am happy, have never been depressed, never drank, don't fight with my husband except over the remote control, love my life and hope to continue my work at the university and perhaps even learn to play bridge. I have almost given up on golf ... but who knows. That really doesn't fit my personality. I'll give it another try or two! 70 isn't half as bad as it is cracked up to be. In fact, this age does have many perks. I usually get a seat on the subway and no longer have to smile at everyone. Of course construction workers never whistle or make rude comments. I suppose that like my mom, fantasy life reigns supreme.

Feelings toward my mother continue to vary between rage and guilt. Sometimes I dream of punching her in the mouth or biting off her lips. These dreams concern her ability to speak. (The lies of my childhood and the rage of being unprotected.) At other times, I am consumed with guilt at not being a better daughter. The loving feelings are there as well. I do miss her humor and affection. Many times since my father's death, we had so much fun traveling and the like. Today, very near the end, her world is about survival. I will be so saddened by loss.

The road I walked was thorny ... so I learned to "walk fast and carry a big stick."

Index

Abreaction, 140
ACOA. *See* Adult Children of Alcoholics
Acting out child, 11
Adderall, for ADHD, 90, 229
Adolescent Mentalization-Based
    Integrative Therapy
    (AMBIT), 41
Adolescent children of substance-
    abusing parents (COSAPs), 13
  characteristics of, prenatally
     exposed to ATOD, 83–84
  core interventions, 208
    awareness activities, 208–210
    counseling for emotional and
     behavioral issues, 213–215
    skill building, 212–213
    substance abuse education,
     210–211
    supplementary resources,
     use of, 215
    support for substance-abuse–
     specific concerns, 211–212
  guidelines for prevention and
    intervention, 220–221
  impact of parental substance
    use, 13–16
  mentalization-based family therapy
    for, 40–41
  parental consent issues, 217
  residential-based interventions, 219
  Residential Student Assistance
    Program (RSAP), 220
  school-based interventions, 218
  staff qualifications, training, and
    responsibilities, 216–217
  Student Assistance Programs, 219

Adolescents with substance-abusing
    parents, 127
  assessment, 134
  case example, 144–145
  health, mental health, and
    behavioral consequences,
    128–129
  interventions, 138–140
    for families, 141–143
    group interventions, 143–144
    individual-level intervention
     strategies for adolescents,
     140–141
  issues, 135–137
  risk factors, 130
    environmental and cultural
     factors, 131–132
    familial factors, 131
    individual characteristics, 131
  screening, 134–135
  teens, positive outcomes in, 129
Adoption and Safe Families Act
    (ASFA) of 1997, 194–195, 257
Adult Attachment Interview, 33
Adult Children of Alcoholics
    (ACOAs), 18, 19, 21, 153,
    224–225
Adult children of substance-abusing
    parents (COSAPs)
  interventions with, 163–164
  psychodrama, 164–168
AEP. *See* Alcohol-exposed pregnancy
AIDS, impact of, 6
Al-Anon program, 14, 21, 144
Alateen self-help groups, 14, 144,
    211, 215

Alcohol, tobacco, or other drugs
    (ATOD), 81
  ATOD-exposed adolescents, 83–84
  ATOD-exposed newborns and
    infants, 82
  ATOD-exposed school-aged
    children, 82–83
Alcohol-abusing individuals, 5
Alcohol- and drug-abusing families,
    attachment and mentalization
    in, 36–37
Alcohol consumption by pregnant
    women, 8, 78–79
Alcohol-exposed pregnancy (AEP), 79,
    173–174
Alcohol-related birth effects
    (ARBD), 79
Alcohol-related neurodevelopmental
    disorder (ARND), 79
Alcohol use, parental, 18–21
AMBIT. *See* Adolescent Mentalization-
    Based Integrative Therapy
Amygdala, 13, 155
Antisocial Personality Disorder, 54
ARBD. *See* Alcohol-related
    birth effects
ARC Community Services, 202
ARND. *See* Alcohol-related
    neurodevelopmental disorder
    (ARND)
ATOD. *See* Alcohol, tobacco, or other
    drugs (ATOD)
Attachment, in adolescence, 31, 33–34
Attachment and mentalization,
    in alcohol- and drug-abusing
    families, 36–37
Attachment and mentalization-based
    prevention and intervention
    programs, 37
  for adults in individual treatment,
    41–42
  for children and adolescents,
    40–41
  for parents, 39–40
Attachment patterns, 30
  in adulthood, 32, 34
  in childhood, 32–33

Attachment theory, 31
  attachment and mentalization, 34
  childhood, attachment patterns
    in, 32–33
  lifespan, attachment through, 33–34
  mentalization, role of parenting
    in, 35
Attention Deficit Hyperactivity
    Disorder and Conduct
    Disorder, 9
Authoritarian parenting, 35

Behavioral couples therapy, 61–63
Betty Ford Children's Program,
    109, 110
Binge drinking, 228
Brief motivational intervention (BMI),
    177–178
Brief Strategic Family Therapy (BSFT),
    60, 143
BSFT. *See* Brief Strategic Family
    Therapy (BSFT)
Buprenorphine, 10

Cannabis, 84, 130
Caring for children of incarcerated
    parents, 253–254
CASA. *See* National Center for
    Addiction and Substance
    Abuse
CAST. *See* Children of Alcoholics
    Screening Test
Celebrating Families!, 12, 16, 109, 142
Center for Substance Abuse Prevention
    (CSAP), 185
Center for Substance Abuse Treatment
    (CSAT), 185
Centers for Disease Control and
    Prevention (CDC), 179
Child abuse and partner violence,
    54–55
Child adjustment and parental
    substance abuse, 53
Child Protective Services, 65
Child–parent psychotherapy, 92

Childhood attachment patterns,
32–33
Children living with substance-
abusing parents, 102–104
Children of Alcoholics (COA), 103,
104, 231
Children of Alcoholics Screening Test
(CAST), 12–13, 14, 135
Children of substance-abusing parents
(COSAPs), 2, 7, 12, 13, 17, 20,
21, 50, 52, 53, 55, 101–102,
106–108, 233.
See also Adolescents; College
students with substance-
abusing parents
adult, 163
resilience in, 163
use of psychodrama, 164–168
developmental processes, 104–105
developmental psychopathology,
105–108
and dysfunctional family dynamics,
156–157
high-riskbehaviors in, 159
intervention programs for, 108–110
substance-abusing parents, children
living with, 102–104
symptoms and dynamics in,
157–162
Chrysalis Center, 201
Circle Park Behavioral Health
Services, 201
Clozarile, 90
Co-Anon program, 21
COA. *See* Children of Alcoholics
Cocaine use, 6
during pregnancy, 80
prenatal, 9
Cognitive therapy and cognitive-
behavioral therapy, 15,
140–141
College COSAPs, 17
College students with substance-
abusing parents, 16–18, 37
interventions with, 223
case study, 233–240
college environment, 228–229

community and internet
resources, 231–232
epidemiology, 224–225
risk factors for COSAPs in
college, 225–227
support for COSAPs, 230–231
Comorbid parental psychopathology,
55–56
Concerta, for ADHD, 90
Conduct disorder, 52
Constructivist theory
of equilibrium, 105
Co-occurring mental health disorders,
20, 162
COSA. *See* Children of Substance
Abusers
COSAPs and dysfunctional family
dynamics, 156–157
Crack, use of, 7
Crack babies, 9
CRAFFT, 14
"Crank babies," 9
CSAP. *See* Center for Substance Abuse
Prevention
CSAT. *See* Center for Substance Abuse
Treatment

DDCs. *See* Dependency Drug Courts
Dependency Drug Courts (DDCs),
256–257
Developmental fluctuation, 105
Developmental processes, 104–105
Developmental psychopathology,
105, 108
for prevention and intervention
with young COSAPs, 106–108
Dexedrine, for ADHD, 90
*Diagnostic and Statistical Manual
of Mental Disorders* (DSM-IV),
2, 137
Disorganized attachment pattern,
of infancy, 33
Distorted reasoning, 160
Dynamics of substance-abusing
families. *See* Substance-
abusing families, dynamics of

EAPs. *See* Employee Assistance
  Programs
Early adolescents, 139
East Coast Solutions, 201
Elementary school-aged children,
  group intervention of, 12
Emotional constriction, 158
Emotional dysregulation, problems
  with, 19
Employee Assistance Programs
  (EAPs), 219
Enabling, 5

FABS. *See* Fetal Alcohol Behavior Scale
FAE. *See* Fetal alcohol effects
False self, cultivation of, 158
Family, impact of different substances
  on, 5–7
Family Drinking Survey, 14, 135
Family Drug Treatment Court
  system, 203
Family Support Network, 143
Family system, impact of substance
  abuse on, 3–4
Family therapy, 59–61
FAS. *See* Fetal Alcohol Syndrome
FASD. *See* Fetal Alcohol Spectrum
  Disorder
Father–child relationships, 63
Fetal Alcohol Behavior Scale
  (FABS), 88
Fetal alcohol disorders, 10
Fetal alcohol effects (FAE), 9, 79
Fetal Alcohol Spectrum Disorder
  (FASD), 8–9, 79, 171,
  174–175, 186
Fetal Alcohol Syndrome (FAS), 8, 9,
  79, 171
  diagnostic criteria for, 88

Gaudenzia, Inc., 201
Gay/lesbian families, 4
Grief, unresolved, 158–159
Group intervention, of elementary
  school-aged children, 12

Group treatment, 18
Guilt experience, of survivor, 20

Hallucinogens, 80
Haven Doula Program, 201–202
Haymarket Center, 202
Health Promotion program, 18, 230
Healthy Moms study, 178
Heroin, 6, 10, 80
High-risk behaviors, in traumatized
  COSAPs, 159
HIV/AIDS, 6
Hyperreactivity, 158
Hypervigilance, 19, 158

IEP. *See* Individualized Education Plan
Illicit drug use, during pregnancy, 9,
  80–81
Incarcerated parents, 245
  case example, 259–261
  children of, 253–254
  intervention impact factors, 257–259
  jails versus prisons, 245–246
  parental caretaking disruption, 254
  parental contact needs of children
    during parental incarceration,
    255–256
  parents as prison inmates, 246–247
  practice implications, 255
    programs for, 256–257
  pregnant mothers and substance-
    related incarceration, 252–253
  substance abuse services in jails and
    prisons, 248–251
  substitute care, 254–255
Individual counseling, 18
Individual treatment, 41–43
Individualized Education Plan
  (IEP), 91
Inhalants, 80
Insecure ambivalent attachment, 32
Insecure avoidant attachment, 32
"Internalizing" behaviors
  and feelings, 11
Interparental conflict, 53–54

Intravenous drug abuse (IVDA), 6
Isolate, tendency to, 160–161
IVDA. *See* Intravenous drug abuse

Jails, parents in, 247
Jails and prisons, 244, 245–246
  substance abuse services in,
    248–251
Joint Commission on Accreditation of
    Health Care Organization, 59

Learned helplessness, 159
Lesbian/gay families, 4
Lifespan, attachment through,
    33–34
Living with substance-abusing
    parents, effects of, 102–104

March of Dimes, 197
Marijuana, 229
  during pregnancy, 9, 80, 81
Maternal and Child Health Bureau
    (MCHB), 184
Maternal Substance Abuse Checklist
    (MSAC), 173
Maternal substance abuse during
    pregnancy, 8
MBT. *See* Mentalization-based
    treatment
MCHB. *See* Maternal and Child Health
    Bureau (MCHB)
MDFT. *See* Multidimensional Family
    Therapy
Mentalization, 30
  attachment and, 34
  role of parenting in, 35
  trauma and, 35–36
Mentalization-based family therapy
    for children and adolescents,
    40–41
Mentalization-based programs for
    parents, 39–40
Mentalization-based treatment (MBT),
    38–39, 41–43

Methadone, 10
Methamphetamine, 107, 130
  prenatal, 9
Middle stage of adolescence, 139
Modified therapeutic communities
    (MTC), 198
Mothers and Toddlers Program
    (MTP), 39
MSAC. *See* Maternal Substance Abuse
    Checklist
MTC. *See* Modified therapeutic
    communities
MTP. *See* Mothers and Toddlers
    Program
Multidimensional Family Therapy
    (MDFT), 60, 143
Multisystemic therapy, 143

NACoA. *See* National Association
    of Children of Alcoholics
    (NACoA)
Nar-Anon program, 21
Narcotic Treatment Program
    (NTP), 40
National Association of Children of
    Alcoholics (NACoA), 14,
    16, 144
National Center for Addiction and
    Substance Abuse (CASA),
    194, 195
National Survey on Drug Use and
    Health (NSDUH), 51, 78, 172,
    193, 225
National Treatment Improvement
    Evaluation Study
    (NTIES), 255
No Safe Haven: Children of Substance-
    Abusing Parents, 195–196
Nonprescription opiate use, 6
NSDUH. *See* National Survey on Drug
    Use and Health
NTIES. *See* National Treatment
    Improvement Evaluation
    Study
NTP. *See* Narcotic Treatment
    Program

Odyssey House, Inc., 200–201
Opiate abusers, 6
Orofacial clefts, 9

Parent skills training with
    behavioralcouples therapy
    (PSBCT), 63, 65
Parental alcoholism
    effects on adult children, 18–21
    effects on children, 102
Parental and adolescent substance
    abuse, relationship between,
    132–133
Parental caretaking disrupted by
    incarceration, 254
Parental consent issues, 217
Parental substance abuse
    adolescents, effect on, 13–16,
        129–130
    child adjustment, 53
    college students, effect on, 16–18
    family system, impact of substance
        abuse on, 3–7
    health, mental health, and
        behavioral consequences,
        128–129
    prenatal substance use, impact
        of, 8–10
    prevalence of, 51
    school-aged children, effect on, 11–13
    substance-use disorders,
        understanding, 2–3
Parenting, 55
    role in mentalization, 35
Parents
    incarcerated parents and their
        substance problems, 247–248
    in jails, 247
    mentalization-based programs
        for, 39–40
    as prison inmates, 246–247
Parents First, 40
Partner violence and child abuse,
    54–55
Paternal substance use, 8
Patriarchal terrorism, 54

Pediatric occupational therapy, 10
Posttraumatic stress disorder
    (PTSD), 156
PPWI. *See* Pregnant and postpartum
    women and their infants
PRAMS. *See* Pregnancy Risk
    Assessment Monitoring
    System
Prefrontal cortex, 155
Pregnancy, substance use during, 8–10,
    80–81
    alcohol, 78–79
    cocaine, prenatal, 9
    heroin, 9
    illicit drug use during, 80–81
    methamphetamine, prenatal, 9
    smoking, prenatal, 9
Pregnancy Risk Assessment Monitoring
    System (PRAMS), 172
Pregnant and postpartum women and
    their infants (PPWI), 184
Pregnant mothers and substance-
    related incarceration, 252–253
Pregnant substance-abusing women,
    treatment for, 10
Prenatal clinic, brief interventions in,
    177–178
Prenatal impact of alcohol and drugs,
    8–10, 77
    alcohol use during pregnancy, 78–79
    ATOD-exposed adolescents, 83–84
    ATOD-exposed newborns and
        infants, 82
    ATOD-exposed school-aged
        children, 82–83
    behavioral and educational
        services, 90–91
    case study, 93–94
    fetal alcohol syndrome (FAS), 88
    identification and assessment, 81
    illicit drug use during pregnancy,
        80–81
    legal and ethical issues, 84–85
    medical interventions, 89–90
    mental health and
        psychopharmacological
        interventions, 90

parenting and family-based
interventions, 91–93
tobacco use during pregnancy, 80
Prison inmates, parents as, 246–247
Project CHOICES, 180
Prostitution, 6
PSBCT. *See* Parent skills training with
behavioralcouples therapy
Psychodrama, 41
use of, with adult COSAPs,
164–168
Psychoeducational programming, 18
Psychostimulants, 229
PTSD. *See* Posttraumatic stress disorder
Puerto Rican teens, 132

Quasi-experimental designs, 108

Relationship dysfunction, 56
Repetition compulsion, 162
Residential-based interventions, 219
Residential Student Assistance
Program (RSAP), 220
Risperdal, 90
Ritalin, for ADHD, 90, 229
RSAP. *See* Residential Student
Assistance Program
Rubicon, Inc., 201

S.E.A.R.I.S.E. program, 2
SAMHSA. *See* Substance Abuse
and Mental Health Services
Administration
School-aged children
with alcoholic parents, 37
impact of parental substance
abuse on, 11–13
School and residential settings, helping
adolescents in, 215
parental consent issues, 217
residential-based interventions, 219
Residential Student Assistance
Program (RSAP), 219
school-based interventions, 218

staff qualifications, training, and
responsibilities, 216–217
Student Assistance Programs, 219
School-based interventions, 218
Secure attachment, 32, 34
Self-medication, 20, 162
Self-regulation, 105, 157
SFP. *See* Strengthening Families Program
Shame, 20, 160
Short-term mentalization and relational
therapy (SMART), 40
SIDS. *See* Sudden infant death
syndrome
SMART. *See* Short-term mentalization
and relational therapy
Smoking during pregnancy, 9, 78
Somatic disturbances, 159
Somatization of feelings, 20
Stages of Change Model, 41
Strattera, for ADHD, 90
Strengthening Families Program (SFP),
12, 15, 109, 142
Student Assistance Counselor, 218
Student Assistance Program, 12, 109,
218, 219
Substance abuse, impact on family
system, 3–4
Substance Abuse and Mental Health
Services Administration
(SAMHSA), 199
Substance-abusing families, dynamics
of, 49
assessment issues, 56–59
case example, 65–67
children of substance abusers, 52
comorbid parental
psychopathology, 55–56
future directions, 67–68
interparental conflict, 53–54
interventions, 59
Behavioral Couples Therapy, 61–63
family therapy, 59–61
parent training, 63–65
parental substance abuse and child
adjustment, 53
partner violence and child abuse,
54–55

Substance-use disorders,
        understanding, 2–3
Sudden infant death syndrome (SIDS),
        9, 80
*Supporting Jails in Providing Women
        with Substance Abuse Services
        project*, 247, 248, 250
Survivor's guilt, 159–160

T-ACE, 173
Teenage drinking, 130
Teens with substance-abusing
        parents, 129

Tobacco use during pregnancy, 9, 80
Trauma and mentalization,
        35–36
Traumatic bonding, 161
Traumatized adult COSAPs, 20
TWEAK, 173
12-step programs, 21

"Wellness" program, 18, 230
Women-specific programs, 197–198

Yale Child Study Center, 39